PUBLIC HEALTH: PRACTICES, METHODS AND POLICIES

ADVANCES IN CHINESE CHILDREN, ADOLESCENT AND FAMILY RESEARCH

PUBLIC HEALTH: PRACTICES, METHODS AND POLICIES

JOAV MERRICK - SERIES EDITOR

MEDICAL DIRECTOR, HEALTH SERVICES, DIVISION FOR INTELLECTUAL AND DEVELOPMENTAL DISABILITIES, MINISTRY OF SOCIAL AFFAIRS AND SOCIAL SERVICES, JERUSALEM, ISRAEL

Advances in Chinese Children, Adolescent and Family Research
Ariel Tenenbaum,
Daniel T.L. Shek,
Moon YM Law and Joav Merrick
(Editors)
2020. ISBN: 978-1-53617-870-8
(Hardcover)
2020. ISBN. 978-1-53617-871-5
(e-book)

Child Environmental Health Disparities: Looking at the Present and Facing the Future
I. Leslie Rubin and Joav Merrick
(Editors)
2020. ISBN: 978-1-53617-823-4
(Hardcover)
2020. ISBN. 978-1-53617-824-1
(e-book)

Positive Youth Development: Digital Game-Based Learning
Ty Lee, Daniel T.L. Shek,
Sarah Sw Lee, and Joav Merrick
(Editors)
2020. ISBN: 978-1-53617-795-4
(Hardcover)
2020. ISBN. 978-1-53617-796-1
(e-book)

Service Leadership Education in an Era of Service Economy
Daniel TL Shek, Xiaoqin Zhu,
and Joav Merrick
(Editors)
2020. ISBN: 978-1-53617-514-1
(Hardcover)
2020. ISBN: 978-1-53617-515-8
(e-book)

Parenting and Family Life in a Chinese Society
Daniel TL Shek, Moon YM Law,
Joav Merrick
(Editors)
2020. ISBN: 978-1-53616-705-4
(Softcover)
2020. ISBN: 978-1-53616-706-1
(e-book)

Public Health: Topics, Themes and Trends
Satesh Bidaisee, Sadik Uddin Emmanuel Keku, Joav Merrick (Editors)
2020. ISBN: 978-1-53616-655-2 (Softcover)
2020. ISBN: 978-1-53616-656-9

Public Health: Environment and Child Health in a Changing World
I. Leslie Rubin and Joav Merrick (Editors)
2019. ISBN: 978-1-53615-394-1 (Hardcover)
2019. ISBN: 978-1-53615395-8 (e-book)

Service Leadership: Tools to Assess Knowledge, Attitude and Behavior
Daniel TL Shek, Xiaoqin Zhu, Li Lin and Joav Merrick (Editors)
2019. ISBN: 978-1-53614-852-7 (Hardcover)
2019. ISBN: 978-1-53614-853-4 (e-book)

Public Health Yearbook 2017
Joav Merrick (Editor)
2018. ISBN: 978-1-53613-792-7 (Hardcover)
2018. ISBN: 978-1-53613-793-4 (e-book)

Resilience and Health: A Potent Dynamic
I Leslie Rubin and Joav Merrick (Editors)
2018. ISBN: 978-1-53613-412-4 (Hardcover)
2018. ISBN: 978-1-53613-413-1 (e-book)

Medical History: Some Perspectives Second Edition
Donald E. Greydanus and Joav Merrick, (Editors)
2018. ISBN: 978-1-53613-319-6 (Hardcover)
2018. ISBN: 978-1-53613-320-2 (e-book)

University Students: Promotion of Holistic Development in Hong Kong
Daniel TL Shek, Lu Yu and Joav Merrick (Editors)
2017. ISBN: 978-1-53612-535-1 (Hardcover)
2017. ISBN: 978-1-53612-537-5 (e-book)

Alzheimer's Disease: Awareness among Young Adults
Ronald Chow, Drew Hollenberg, Michael Borean and Joav Merrick (Editors)
2017. ISBN: 978-1-53612-456-9 (Softcover)
2017. ISBN: 978-1-53612-457-6 (e-book)

Service Leadership Education for University Students
Daniel TL Shek, Po Chung, Li Lin and Joav Merrick (Editors)
2017. ISBN: 978-1-53611-949-7 (Hardcover)
2017. ISBN: 978-1-53611-969-5 (e-book)

Leadership: Promoting Leadership and Intrapersonal Development in University Students
Daniel TL Shek, Cecilia MS Ma and Joav Merrick (Editors)
2017. ISBN: 978-1-53611-950-3 (Hardcover)
2017. ISBN: 978-1-53611-970-1 (e-book)

Caribbean Adolescents: Misuse and Abuse of Alcohol
Cecilia Hegamin-Younger and Joav Merrick (Editors)
2017. ISBN: 978-1-63485-880-9 (Hardcover)
2016. ISBN: 978-1-63485-894-6 (e-book)

Public Health: An Ecological Framework for Child Environmental Health Interventions
I. Leslie Rubin and Joav Merrick (Editors)
2017. ISBN: 978-1-53610-700-5 (Hardcover)
2017. ISBN: 978-1-53610-714-2 (e-book)

Diabetes Mellitus: A Medical History Journey
Donald E. Greydanus and Joav Merrick
2016. ISBN: 978-1-53610-094-5 (Softcover)
2016. ISBN: 978-1-53610-103-4 (e-book)

Education in Hong Kong: Service Leadership for University Students
Daniel TL Shek, Cecilia MS Ma, Li Lin and Joav Merrick (Editors)
2016. ISBN: 978-1-63484-928-9 (Hardcover)
2016. ISBN: 978-1-63484-960-9 (e-book)

Environmental Health Disparities: Costs and Benefits of Breaking the Cycle
I. Leslie Rubin and Joav Merrick (Editors)
2016. ISBN: 978-1-63484-211-2 (Hardcover)
2016. ISBN: 978-1-63484-212-9 (e-book)

Higher Education in Hong Kong: Nurturing Students to be Caring Service Leaders
Daniel TL Shek, Andrew MH Siu, Hildie Leung and Joav Merrick (Editors)
2016. ISBN: 978-1-63484-980-7 (Hardcover)
2016. ISBN: 978-1-63485-009-4 (e-book)

Measles: Epidemiology and Control of Measles in the Gweru Urban District in Zimbabwe
Tawanda Marufu, Seter Siziya, Mazyanga L. Mazaba and Joav Merrick (Editors)
2016. ISBN: 978-1-63485-559-4 (Hardcover)
2016. ISBN: 978-1-63485-573-0 (e-book)

Medical History: Some Perspectives
Donald E. Greydanus and Joav Merrick
2016. ISBN: 978-1-63484-747-6 (Hardcover)
2016. ISBN: 978-1-63484-849-7 (e-book)

Public Health: Some International Aspects
Joav Merrick (Editor)
2016. ISBN: 978-1-63484-612-7 (Hardcover)
2016. ISBN: 978-1-63484-630-1 (e-book)

Public Health: International Aspects on Environment and Health
I. Leslie Rubin and Joav Merrick (Editors)
2016. ISBN: 978-1-63484-834-3 (Hardcover)
2016. ISBN: 978-1-63484-849-7 (e-book)

Smoking and Adolescence: International Public Health Experiences
Mazyanga L. Mazaba, Seter Siziya and Joav Merrick (Editors)
2016. ISBN: 978-1-63484-311-9 (Hardcover)
2016. ISBN: 978-1-63484-312-6 (e-book)

Arbovirus: Public Health Experience from Zambia
Seter Siziya, Mazyanga L. Mazaba, and Joav Merrick (Editors)
2015. ISBN: 978-1-63463-601-8 (Hardcover)
2015. ISBN: 978-1-63463-618-6 (e-book)

Health Issues in Diverse Cultures
Cecilia Obeng, Samuel Gyasi Obeng and Joav Merrick (Editors)
2015. ISBN: 978-1-63463-613-1 (Hardcover)
2015. ISBN: 978-1-63463-619-3 (e-book)

Public Health, Social Work and Health Inequalities
Bruce D. Friedman and Joav Merrick (Editors)
2015. ISBN: 978-1-63482-838-3 (Hardcover)
2015. ISBN: 978-1-63482-850-5 (e-book)

Patient Dumping: Background, Protections, and the Mentally Ill
Tabitha E. Rivers (Editor)
2015. ISBN: 978-1-63483-726-2 (Hardcover)
2015. ISBN: 978-1-63483-727-9 (e-book)

Tomorrow's Leaders: Service Leadership and Holistic Development in Chinese University Students
Daniel TL Shek, Andrew MH Siu and Joav Merrick (Editors)
2015. ISBN: 978-1-63321-880-2 (Hardcover)
2014. ISBN: 978-1-63321-943-4 (e-book)

Environment and Public Health: Environmental Health, Law and International Perspectives
I. Leslie Rubin and Joav Merrick (Editors)
2014. ISBN: 978-1-63463-167-9 (Hardcover)
2014. ISBN: 978-1-63463-189-1 (e-book)

PUBLIC HEALTH: PRACTICES, METHODS AND POLICIES

ADVANCES IN CHINESE CHILDREN, ADOLESCENT AND FAMILY RESEARCH

ARIEL TENENBAUM, MD
DANIEL T.L. SHEK, PHD
MOON YM LAW
AND
JOAV MERRICK, MD, MMEDSCI, DMSC
EDITORS

nova
Medicine & Health
New York

Library of Congress Cataloging-in-Publication Data

Names: Tenenbaum, Ariel, editor. | Shek, Daniel T. L., editor. | Law, Moon Y. M., editor. | Merrick, Joav, 1950- editor.
Title: Advances in Chinese children, adolescent and family research / Ariel Tenenbaum, Daniel T.L. Shek, Moon YM Law, Joav Merrick, editors. Description: New York : Nova Science Publishers, [2020] | Series: Public health: practices, methods and policies | Includes bibliographical references and index. | Summary: "A survey of the literature showed that most research studies in children, adolescents and families have been conducted in Western contexts, which may not be applicable to non-Western contexts. Hence, research on children, adolescents and families in non-Western contexts is particularly important and we therefore need to enrich human development and family research in the Chinese context. In this book, we included 16 chapters to demonstrate the advances in Chinese children, adolescents, and family research. And it is our sincere hope that through this book, we can attempt to conduct more empirical studies that can help to promote the research atmosphere and enrich the knowledge of Chinese children, adolescent, and family research in a larger context"-- Provided by publisher. Identifiers: LCCN 2020016644 (print) | LCCN 2020016645 (ebook) | ISBN 9781536178708 (hardcover) | ISBN 9781536178715 (adobe pdf) Subjects: LCSH: Children--Health and hygiene--China. | Teenagers--Health and hygiene--China. | Families--Health and hygiene--China. Classification: LCC RJ103.C6 A38 2020 (print) | LCC RJ103.C6 (ebook) | DDC 362.19892000951--dc23
LC record available at https://lccn.loc.gov/2020016644
LC ebook record available at https://lccn.loc.gov/2020016645

Published by Nova Science Publishers, Inc. † New York

CONTENTS

Introduction		**1**
Chapter 1	Advances in Chinese children, adolescent and family research *Moon Law, Daniel TL Shek, Ariel Tenenbaum and Joav Merrick*	**3**
Section one: Child and adolescent development		**9**
Chapter 2	Reliability and validity of the Chinese version of the psycho-educational profile (third edition) for Children with Developmental Problems *Daniel TL Shek and Lu Yu*	**11**
Chapter 3	The impacts of a UNICEF health promotion project on primary health care in Western China: A comprehensive evaluation at provincial level *Yuxue Bi, Dejian Lai and Hong Yan*	**37**
Chapter 4	Materialism in Chinese adolescents in Hong Kong: Profiles and socio-demographic correlates *Daniel TL Shek, Li Lin, Andrew MH Siu and Britta M Lee*	**55**

Chapter 5	Materialism and egocentrism in Chinese adolescents in Hong Kong: Perceptions of teachers *Daniel TL Shek, Cecilia Ma, Andrew MH Siu and Britta M Lee*	**77**
Section two: Family environment		**97**
Chapter 6	Family mealtime environment and child behavior outcomes in Chinese preschool children *Cynthia Leung, Sandra Tsang, Sing Kai Lo and Ruth Chan*	**99**
Chapter 7	Families in transition in Hong Kong: Implications to family research and practice *Janet TY Leung and Daniel TL Shek*	**115**
Chapter 8	Subjective outcome evaluation of the Tin Ka Ping P.A.T.H.S. Project in China: View of the students *Daniel TL Shek, Tak Yan Lee, Xiaoqin Zhu and Lawrence K Ma*	**141**
Chapter 9	Evaluation of the Project P.A.T.H.S. in Mainland China: Views of the program implementers in senior high schools *Daniel TL Shek, Florence KY Wu, Rachel CF Sun and Mengtong Chen*	**157**
Chapter 10	Evaluation of the training program of a positive youth development program: Tin Ka Ping P.A.T.H.S. project in China *Daniel TL Shek, Janet TY Leung, Rachel CF Sun, Mengtong Chen and Chi Kin Chung*	**175**
Chapter 11	Tin Ka Ping P.A.T.H.S. project in Mainland China: Preliminary evaluation findings *Daniel TL Shek, Tak-Yan Lee, Rachel CF Sun, Florence KY Wu and Janet TY Leung*	**197**

Chapter 12 Evaluation findings of Tin Ka Ping P.A.T.H.S. Project implemented in junior secondary schools: Implementers' views **213**
Daniel TL Shek, Xiaoqin Zhu and Janet TY Leung

Chapter 13 Subjective outcome evaluation of the Tin Ka Ping P.A.T.H.S. Project: Views of senior secondary school students **231**
Daniel TL Shek, Rachel CF Sun, Irene Wu and Moon YM Law

Chapter 14 Implementation of the Tin Ka Pin Project in two Chinese cities: Students' subjective outcome evaluation **249**
Lu Yu and Esther YW Shek

Chapter 15 Subjective outcome evaluation of a service leadership subject: Findings based on university students in Hong Kong **267**
Janet TY Leung and Daniel TL Shek

Chapter 16 Student development under a new general education program in Hong Kong: A 3-Year longitudinal assessment **289**
Daniel TL Shek, Lu Yu and Xiaoqin Zhu

Chapter 17 Promotion of service leadership qualities in Chinese university students: Objective outcome evaluation based on six waves of data **313**
Hildie Leung, Daniel TL Shek and Li Lin

Section two: Acknowledgments **331**

Chapter 18 About the editors **333**

Chapter 19 About the Center for Children with Chronic Diseases and Down Syndrome Center Jerusalem, Israel, Department of Pediatrics, Mt Scopus Campus, Hadassah Hebrew University Medical Center, Jerusalem, Israel **337**

Chapter 20 About the Department of Applied Social Sciences, The Hong Kong Polytechnic University, Hung Hom, Hong Kong **341**

Chapter 21 About the National Institute of Child Health and Human Development in Israel **345**

Chapter 22 About the book series "Public health: Practices, methods and policies" **349**

Section three: Index **353**

Index **355**

INTRODUCTION

In: Advances in Chinese Children … ISBN: 978-1-53617-870-8
Editors: Ariel Tenenbaum et al.

Chapter 1

ADVANCES IN CHINESE CHILDREN, ADOLESCENT AND FAMILY RESEARCH

Moon Law[1,*], BSW, MSW, DSW, RSW,
Daniel TL Shek[2], PhD, FHKPS, BBS, SBS, JP,
Ariel Tenenbaum[3-5], MD
and Joav Merrick[4-7], MD, MMedSci, DMSc
[1]School of Social Sciences, Caritas Institute of Higher Education, Hong Kong, PR China
[2]Department of Applied Social Sciences, The Hong Kong Polytechnic University, Hung Hom, Hong Kong, PR China
[3]Center for Children with Chronic Diseases and Down Syndrome Center Jerusalem, Israel
[4]Department of Pediatrics, Mt Scopus Campus, Hadassah Hebrew University Medical Center, Jerusalem, Israel
[5]National Institute of Child Health and Human Development, Jerusalem, Israel

---

* Corresponding Author: Moon YM Law, BSW, MSW, DSW, RSW, Assistant Professor of School of Social Sciences, Caritas Institue of Higher Education, Hong Kong PRChina. E-mail: mlaw@cihe.edu.hk.

[6]Kentucky Children's Hospital, University of Kentucky, Lexington, Kentucky, United States
[7]Center for Healthy Development, School of Public Health, Georgia State University, Atlanta, Georgia, United States

ABSTRACT

A survey of the literature showed that most research studies in children, adolescents and families have been conducted in Western contexts, which may not be applicable to non-Western contexts. Hence, research on children, adolescents and families in non-Western contexts is particularly important and we therefore need to enrich human development and family research in the Chinese context. In this book, we included 16 chapters to demonstrate the advances in Chinese children, adolescents, and family research. And it is our sincere hope that through this book, we can attempt to conduct more empirical studies that can help to promote the research atmosphere and enrich the knowledge of Chinese children, adolescent, and family research in a larger context.

INTRODUCTION

A survey of the literature showed that most research studies in children, adolescents and families have been conducted in Western contexts. One major limitation is that the related theories and findings may not be applicable to non-Western contexts. Hence, research on children, adolescents and families in non-Western contexts is particularly important. As roughly one-fifth of the world's population are Chinese, the development of research on human development and families in the Chinese context is very important. Although more Chinese research studies have been conducted in the past decades, most of the studies were based on Western theories and tools. Due to cultural differences, it is argued that researchers and practitioners should develop their own theories, programs and measurements (1-3).

There are several areas that require more Chinese research. The first area is the prevention intervention research. For example, by adopting fifteen positive youth development constructs from the West, the first local positive youth development program ("Project P.A.T.H.S.") has been developed for Hong Kong junior secondary students since 2005. Since the implementation, the research team employed multiple evaluation strategies to ensure the quality of the program implementation, such as subjective and outcome evaluation, process evaluation, and focus group and individual interviews. Also, based on the results of the evaluation, the program materials have been updated and revamped based on the results of the evaluations during the 15-year program (4-5).

Mainland China

Based on the positive feedback and effectiveness of the Project P.A.T.H.S. in Hong Kong, the program has been introduced into mainland China ("Tin Ka Ping P.A.T.H.S. Project") since 2011 for more than 28 mainland China cities. However, due to the cultural differences between Hong Kong and mainland China, there is a need to have ongoing feedback from different stakeholders. Normally speaking, the teaching style of Hong Kong teachers is more interactive when compared with the style of mainland Chinese teachers. For positive youth development programs, like Project P.A.T.H.S., interaction and students' participation are key factors for promoting students' reflection and learning. Therefore, apart from providing trainings for teachers and program implementers, feedback from both participants and program implementers can not only help researchers to have a full picture of the program effectiveness, but also facilitate program implementers' reflection on their teaching performance and improvement. This example proved that ongoing evaluations and researches are needed for adopted programs for better program effectiveness. In this book, we included some related papers on the Tin Ka Ping Project in China.

EVALUATION

Second, we need more research on the evaluation of holistic adolescent development programs. In order to have a comprehensive picture of the program's effectiveness, it is suggested to collect feedback from both participants and different stakeholders, including program implementers. Besides collecting participants' feedback, it is also important to collect feedback from the program implementers for several reasons: (i) program implementers are more experienced than participants, and they can provide more "accurate" views towards the programs; (ii) it can facilitate reflective practice and to enhance the quality of the programs; (iii) it can provide a better understanding about the implementation process across different settings/schools, especially for those programs which are implemented in different schools; (iv) according to the principle of triangulation, collecting data from different sources can help researchers to generate the same picture and further examine if there are different views among participants and stakeholders. In this book, we included some papers on evaluation based on different evaluation strategies.

Beside intervention research, it is also important to understand adolescent development. As there are few studies on adolescent materialism and egocentrism, there is a need to conduct more studies in this area. Furthermore, there is a need to conduct more longitudinal studies. Although there is an increase of longitudinal studies in adolescents' development, longitudinal studies about late adolescents' well-being (e.g., university students) are still lacking in number, especially in the Chinese context (6). University life should be regarded as an important transition period from adolescence to adulthood. However, there is a myth in the Chinese society that university students need less support and concern as they are "old" enough to face different challenges. In this book, several papers on adolescent materialism and egocentrism are included. Also, some papers on the development of university students are covered.

FAMILY RESEARCH

Finally, several points should be noted when conducting family research: (i) cultural differences should be taken into consideration, (ii) there is a need to examine the differential paternal and maternal influences when examining a factor on children and adolescent; and (iii) both parents' and children' views should be included in a single study. Because of the unique historical backgrounds between the West and East, cultural differences should always be considered when studying family factors in the Chinese context. Besides, to have a complete understanding of different sides, it would be good to include both parents' and children's views in a single study.

THIS BOOK

Based on the above discussion, there is a need to enrich human development and family research in the Chinese context. In this book, we included 16 chapters to demonstrate the advances in Chinese children, adolescents, and family research. And it is our sincere hope that through this special issue, we can attempt to conduct more empirical studies that can help to promote the research atmosphere and enrich the knowledge of Chinese children, adolescent, and family research.

ACKNOWLEDGMENTS

In this book we have gathered single papers published earlier in several of Nova journals with permisssion releavnt to the topic of the book.

REFERENCES

[1] Shek DTL, Law MYM. Factors influencing the quality of implementation of a positive youth development program in Hong Kong. Int J Adolesc Med Health 2013;25:363-72. doi: 10.1515/ijamh-2013-0034.

[2] Shek DTL, Law MYM. Parental behavioral control, parental psychological control and parent-child relational qualities: Relationships to Chinese adolescent risk behavior. In: Shek DTL, Sun RCF, Ma CMS, eds. Chinese adolescents in Hong Kong: Family life, psychological well-being and risk behavior. Quality of Life in Asia, vol 5. Singapore: Springer, 2014:51-69.

[3] Shek DTL, Law MYM. Assessment of parent-child subsystem qualities in Chinese adolescents: Behavioral control, psychological control and parent-child relational qualities. Int J Disabil Hum Dev 2015;8:207-17.

[4] Shek DTL, Sun RCF, eds. Development and evaluation of positive adolescent training through holistic social programs (P.A.T.H.S.). Heidelberg: Springer, 2013.

[5] Shek DTL, Sun RCF. The Project P.A.T.H.S. in Hong Kong: Development, training, implementation, and evaluation. J Pediatr Adolesc Gynec 2013;26(3S):S2-9. doi: 10.1016/j.jpag.2013.03.009.

[6] Shek DTL, Yu L, Wu FKY, Zhu JXQ, Chan KHY. A 4-year longitudinal study of well-being of Chinese university students in Hong Kong. Appl Res Qual Life 2017;12:867-84. doi: 10.1007/s11482-016-9493-4.

SECTION ONE:
CHILD AND ADOLESCENT DEVELOPMENT

In: Advances in Chinese Children … ISBN: 978-1-53617-870-8
Editors: Ariel Tenenbaum et al.

Chapter 2

RELIABILITY AND VALIDITY OF THE CHINESE VERSION OF THE PSYCHO-EDUCATIONAL PROFILE (THIRD EDITION) FOR CHILDREN WITH DEVELOPMENTAL PROBLEMS

Daniel TL Shek*[*], PhD, FHKPS, BBS, JP
and Lu Yu, PhD
Department of Applied Social Sciences,
The Hong Kong Polytechnic University, Hong Kong, PR China

ABSTRACT

The Psycho-Educational Profile-3rd edition (PEP-3) is a popular instrument that assesses the skills and behaviors of children with autism and

[*] Corresponding Author: Professor Daniel TL Shek, PhD, FHKPS, BBS, JP, Chair Professor of Applied Social Sciences, Faculty of Health and Social Sciences, Department of Applied Social Sciences, The Hong Kong Polytechnic University, Room HJ407, Core H, Hunghom, Hong Kong. E-mail: daniel.shek@polyu.edu.hk.

communicative disabilities, while its application in Chinese population has not been systematically examined. Based on the data collected from a clinical sample of children ($N = 455$) diagnosed as having autism spectrum disorder (ASD) and other pervasive developmental disorders (PPDs) as well as a sample of healthy controls ($N = 281$) in Hong Kong, this study examined the psychometric properties of the Performance Test of the Chinese version of the PEP-3 (CPEP-3). Different types of evidence on the reliability (internal consistency, test-retest reliability and inter-rater reliability) and validity (content validity and criterion-related validity) of the test were examined. It was found that the Performance Test of CPEP-3 possessed sound psychometric properties in assessing the developmental level of Chinese children with autism spectrum disorder in Hong Kong. The translated CPEP-3 Performance Test is a reliable and valid measure for assessing Chinese children with autism.

INTRODUCTION

Autism spectrum disorder (ASD) refers to a group of developmental disabilities, characterized by unreciprocated interpersonal and emotional interactions, disordered language and communication, and repetitive and stereotypic behaviors (1-3). Although earlier studies had suggested the prevalence of autism was low, the global prevalence of ASD increased tremendously in the global context in the past decades (4-8). While children with ASD share similar symptoms, the age of onset, nature and severity of the problems are highly variable, which require different treatment approaches (9). Hence, psychometrically sound instruments that can help professionals to objectively assess children with ASD are of great importance to ensure accurate diagnosis and appropriate educational programming (10).

According to Shriver, Allen and Mathew (11), assessment is considered as core components in treating children with ASD in terms of three aspects. First, assessment helps to obtain an accurate verification for the diagnosis and special education eligibility. Second, assessment can guide the development of appropriate interventions by providing a descriptive profile on children's development in different areas. Third, assessment enables researchers to establish baselines against which evaluation of different intervention programs could be conducted.

Among different types of assessments measuring children with ASD, the Psycho-Educational Profile-3rd edition (PEP-3) is a standardized observation tool primarily designed for planning educational program for children with ASD from 2 to 7 years of age (12). It is the revised version of the Psycho-Educational Profile-Revised (PEP-R) which has been widely used in different parts of the world for the assessment of children with ASD in terms of their developmental skills and behaviors (13-17). Compared with the PEP-R, there are several significant improvements in the PEP-3. First, the measured function domains have been revised by incorporating the most recent research findings, such as the social and communication aspects. Second, normative data from both a sample with autism and a typically developing sample were provided which makes it possible to compare the two groups of children on their developmental profiles. Third, a Caregiver Report, which utilizes information reported by parents and other caregivers about the child's development and behavior in daily lives, has been added to help professionals have a fuller understanding about the child. Fourth, new items and important subtests were added into the PEP-3 while obsolete items were deleted. The validity of the revised instrument has been examined in the West (18).

Specifically, the PEP-3 consists of two complementary parts. The first part is a norm-referenced performance scale (Performance Test) which measures autistic children's development in three areas: communication, motor skills, and maladaptive behaviors. The second part is a parent or caregiver reported form (Caregiver Report). Children's development and performance in communication, motor and social functioning, adaptive behaviors and thinking are rated by their caregivers based on their daily observation. As autistic children's symptoms vary across settings (such as people, places, and things the child interacts with), using both professional observers' ratings on children's performance in the laboratory and caregivers' ratings on children's daily lives helps to obtain a richer and comprehensive developmental profile of the child with reference to the strengths and weaknesses of the child in different environment. This could be very useful for professionals to design individualized educational and behavioral intervention programs in different settings.

Based on a normative sample of 407 children with ASD and 148 children with typical development in the United States, Schopler et al. (18) reported the reliability and validity of the PEP-3 in its user manual. As far as reliability is concerned, the PEP-3 showed high reliability, with all subtests showing high internal consistency (alphas ranged from 0.84 to 0.90) and temporal stability (test-retest coefficients over a period of two weeks ranged from 0.94 to 0.99). Besides, for the inter-rater reliability for the Caregiver Report, the polychoric correlation coefficients ranged from 0.52 to 1.00. In terms of validity, consistent with the expectations, autistic children's scores on PEP-3 Performance subtests were negatively correlated with their scores on measures of symptom severity in autistic children, including the Childhood Autism Rating Scales (CARS) (19) and the Autism Behavior Checklist-Second Edition (ABC) (20). For the Caregiver Report, positive correlation coefficients were found between the Vineland Adaptive Behavior Scales (VABS) (21) which assess parent-reported adaptive behavior of children and PEP-3. These findings provide sound support for the good psychometric properties of the PEP-3 when applied to children with ASDs in the United States.

The PEP-R has been translated into several languages and research findings supporting the psychometric properties of the translated measures have been reported (14, 15, 22). In contrast, there are very few reports on the application of PEP-3 in countries other than the United States (23). As Chinese people constitute roughly one-fifth of the world's population, translation of PEP-3 to Chinese and establishment of the related psychometric properties should be conducted. Actually, a Chinese version of the PEP-R (CPEP-R) was validated and used in assessing children with ASD in Hong Kong since 2005 which has largely facilitated the diagnoses and treatment of autistic children (14). Nevertheless, very few reports have been published on the Chinese version of PEP-3 and its psychometric properties. In Taiwan, researchers translated the PEP-3 into Chinese and reported the reliability and validity of the instrument based on Taiwanese children with autism. While the preliminary findings supported the application of PEP-3 in Chinese children, the published studies were mostly based on small samples (ranged from 42 to 64 participants), which makes the generalization of the findings to other Chinese population questionable (22-24).

Against the above background, Heep Hong Society, the biggest organization in Hong Kong that provides professional training and education to children with developmental and learning problems and their families, invited a group of experts consisting of psychologists, occupational therapists, special educators, and special child-care workers to translate the PEP-3 into Chinese (25) and conduct a validation study to examine the psychometric properties of the instrument. Based on a sample of 455 children with ASD and a comparison group of 281 children with typical development, the construct validity of the Chinese version of PEP-3 (CPEP-3) was examined. It was found that older children scored higher than younger children for both groups on different subsets of CPEP-3, while no gender difference was identified within the autistic group. The results of confirmatory factor analysis further showed the three-factor theoretical model of the Performance Test fitted well. These findings provide important evidence for the construct validity of the CPEP-3 (25. However, besides construct validity, there is a need to further understand the reliability as well as other types of validity of the CPEP-3.

As far as reliability is concerned, three types of reliability are commonly assessed for an assessment tool (26). First, Cronbach's alphas are usually computed to examine the internal consistency of the scale to see whether the items measure something which is homogenous in nature. Second, temporal stability of the test scores (i.e., test-retest reliability) is typically examined by getting the test scores at two different time points. Finally, if the test is completed by different raters, consistency across raters is examined by inter-rater reliability.

Regarding validity, besides construct validity which was examined in the study of Shek and Yu (25), two additional forms of validity evidence were examined in the present study. First, evidence about content validity was explored, which refers to "the systematic examination of the test content to determine whether it covers a representative sample of the behavior domain to be measured" (27). Based on the method adopted by the original author of PEP-3 (12), conventional item analyses were performed to provide evidence for content validity, including item discrimination and item difficulty analyses. Second, criterion-related validity was investigated, which was defined as the correlation between a test and an (or a series of) external criterion variable(s) taken as representative of the construct, for example, measures that have previously been validated assessing presumably related constructs (27). In this study, it was hypothesized that the Performance Test of CPEP-3 should correlate well with previously validated tests that measure developmental skills and behavioral symptoms in children with autistic disorders.

The primary purpose of this paper is to report the reliability and validity of the Performance Test of the Chinese version of PEP-3 (CPEP-3) based on further data collected from the same samples of children as reported in Shek and Yu's (25) paper. Psychometric properties of the Caregiver Report will be presented elsewhere (28). Specifically, the current study attempted to assess the reliability (internal consistency, test-retest reliability and inter-rater reliability) and validity (content validity and criterion-related validity) of the CPEP-3 Performance Test as a measure to estimate the developmental level among children with ASD in Hong Kong.

OUR STUDY

Prior to the study, approval to conduct the study (including ethics approval) was obtained from the Executive Committee of Heep Hong Society. The primary caregivers of the participated children have given their written informed consents to the research team. Participants were ensured that the data collected in the study would be kept confidential.

Participants

As described in Shek and Yu's (25) paper, 455 children who were diagnosed as having autism or other pervasive developmental disorders (PDDs) in 25 service units in Heep Hong Society including special child care centers, early education and training centers, and parent resource center were recruited to participate in the study. Another sample of 281 children without developmental problems was selected as the "healthy control" from 13 local kindergartens matched for age with the autistic sample for comparison. The diagnoses of the autistic sample were made based on ICD-10/DSM-IV by consultant psychiatrists and endorsed by a multidisciplinary team consisting of clinical psychologists, special educators, and other helping professionals. Several subgroups of participants were randomly selected for the analyses of test-retest reliability, inter-rater reliability, and criterion-prediction validity.

Table 1. Demographic characteristic of the samples

Age group	**2**	**3**	**4**	**5**	**6**	**7**	
Age range in years	2.0-2.9	3.0-3.9	4.0-4.9	5.0-5.9	6.0-6.9	7.0-7.9	Total
Sample with autism							
No. of participants	32	79	140	161	37	6	455
Percentage	7.0%	17.4%	30.8%	35.4%	8.1%	1.3%	100%
No. of girls	6	11	22	22	5	0	66
No. of boys	26	68	118	139	32	6	389
Typically developing sample							
No. of participants	67	60	60	62	30	2	281
Percentage	23.8%	21.4%	21.4%	22.1%	10.7%	0.7%	100%
No. of girls	34	37	36	30	14	1	152
No. of boys	33	23	24	32	16	1	129

Participants' age ranges from 2.0 to 7.9 years. The characteristics of the two samples in terms of age and gender can be seen in Table 1. For the autistic sample, the ratio of boys to girls is 6:1, which is consistent with the reflecting the fact that boys have a higher risk of autistic disorders than girls. While this figure is higher than the related ratio (4:1); in the sample reported in Schopler et al. (12), it is highly similar to the findings of a large epidemiological study of autistic spectrum disorder in which the male to female ratio was found to be 6.58:1 in Hong Kong children (8). Scores of the sample with ASD and the typically developing sample were compared as an indication of criterion-related validity.

Procedures

The translation of the CPEP-3 followed standard procedure in questionnaire adaptation, of which the details were reported in Shek and Yu's (25) paper. A group of professionals including speech therapists, occupational therapists, educational psychologists, and preschool teachers administered the tests and rated the participants' performance. All of the raters had experience working with and testing young children. Before the formal launching of the validation study, training sessions were conducted so that the raters worked together to clarify and get familiar with general testing, scoring and interpreting procedures of the CPEP-3 to ensure consistency in the test administration.

To investigate whether the participants' test performance is consistent over time, test-retest reliability was examined on a subsample of 42 children with autism. Six girls and 36 boys between 2.3 and 5.9 years of age were tested twice over a period of time that ranged from 6 weeks to 3 months. The variation of the interval was due to difficulties in the arrangement involved.

Besides, inter-rater reliability was conducted on a subsample of 46 children randomly selected from the autistic group with age ranging from 2 to 5 years (5 girls and 41 boys) to understand whether the test would be affected by subjective ratings of different raters. Each subject was administered the CPEP-3 Performance Test independently by one administrator and two co-raters as observers. The administrator-co-raters grouping was randomly assigned by a research assistant who was blind to the characteristics of the subjects. In order to keep neutrality throughout the process, testing conditions were similar for all the children and the researchers involved in the case would rate the child's performance independently and handed the protocols to the research assistant directly for data entry.

To test the criterion-related validity of CPEP-3 Performance Test, two established measures related to developmental problems were administered on a subsample of 64 children with autism (56 boys and 8 girls) aged 2 to 6 years. The two measures included the Merrill-Palmer Revised Scales of Development (MPR) (29) and the Childhood Autism Rating Scale (CARS) (18). Both measures were administered by the raters and the participants were randomly assigned to the researchers. The correlations between the criterion measures and CPEP-3 Performance Test would serve as an index of criterion-related validity.

Instruments

The Chinese version of Psycho-Educational Profile—3rd Edition (CPEP-3)

The PEP-3 has two major parts: Performance Test and Caregiver Report. The 172-item Performance Test is composed of 10 subtests. Three subtests measure communication ability including Cognitive Verbal/Preverbal (34 items), Expressive Language (25 items), and Receptive Language (19 items). Another three subtests measure motor ability: Fine Motor (20 items), Gross Motor (15 items), and Visual-Motor Imitation (10 items). These six subtests focus on the child's developmental level. The rest four subtests measure maladaptive behaviors, including Affective Expression (11 items), Social Reciprocity (12 items), Characteristic Motor Behaviors (15 items), and Characteristic Verbal Behaviors (11 items). The Caregiver Report consists of 38 items which are combined into three subtests: Problem Behavior (10 items), Personal Self-Care (13 items), and Adaptive Behavior (15 items). The current study focuses on examining the Performance section.

Authorized by the PEP-3 developers, Heep Hong Society organized a working group comprising clinical, developmental and educational psychologists to translate the PEP-3 items into Chinese. The translated draft was then reviewed and modified by the group after discussion. Compared with the English version of PEP-3, changes in the CPEP-3 were made in the areas of language and use of stimuli. Adaptation and modifications were conducted taking into account the cultural and language factors. Chinese words were used to replace the English ones in the items for letter matching, naming and sorting, and a few more culturally suitable pictures were used to replace the original ones. The scoring of items has been quantified as 0, 1, and 2, with "Pass" = 2, "Emerge" = 1, and "Fail" = 0.

To assess the convergent validity of the CPEP-3, the following measures were employed:

Merrill–Palmer Revised Scales of Development (MPR)

The MPR is an individually-administered, norm-referenced measure of children's development in cognitive, language, motor, self-help, and social-emotional domains (29). It is characterized by a wide range of visual-motor tasks and a few verbal items. This instrument has been widely used by practitioners in assessing the cognitive functioning of pre-school children with language and cognitive delays, with high scores suggesting high cognitive functioning. There are seven subscales in the MPR: development, cognitive, fine motor, infant language/receptive language, infant memory/memory, speed, and visual motor, measuring different areas of cognitive functioning. It was hypothesized that positive correlation would be found between MPR scores and CPEP-3 Performance subtest scores.

Childhood Autism Rating Scale (CARS)

The CARS is a behavioral rating scale developed by the TEACCH Division (18). The CARS consists of ratings in 15 different areas of functioning significant for autism: Relating to People, Imitation, Emotional Response, Body Use, Object Use, Adaptation to Change, Visual Response, Listening Response, Taste, Smell, and Touch Response and Use, Fear or Nervousness, Verbal Communication, Nonverbal Communication, Activity Level, Level and Consistency of Intellectual Response and General Impressions. Children's behaviors were observed and rated on a 7-point scale (4 anchor points and 3 half steps) with clear behavioral anchors. High scores on the CARS are considered more maladaptive. Both total score and subscale scores of the CARS were used in the current validity test. It is expected that negative correlation would be found between the CARS and the CPEP-3. On a sample of Hong Kong children with autism, Shek et al. (16) reported a significant correlation coefficient of 0.70 between the Behavioral Scale of CPEP-R and the total score of CARS.

Table 2. Cronbach's alpha coefficients and mean inter-item correlation coefficients for the CPEP-3 performance subtests and composites

Age Group	2	3	4	5	6	7	Average	Mean inter-item correlation coefficients	No. of items
Performance Subtests									
CVP	0.92	0.96	0.96	0.97	0.93	0.60	0.97	0.48	34
EL	0.91	0.96	0.96	0.97	0.94	0.92	0.97	0.53	25
RL	0.92	0.96	0.96	0.97	0.92	0.60	0.97	0.62	19
FM	0.84	0.89	0.88	0.90	0.77	0.52	0.91	0.32	20
GM	0.82	0.88	0.86	0.89	0.62	-	0.90	0.38	15
VMI	0.85	0.90	0.88	0.88	0.71	-	0.90	0.48	10
AE	0.88	0.87	0.91	0.90	0.45	0.72	0.89	0.43	11
SR	0.86	0.86	0.89	0.91	0.81	0.87	0.90	0.45	12
CMB	0.89	0.92	0.91	0.92	0.89	-	0.92	0.41	15
CVB	0.94	0.95	0.93	0.95	0.84	0.64	0.95	0.62	11
Composites									
Communication	0.97	0.98	0.99	0.99	0.97	0.93	0.99	0.51	78
Motor	0.93	0.96	0.95	0.96	0.87	0.82	0.96	0.36	45
Maladaptive Behaviors	0.96	0.97	0.97	0.97	0.93	0.89	0.97	0.40	49

Note. CVP = cognitive verbal/preverbal; EL = expressive language; RL = receptive language; FM = fine motor; GM = gross motor; VMI = visual-motor imitation; AE = affective expression; SR = social reciprocity; CMB = characteristic motor behaviors; CVB = characteristic verbal behaviors.

Data analyses

Preliminary data screening was performed to verify the suitability of the current data for parametric analyses. The psychometric properties of CPEP-3 were examined at both the subtests and composite levels. First, three types of reliability tests were conducted to examine the consistency of CPEP-3 subtests and composites on the current samples of Hong Kong children. These included internal consistency, test-retest reliability, and inter-rater reliability. Second, conventional item analyses including both item difficulty and item discrimination were performed to provide evidence for the content validity. Third, convergent validity of CPEP-3 was examined by testing the correlation coefficients between CPEP-3 and the two criterion scales, MPR and CARS, which measure similar domains of development as measured by CPEP-3.

FINDINGS

Internal consistency was first examined for the subtests and composites of CPEP-3 Performance Test using the total autistic sample and the subsamples at six age intervals separately. The Cronbach's alpha coefficients and mean inter-item correlation coefficients are reported in Table 2. For the whole autistic sample, the Cronbach's alpha coefficients ranged from 0.89 to 0.97 for the Performance subtests, and ranged from 0.96 to 0.99 for the composites. The values of the mean inter-item correlation coefficients were also acceptable (equaled to or exceeded 0.32 and 0.36 for the Performance subtests and the composites, respectively).

To investigate the temporal stability of the assessment tools, test-retest reliability was examined on a subsample of 42 randomly selected children with autism. The temporal stability of the CPEP-3 was tested on 6 girls and 36 boys between 2.3 and 5.9 years of age over a period of time ranged from 6 weeks to 3 months. Means and standard deviations of participants' scores at the two time points are presented in Table 3. Correlation coefficients between test and retest raw scores for each subtest were computed. Results showed that test-retest correlation coefficients were all above 0.82, indicating a good time sampling reliability of the Chinese version of PEP-3.

Table 3. Test-retest reliability for the CPEP-3 performance subtests

	First Testing		Second Testing		
PEP-3 Values	M	SD	M	SD	r
Performance Subtests					
CVP	38.26	16.89	40.00	17.36	.98
EL	13.07	11.26	13.79	12.30	.99
RL	18.00	11.43	18.76	11.43	.97
FM	31.19	6.46	31.62	6.66	.96
GM	25.38	5.26	26.29	5.20	.92
VMI	12.62	4.70	13.26	5.11	.93
AE	13.43	3.91	14.05	3.40	.84
SR	13.14	4.27	13.74	3.93	.92
CMB	20.71	6.91	21.40	6.69	.95
CVB	7.86	5.99	8.38	5.97	.96

Note. CVP = cognitive verbal/preverbal; EL = expressive language; RL = receptive language; FM = fine motor; GM = gross motor; VMI = visual-motor imitation; AE = affective expression; SR = social reciprocity; CMB = characteristic motor behaviors; CVB = characteristic verbal behaviors.

Table 4. Polychoric correlation coefficients for CPEP-3 performance subtest items

Performance Subtests	Min	Max	Mean	Median
CVP	0.26	1.00	0.78	0.87
EL	0.41	1.00	0.77	0.81
RL	0.47	0.93	0.71	0.77
FM	0.23	0.96	0.60	0.76
GM	0.14	0.95	0.58	0.62
VMI	0.63	0.91	0.78	0.79
AE	0.11	0.59	0.34	0.34
SR	0.25	0.75	0.46	0.41
CMB	0.47	0.61	0.52	0.48
CVB	0.19	0.71	0.48	0.52

Note. CVP = cognitive verbal/preverbal; EL = expressive language; RL = receptive language; FM = fine motor; GM = gross motor; VMI = visual-motor imitation; AE = affective expression; SR = social reciprocity; CMB = characteristic motor behaviors; CVB = characteristic verbal behaviors.

The reliability between raters was also assessed to understand whether the test would be affected by subjective ratings of different raters. The inter-rater reliability was based on a randomly selected subsample of 46 children with age ranging from 2 to 5 years (5 girls and 41 boys). Two experienced raters evaluated the 46 children independently using the 10 Performance subtests of CPEP-3. Polychoric correlation coefficients for each pair of items rated by different examiners were calculated as an indicator of inter-rater reliability (30). Descriptive statistics about the correlation coefficients for ten Performance subtests are summarized in Table 4. Because polychoric correlation requires bivariate normality of data, skewness of items was computed initially. Results revealed that 61 out of 344 items skewed greater than the absolute value of 2. Among these items, 12 items (items 42, 120, 155, 3, 70, 97, 56, 62, 69, 135, 137, and 138) yielded polychoric correlation coefficients that appeared to be significantly biased under the condition of bivariate normality. These correlation coefficients were then excluded in the calculation of the range, mean and median of the polychoric correlation coefficients for their corresponding subtests. As can be seen in Table 4, the mean and median polychoric correlation coefficient for each subtest ranged from 0.34 to 0.78 and from 0.34 to 0.87, respectively. According to Hopkin and Stanley (31), these values can be regarded as evidence showing good inter-rater reliability.

Validity of CPEP-3 Performance Test

Regarding the content validity, the rationales underlying the selection of subtest items were established by the test developers in the United States. In fact, an earlier version of PEP-R in Chinese was used in Hong Kong to assess children with autism (14, 32) and showed sufficient clinical validity (33). The PEP-3 is a modified version of the original PEP-R based on the experience of using this instrument in the United States for more than 20 years. After being translated into Chinese, all test materials and procedures of CPEP-3 were scrutinized by a steering group consisting of local experts including psychologists, occupational therapists and special teachers in Hong Kong. They generally held the expert view that items of the CPEP-3 are representative and highly relevant to the domains assessed.

Besides content validity supported by expert views, tests of item discrimination and item difficulty were conducted. Item discrimination refers to the extent to which success on an item corresponds to success on the whole test, which can be indexed by the correlation between a specific item and the other items of the questionnaire. Consistent with the method used by the original scale developers, item-total score correlation coefficients were calculated on the current autistic samples of children (age 2 through age 7) to represent for the item discrimination of the CPEP-3 items.

Table 5 shows the median item discrimination coefficients for each subtest of CPEP-3. Using the criterion that discrimination indexes of 0.35 or higher are acceptable (34-35), most items can be regarded as having good item-discrimination ability on both the whole sample and different age groups. For children aged at 7 years or older, item-discrimination indices for several subtests (RL, GM, VMI, CMB, and PSC) are either uninterpretable or less than 0.35, which may be due to the limited number of participants in this age group ($N = 6$).

Table 5. Item discrimination for the CPEP-3 performance subtests

Performance subtests	2	3	4	5	6	7	Overall
CVP	0.54	0.62	0.67	0.74	0.61	0.35	0.72
EL	0.63	0.72	0.77	0.81	0.71	0.85	0.83
RL	0.64	0.81	0.75	0.80	0.65	0.22	0.80
FM	0.46	0.58	0.59	0.63	0.48	0.77	0.61
GM	0.46	0.57	0.52	0.58	0.52	-	0.59
VMI	0.60	0.67	0.61	0.66	0.42	-0.33	0.68
AE	0.60	0.59	0.67	0.71	0.21	0.91	0.66
SR	0.56	0.56	0.61	0.66	0.51	0.72	0.63
CMB	0.61	0.63	0.58	0.61	0.59	0.11	0.64
CVB	0.83	0.78	0.73	0.77	0.52	0.60	0.76

Note. CVP = cognitive verbal/preverbal; EL = expressive language; RL = receptive language; FM = fine motor; GM = gross motor; VMI = visual-motor imitation; AE = affective expression; SR = social reciprocity; CMB = characteristic motor behaviors; CVB = characteristic verbal behaviors.

Table 6. Item difficulty for the CPEP-3 performance subtests

Performance Subtests	2	3	4	5	6	7
CVP	18.8%	42.4%	59.3%	69.9%	89.2%	100%
EL	3.1%	19.0%	36.4%	49.7%	75.7%	83.3%
RL	21.9%	45.6%	62.9%	73.9%	89.2%	100%
FM	48.5%	70.3%	87.2%	91.0%	96.0%	100%
GM	53.1%	75.9%	88.6%	93.8%	100%	100%
VMI	14.1%	40.5%	62.5%	67.1%	82.5%	100%
AE	53.1%	46.8%	57.9%	68.3%	73.0%	83.3%
SR	21.9%	22.8%	44.3%	48.1%	63.6%	83.3%
CMB	43.8%	51.9%	64.3%	67.7%	73.0%	100%
CVB	12.5%	20.5%	35.7%	42.2%	64.9%	66.7%

Note. CVP = cognitive verbal/preverbal; EL = expressive language; RL = receptive language; FM = fine motor; GM = gross motor; VMI = visual-motor imitation; AE = affective expression; SR = social reciprocity; CMB = characteristic motor behaviors; CVB = characteristic verbal behaviors.

Item difficulty refers to the percentage of participants who can pass a given item, which helps to identify whether an item is too difficult or too easy. Anastasi and Urbina (27) suggested an average item difficulty of 50%, with a range of 15% to 85% considered acceptable. Table 6 summarizes the median item difficulty for each subscale of CPEP-3 on the autistic sample of children. For most parts of the test, test items satisfy the requirements. Results showed that as age increased, the percentage of children who passed the item also increased. These results are also consistent with the Western findings (12).

To test the criterion-related validity of CPEP-3, two well-known measures, MPR and CARS were used as criterion measures based on a subsample of 64 randomly selected autistic children. Descriptive information about the two measures and their subscales is reported in table 7. As shown in table 8, MPR subscale scores were positively correlated with the subtest scores of CPEP-3 Performance Test. All correlation coefficients were significant with values being moderate to large. This suggests high convergent validity of the Performance subtests of CPEP-3 when applied to Chinese children. For CARS, both its total score and subscale scores were used in the current validity test. As CARS measures malfunctioning in autistic children, it is expected that negative correlation would be found between the CARS and the CPEP-3 Performance subtests. As can be seen in Table 9, with a few exceptions, most correlation coefficients were significant, with the direction of the correlation coefficients consistent with the hypotheses, providing further evidence for the criterion-prediction validity of the CPEP-3. These findings were also comparable favorably with previous validation studies conducted in the United States using the CARS as one criterion measure for PEP-3 (12).

Table 7. Descriptive information on two criterion measures and their subscales

		Mean	SD	Range
MPR	Development	179.27	54.86	38.00-237.00
	Cognitive	82.20	22.22	24.00-110.00
	Fine motor	47.20	12.27	13.00-64.00
	Infant language/receptive language	49.61	21.80	0.00-71.00
	Infant memory/memory	15.95	8.78	0.00-34.00
	Speed	14.72	4.70	2.00-20.00
	Visual motor	44.84	10.42	10.00-55.00
CARS	Relating to people	2.52	0.53	1.50-4.00
	Imitation	2.16	0.82	1.00-4.00
	Emotional response	1.82	0.68	1.00-3.50
	Body use	2.08	0.54	1.00-3.50
	Object use	2.30	0.50	1.00-3.50
	Adaptation to change	2.03	0.68	1.00-3.50
	Visual response	2.23	0.74	1.00-3.50
	Listening response	2.32	0.51	1.00-3.00
	Taste, smell, and touch response and use	1.78	0.68	1.00-3.00
	Fear or nervousness	1.24	0.62	1.00-4.00
	Verbal communication	2.59	0.75	1.00-4.00
	Nonverbal communication	1.95	0.62	1.00-3.00
	Activity level	1.52	0.65	1.00-3.00
	Level and consistency of intellectual response	1.84	0.62	1.00-4.00
	General impressions	2.69	0.63	1.00-4.00
	Total score	31.05	6.03	21.50-46.00

Table 8. Correlation coefficients between CPEP-3 performance subtests and MPR subscales

		Performance subtests									
		CVP	EL	RL	FM	GM	VMI	AE	SR	CMB	CVB
MPR	Development	.93**	.92**	.91**	.81**	.72**	.79**	.70**	.80**	.73**	.81**
	Cognitive	.88**	.89**	.86**	.75**	.63**	.73**	.68**	.79**	.71**	.80**
	Fine motor	.92**	.87**	.88**	.81**	.75**	.80**	.65**	.72**	.65**	.75**
	Infant language/receptive language	.92**	.91**	.91**	.80**	.74**	.82**	.73**	.81**	.75**	.81**
	Infant memory/memory	.84**	.85**	.81**	.68**	.60**	.68**	.63**	.74**	.65**	.74**
	Speed	.95**	.89**	.90**	.85**	.78**	.80**	.66**	.74**	.66**	.76**
	Visual motor	.92**	.89**	.89**	.83**	.74**	.77**	.64**	.74**	.66**	.76**

Note. CVP = cognitive verbal / preverbal; EL = expressive language; RL = receptive language; FM = fine motor; GM = gross motor; VMI = visual-motor imitation; AE = affective expression; SR = social reciprocity; CMB = characteristic motor behaviors; CVB = characteristic verbal behaviors.

** $p < .01$

Table 9. Correlation coefficients between CPEP-3 performance subtests and CARS subscales

	Performance subtests									
CARS subscales	CVP	EL	RL	FM	GM	VMI	AE	SR	CMB	CVB
Relating to people	-.55**	-.59**	-.65**	-.44**	-.42**	-.62**	-.63**	-.69**	-.74**	-.64**
Imitation	-.72**	-.72**	-.74**	-.66**	-.56**	-.72**	-.65**	-.76**	-.66**	-.73**
Emotional response	-.05	-.01	-.05	-.04	-.03	-.11	-.08	-.11	-.20	-.07
Body use	-.39**	-.44**	-.35**	-.32**	-.28*	-.28*	-.27*	-.43**	-.39**	-.32**
Object use	-.05	-.10	-.07	-.03	-.11	-.16	-.15	-.20	-.36**	-.07
Adaptation to change	.07	.08	.08	.12	.20	.01	-.01	-.07	-.11	.13
Visual response	-.24	-.31*	-.33**	-.17	-.17	-.25*	-.20	-.32**	-.34**	-.39**
Listening response	-.33**	-.36**	-.38**	-.28*	-.30*	-.30*	-.36**	-.43**	-.52**	-.40**
Taste, smell, touch response and use	-.37**	-.45**	-.40**	-.27*	-.23	-.39**	-.48**	-.59**	-.61**	-.50**
Fear or nervousness	.04	.02	.06	.08	.06	.00	.00	.19	.13	-.08
Verbal communication	-.67**	-.72**	-.75**	-.55**	-.47**	-.67**	-.68**	-.72**	-.77**	-.77**
Nonverbal communication	-.63**	-.71**	-.72**	-.49**	-.46**	-.46**	-.66**	-.70**	-.71**	-.76**
Activity level	-.49**	-.50**	-.47**	-.39**	-.31*	-.48**	-.56**	-.65**	-.66**	-.49**
Level& consistency of intellectual response	-.39**	-.43**	-.39**	-.27*	-.20	-.31*	-.53**	-.48**	-.51**	-.51**
General impressions	-.56**	-.62**	-.64**	-.43**	-.38**	-.57**	-.59**	-.70**	-.73**	-.64**
Total score	-.60**	-.65**	-.64**	-.46**	-.39**	-.60**	-.63**	-.77**	-.79**	-.68**

Note. CVP = cognitive verbal/preverbal; EL = expressive language; RL = receptive language; FM = fine motor; GM = gross motor; VMI = visual-motor imitation; AE = affective expression; SR = social reciprocity; CMB = characteristic motor behaviors; CVB = characteristic verbal behaviors. ** $p < .01$; * $p < .05$.

Table 10. Comparison of the psychometric findings on CPEP-3 performance subtests and the findings in the PEP-3 manual

Performance subtests	No. of items	Average Cronbach's alpha		Test-retest reliability		Median Inter-rater reliability		Correlation with CARS	
		Chinese ($N = 455$)	American ($N = 407$)	Chinese ($N = 42$)	American ($N = 33$)	Chinese ($N = 46$)	American (N.A.)	Chinese ($N = 64$)	American ($N = 68$)
CVP	34	0.97	0.97	0.98	0.99	0.87	-	-.060	-0.75
EL	25	0.97	0.97	0.99	0.99	0.81	-	-0.65	-0.63
RL	19	0.97	0.97	0.97	0.99	0.77	-	-0.64	-0.76
FM	20	0.91	0.93	0.96	0.98	0.76	-	-0.46	-0.78
GM	15	0.90	0.92	0.92	0.99	0.62	-	-0.39	-0.70
VMI	10	0.90	0.95	0.93	0.97	0.79	-	-0.60	-0.78
AE	11	0.89	0.90	0.84	0.94	0.34	-	-0.63	-0.74
SR	12	0.90	0.91	0.92	0.97	0.41	-	-0.77	-0.68
CMB	15	0.92	0.91	0.95	0.98	0.48	-	-0.79	-0.71
CVB	11	0.95	0.93	0.96	0.95	0.52	-	-0.68	-0.65

Note. CVP = cognitive verbal / preverbal; EL = expressive language; RL = receptive language; FM = fine motor; GM = gross motor; VMI = visual-motor imitation; AE = affective expression; SR = social reciprocity; CMB = characteristic motor behaviors; CVB = characteristic verbal behaviors.

Findings of the American sample were excerpted from the PEP-3 manual (Schopler et al., 2005).

Finally, Table 10 summarizes the psychometric findings of CPEP-3 on the present sample of Chinese children and corresponding results of PEP-3 available in the PEP-3 user manual. It can be found that the psychometric properties of CPEP-3 compared favorably with those of PEP-3 reported by the test developers (12).

DISCUSSION

The aim of the present study was to further report evidence on the reliability and validity of the Performance Test of the Chinese version of Psycho-Educational Profile-3rd Edition (CPEP-3) in the assessment of developmental disorders in a Chinese context. The findings showed that the Performance Test of the CPEP-3 has good psychometric properties when applied to Chinese population, which lends support to the cross-cultural applicability and stability of the CPEP-3.

There are several unique features of this study. First, this is a pioneering scientific study of the PEP-3 on a large sample of Chinese children who are under-represented in the scientific literature on ASD. Second, consistent with the approaches adopted in Schopler et al. (12), different types of reliability and validity were examined in this study. Third, the present findings are on par or even better than those reported in the original study. Finally, the sample size of the current study was quite large considering the relatively low incidence of ASD in children.

Three different types of reliability were examined. The internal consistency of each subtest measured by Cronbach's alpha coefficient for the whole sample of children (ranging from 0.89 to 0.97) was high in this study and is comparable with the findings (Cronbach's alpha coefficients ranging from 0.90 to 0.97) reported by Schopler et al. (12) on American samples. The values of the reliability measures appeared to be higher than the previous reports on the Chinese version of PEP-R (ranging from 0.74 to 0.98) in Hong Kong context (14), which suggests that the items of CPEP-3 are more homogeneous than CPEP-R in measuring their latent constructs. For the composites, their internal consistency was also high (ranging from

0.96 to 0.99). When the Cronbach's alpha coefficients were calculated for children at different ages, it was found that all values are high, except for participants of 7 to 7.9 years of age. This may be due to the limited number of cases ($N = 6$) at this age group and the lack of variance for a few items, which make it impossible to calculate any error variance.

For test-retest reliability, a subsample of children with autism was rated twice on the Performance Test of CPEP-3 over six weeks to three months. The correlation coefficients for each subtest at the two time points ranged from 0.84 to 0.99, suggesting high test-retest reliability. In other words, the participants' scores on CPEP-3 are unlikely to be influenced by random factors in the conditions of the participants or the testing environment over time. Inter-rater reliability was assessed for 46 children with ASDs. According to the criterion suggested by Hopkin and Stanley (31) for determining the size of correlation coefficients ($0 < r < 0.1$ means very small correlation; $0.1 < r < 0.3$ means small correlation; $0.3 < r < 0.5$ means moderate correlation; $0.5 < r < 0.7$ means large correlation; and $0.7 < r < 0.9$ means very large correlation), the mean and median polychoric correlation coefficients for each Performance subtest ranged from moderate to very large. This provides support for the inter-rater reliability of the CPEP-3 Performance subtests. The findings suggest that using the CPEP-3, different examiners rated the items in a consistent way.

Consistent with western findings, traditional item analyses on the CPEP-3 Performance Test showed that both item discrimination and item difficulty were at an acceptable range, and with age increased, the percentage of participants who passed a particular item also increased. These findings support the content validity of the instrument. The evaluation of the criterion-related validity as a measure to estimate the developmental level in comparison with two standardized developmental assessment measures (MPR and CARS) on a subsample of 64 autistic children demonstrated that CPEP-3 can be well used to effectively quantify the developmental level of children with ASDs. Significant correlations were found between CPEP-3 and the two criterion measures, MPR and CARS. These findings echo with the findings reported by Schopler et al. (12) on samples of children in the

United States and provide evidence for the criterion-related validity of CPEP-3.

Overall, the above findings support that the CPEP-3 Performance Test had good reliability and validity when applied to Hong Kong samples, which compared favorably with previous findings based on American samples. The summary shown in Table 10 clearly suggests that the translated CPEP-3 Performance Test is a reliable and valid measure for assessing Chinese children with autism and its results can be regarded as consistent.

It should be noted that there are several limitations in the present study. First, the study was conducted in Hong Kong and spoken Cantonese was used as the language for the administration of the test. Therefore, the participants may not be representative of the children with autism in a broader Chinese context, particularly for Mandarin-speaking areas. Further studies must be conducted in other Chinese societies and evaluate the psychometric properties of CPEP-3 when administered in Mandarin. Second, while one significant difference between CPEP-3 and PEP-R is the addition of a Caregiver Report, which rates children's performance based on caregivers' daily observation, the present study only investigated the psychometric properties of the Performance Test. As the adaptive behaviors and symptom severities of children with ASDs vary across different environments, the Caregiver Report would provide important information on children's development in different contexts. To obtain a full picture of the development of children with ASDs in Chinese contexts, the reliability and validity of the Caregiver Report must be investigated. Third, although the group with autism and the control group were matched on participants' age in the present study, other factors that contribute to children's development were not taken into account, such as gender and IQ. Future study shall consider these factors when setting up the inclusion criterion in participants recruitment. Nevertheless, as a promising assessment tool for children with ASD, the psychometric properties of CPEP-3 need to be established before they can be used to guide the development of intervention programs. Researchers and practitioners are most interested in obtaining scores that are accurate, reliable, and can best estimate the child's true level of development. The present study clearly suggests that the Chinese version of the Psycho-Educational Profile-3rd edition (CPEP-3) Performance Test has good reliability and validity when it is used to measure the developmental level of children with autism spectrum disorders in a Chinese context. In future, more evidence on the construct validity of the Performance Test and the psychometric properties of the Caregiver Report of the CPEP-3 need to be further established.

ACKNOWLEDGMENTS

The study was conducted by Heep Hong Society in Hong Kong. We thank colleagues of Heep Hong Society for collecting the data for the validation study. The authorship of the paper is equally shared by the first author and second author. This chapter is a re-print with minor revision of an earlier published paper in the *International Public Health Journal* 2018;10(1) issue with permission.

REFERENCES

[1] American Psychiatric Association. Diagnostic and statistical manual of mental disorders: DSM-4. Washington, DC: American Psychiatric Association, 1994.

[2] American Psychiatric Association. Diagnostic and Statistical Manual of Mental Health Disorders: DSM-5. Washington, DC: American Psychiatric Publishing, 2013.

[3] Rapin I, Katzman, R. Neurobiology of autism. Ann Neurol 1998;43:7-14.

[4] Bertrand J, Mars A, Boyle C, Bove F, Yeargin-Allsopp M, Decoufle P. Prevalence of autism in a United States population: the Brick Township, New Jersey, investigation. Pediatrics 2001;108:1155-61.

[5] Kielinen M, Linna SL, Moilanen I. Autism in Finland. Eur Child Adolesc Psychiatry 2000;9(3):162-7.

[6] Matson JL, Kozlowski AM. The increasing prevalence of autism spectrum disorders. Res Autism Spectr Disord 2011;5(1):418-25.

[7] Scott FJ, Baron-Cohen S, Bolton P, Brayne C. Brief report: prevalence of autism spectrum conditions in children aged 5-11 years in Cambridgeshire, UK. Autism 2002;6:231-7.

[8] Wong VCN, Hui SLH. Epidemiological study of autism spectrum disorder in China. J Child Neurol 2008;23:67-72.

[9] Volkmar F, Cook EH, Pomeroy J, Realmuto G, Tanguay, P. Practice parameters for the assessment and treatment of children, adolescents, and adults with autism and other pervasive developmental disorders. American Academy of Child and Adolescent Psychiatry Working Group on Quality Issues. J Am Acad Child Adolesc Psychiatry 1999;38:32S-54S.

[10] Salvia JA, Ysseldyke JE. Assessment in special and remedial education, 6th ed. Boston, MA: Houghton-Mifflin, 1995.

[11] Shriver MD, Allen KD, Mathews JR. Effective assessment of the shared and unique characteristics of children with autism. Sch Psychol Rev 1999;28:538-58.

[12] Schopler E, Lansing MD, Reichler RJ, Marcus LM. Psychoeducational profile: TEACCH individualized psychoeducational assessment for children with autism spectrum disorders, 3rd ed. Austin, TX: Pro-Ed, 2005.

[13] De Leon C. Psychoeducational profile revised (PEP-R): the Brazilian version elaboration. Autism 2005; 9:450-1.

[14] Portoghese C, Buttiglione M, Pavone F, Lozito V, De Giacomo A, Martinelli D, Margari Li. The usefulness of the revised psychoeducational profile for the assessment of preschool children with pervasive developmental disorders. Autism 2009;13:179-91.

[15] Schopler E, Reichler RJ, Bashford A, Lansing MD, Marcus LM. Psychoeducational Profile-Revised (PEP-R), individualized assessment and treatment for autistic and developmentally disabled children, vol 1. Austin, TX: Pro-Ed, 1990.

[16] Shek DTL, Tsang SKM, Lam LL, Tang FLY, Cheung, PMP. Psychometric properties of the Chinese version of the Psycho-Educational Profile-Revised (CPEP-R). J Autism Dev Disord 2005;35:37-44.

[17] Villa S, Micheli E, Villa L, Pastore V, Crippa A, Molteni, M. Further empirical data on the psychoeducational profile-revised (PEP-R): reliability and validation with the Vineland adaptive behavior scales. J Autism Dev Disord 2001;40:334-41.

[18] Schopler E, Reichler RJ, Renner BR. The Childhood Autism Rating Scale (CARS). Los Angeles, CA: Western Psychological Services, 1988.

[19] Krug D, Arick J, Almond P. Autism Behavior Checklist—ABC. In: Krug DA, Arick J, Almond P, eds. Autism screening instrument for educational planning—ASIEP-2. Austin, TX: Pro-Ed, 1993.

[20] Sparrow SS, Balla D, Cicchetti, DV. Vineland Adaptive Behavior Scales. Circle Pines, MN: American Guidance Services, 1984.

[21] Kikas E, Häidkind P. Developing an Estonian version of the psychoeducational profile revised (PEP-R). J Autism Dev Disord 2003;33:217.

[22] Chen KL, Chiang FM, Tseng MH, Fu CP, Hsieh, CL. Responsiveness of the Psychoeducational profile-third edition for children with autism spectrum disorders. J Autism Dev Disord 2011;41:1658-64.

[23] Fu CP, Chen KL, Tseng MH, Chiang FM, Hsieh CL. Reliability and validity of the psychoeducational profile-third edition caregiver report in children with autism spectrum disorders. Res Autism Spectr Disord 2011;6:115-22.

[24] Fu CP, Hsieh CL, Tseng MH, Chen YL, Huang WT, Wu PC, Chiang FM. Inter-rater reliability and smallest real difference of the Chinese Psychoeducational Profile-third edition for children with ASD. Res Autism Spectr Disord 2010;4:89-94.

[25] Shek DTL, Yu L. Construct validity of the Chinese version of the Psycho-Educational Profile-3rd Edition (CPEP-3). J Autism Dev Disord 2014;44: 2832-43.

[26] Carmines EG, Zeller RA. Reliability and validity assessment. Beverly Hills, CA: Sage, 1979.

[27] Anastasi A, Urbina S. Psychological testing, 7th ed. Upper Saddle River, NJ: Prentice Hall, 1997.

[28] Shek DTL & Yu L. Psychometric properties of the Chinese version of the Psychoeducational Profile-3rd edition-Caregiver Report. J Intellect Dev Disabil, in press.

[29] Roid GH, Sampers J. Merrill-Palmer Developmental Scale—Revised manual. Wood Dale, IL: Stoelting, 2004.

[30] Jöreskog KG, Sörbom D. LISREL 7: A guide to the program and applications. Chicago, IL: SPSS, 1988.

[31] Hopkins K, Stanley J. Educational and psychological measurement and evaluation, 6th ed. Englewood, NJ: Prentice Hall, 1981.

[32] Lam MK, Rao N. Developing a Chinese version of the psychoeducational profile (CPEP) to assess children in Hong Kong. J Autism Dev Disord 1993;23: 273-9.

[33] Tsang SKM, Shek DTL, Lam LL, Tang FLY, Cheung, PMP. Application of the TEACCH Program on Chinese pre-school children with autism—Does culture make a difference? J Autism Dev Disord 2007;37:390-6.

[34] Ebel RL. Essentials of educational measurement, 2nd ed. Englewood Cliffs, NJ: Prentice Hall, 1972.

[35] Pyrczak F. Validity of the discrimination index as a measure of item validity. J Educ Meas 1973;10:227-31.

In: Advances in Chinese Children … ISBN: 978-1-53617-870-8
Editors: Ariel Tenenbaum et al.

Chapter 3

THE IMPACTS OF A UNICEF HEALTH PROMOTION PROJECT ON PRIMARY HEALTH CARE IN WESTERN CHINA: A COMPREHENSIVE EVALUATION AT PROVINCIAL LEVEL

Yuxue Bi[1], PhD, Dejian Lai[2], PhD and Hong Yan[1,*], MD, PhD

[1]Department of Epidemiology and Health Statistics, School of Public Health, Xi'an Jiaotong University School of Medicine, Xi'an, Shaanxi, PRChina

[2]School of Public Health, The University of Texas Health Science Center at Houston, Houston, Texas, United States

---

* Corresponding Author: Hong Yan, Department of Epidemiology and Health Statistics, School of Public Health, Xi'an Jiaotong University School of Medicine, Xi'an, Shaanxi 710061, PR China. E-mail: byx@mail.xjtu.edu.cn.

ABSTRACT

In order to improve the health care service in poor rural western region of China, the Ministry of Health of the People's Republic of China and UNICEF had implemented "the Health Management Pilot County Project" in five provinces of western China. The purpose of this article is to evaluate the impacts of the project at provincial level. We collected data through two cross-sectional surveys in 1999, 2000, and used the analytic hierarchy process, the technique for order preference by similarity to ideal solution and linear weighting to analyze the data. The difference of the measurements between the two surveys was tested by paired-samples t test. All synthetic values of the five provinces in 2000 were higher than those in 1999 ($t = 6.62$, $P = 0.003$). The ranks of five provinces from highest to lowest were Xinjiang, Gansu, Qinghai, Ningxia and Guizhou. However, we also found disturbing facts that 10-20% of pregnant women had no prenatal care before child delivery. The project significantly improved the health service from shortly point of view, but there is still much to be done.

INTRODUCTION

Mainland China consists of 31 provincial-level administrative regions under the central government of China, including 22 provinces, five autonomous regions, four municipalities. In general, urban areas are more developed than the rural areas. Villages in the eastern region are generally more developed than the villages in the western region. In rural China, administrative households are nested in villages, which are grouped to form townships, a cluster of townships are governed by a county, tens or even hundreds of counties/cities become a provincial region. The rural health service system of China includes county hospitals such as the main county hospital, maternal and child healthcare hospital, Chinese medicine hospital, township hospitals and village health clinics. We called it "three-tier health service network." The western region of China is a less developed social and economic area with multi-ethnic culture and diverse geographic conditions, since socio-economic reforms commenced in 1980s, some health service-related issues emerged in this region. For example, most village clinics in the western poor region of China lacked of basic medical facilities (1, 2).

Some village clinics have even used "Three-no" drugs (possibly fake drugs out of the official distribution channel) (3, 4), intravenous injections of antibiotics were overused and the hormone was abused commonly (3-5). Village doctors were unwilling to provide primary health care for the villagers due to no payment (6, 7).

Maternal mortality ratio (MMR) in the western region of China was as high as 200 per 100,000 live births, which was four times the average urban MMR and two times the rural average MMR (8). Infant mortality rates are nearly five times higher in the poorest rural counties than those in the wealthiest counties (9). The growth and nutrition of children are in worrying (9-15). For children under 5 years of age, the percentages of child stunting and child underweight were 22.6% and 12.6% (15) respectively in rural areas, moreover in western region they were 24.0% and 22.1% (13).

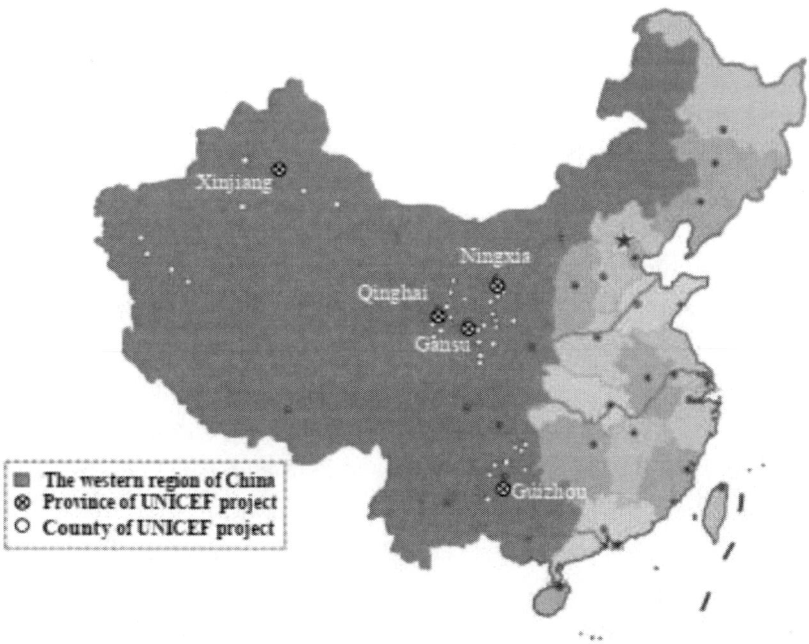

Figure 1. The western region of China and the UNICEF project provinces.

In order to improve the health service especial health care of maternal and children in the poor rural western region of China, the Ministry of Health of the People's Republic of China (MOH) and the United Nations Children's Fund (UNICEF) implemented "the Health Management Pilot County Project" (16) in the forty poor counties of five provinces in the western region of China (Figure 1). In this article, we presented a provincial level analysis on data collected from the project. The counties level analysis was published by Bi, Lai and Yan (17).

OUR STUDY

Two cross-sectional surveys were conducted for the evaluation of the project. A stratified multistage random sampling was used to obtain subjects from each county (17). The sample size was calculated based on the prevalence of anemia in children under the age of 36 months (17). A 4-stage sampling design was adopted for the sample in three different stratums (county, township and village) (17).

The design of the two surveys was developed by three steps (17). The study protocol was reviewed and approved by the Human Research Ethics Committee of the Xi'an Jiaotong University College of Medicine. Ten survey teams were created for five provinces; the team's members consisted of the researchers from Xi'an Jiaotong University a prominent academic institute in west China and the staffs from local healthcare sectors. All questionnaires were filled in through face to face interviews by our professional interviewers trained by Xi'an Jiaotong University. We applied a set of quality control techniques during data collection and used double data entry and logical check procedures to input data (17), and employed EpiInfo to establish the database.

Data analysis

The data in this study came from two surveys. First, in accordance with the objectives of project (16) and the four considerations: purpose, representative, objectivity and comparison (18-22), we selected twenty seven indicators from the questionnaires of the two surveys to evaluate synthetically the effects of the project. These indicators were classified into four aspects: health management, medical treatment condition, maternal health care and child health care (17). Second, we calculated mean or median values for continuous variables and percentages for categorical variables for summary. Next step was the comprehensive evaluation and comparative analysis.

In the comprehensive evaluation, we used the Analytic Hierarchy Process (AHP) (17-19) to determine the weighting coefficients (W_j) of the four aspects, where j is for the four aspects, j = 1 to 4. Then we employed the Technique for Order Preference by Similarity to Ideal Solution (TOPSIS) (17, 20, 21) to compute the D_{jyi} values of the four aspects of the difference year surveys (y = 1999, 2000) in five provinces(i = 1 to 5).

The comprehensive evaluation value was constructed as

$$E_{yi} = \sum_{j=1}^{4} W_j \times D_{jyi} \; .$$

In comparative analysis, paired-samples t test was performed to compare the results of the difference of comprehensive evaluation value between two years, the Chi-square test was employed for each categorical indicator between 2000 and 1999. P-value < 0.05 was used as the threshold of indicating statistical significance for all tests in this study. SPSS was used for all data analysis and Microsoft Excel was used to draw figures.

Table 1. General family information

Province	Sample		Source of family Incoming (%)		Drinking water (%)			Cooking salt (%)	
	n	%	Agriculture	others	Not boiled	Sometimes boiled	boiled	Iodine salt	others
Guizhou	1835	24.9	81.2	18.8	25.4	33.5	41.1	98.1	1.9
Gansu	1812	24.6	86.8	13.2	1.5	16.9	81.6	92.0	8.0
Ningxia	1137	15.4	98.3	1.7	2.1	31.8	66.1	56.6	43.4
Qinghai	1083	14.7	95.1	4.9	0.3	2.5	97.2	83.0	17.0
Xinjiang	1497	20.3	95.0	5.0	7.4	42.2	50.4	87.6	12.4

FINDINGS

The household sample sizes in five provinces were from 1,083 (Qinghai, 14.7%) to 1,835 (Guizhou, 24.9%). Their household incomes were mainly from agriculture 81.2% (Guizhou) to 98.3% (Ningxia). Among the five provinces, Qinghai had the highest percentage of household drinking boiled water (97.2%) and Guizhou was reported with highest percentage (98.1%) of household using iodized salt for cooking. More detail percentages about each province on source of family income, drinking water, and salt are tabulated in Table 1. On average, mothers' illiteracy rates in each province were higher than fathers', the difference of the illiteracy rates between male and female in four provinces except Xinjiang was statistically significant by Chi-square test ($P < 0.05$). Both highest illiteracy rates were observed in Ningxia. More values and percentages about each province are presented in Table 2. The average birth weight in each province was about 3.13(kg) in Qinghai to 3.37(kg) in Guizhou; we observed that Gansu had highest children immunization record (95.4%); More information of children are presented in Table 3. Table 4 showed us that average percentage of children born at home were from 37.2% in Xinjiang to 82.7% in Qinghai, and Qinghai also had highest of percentage of family person, the relatives and the neighbor as midwifes (40.1%). More than 63% of children's families chose the village health clinic for primary care except Xinjiang, there was 46.1% of children's families chose the their village health clinic and 33.9%

of children's families chose the township hospital for primary care in Xinjiang (Table 5).

Table 2. Education of parents

Province	Mother (year)				Father (year)			
	mean	median	maximum	Illiteracy rate (%)	mean	median	maximum	Illiteracy rate (%)
Guizhou	3.91	4.00	14	29.5	6.55	7.00	17	5.2
Gansu	4.63	5.00	15	26.5	6.88	8.00	15	7.2
Ningxia	3.62	3.00	16	41.9	5.81	7.00	17	17.4
Qinghai	3.75	3.00	17	40.4	5.84	6.00	16	15.7
Xinjiang	6.27	5.00	16	3.0	6.77	7.00	16	2.0

Table 3. The information on children

Province	Birth weight(kg)		Sex (%)		Immunization records (%)	
	mean	median	male	female	yes	no
Guizhou	3.37	3.40	60.4	39.6	87.6	12.4
Gansu	3.20	3.05	62.1	37.9	95.4	4.6
Ningxia	3.27	3.25	54.6	45.4	83.3	16.7
Qinghai	3.13	3.00	53.0	47.0	93.9	6.1
Xinjiang	3.18	3.00	49.9	50.1	94.2	5.8

Table 4. The information on children's birth site and their midwives

Province	The birth site of children (%)*						Midwives (%) **					
	1	2	3	4	5	6	1	2	3	4	5	6
Guizhou	75.3	6.7	10.4	2.5	2.6	2.2	32.6	13.8	12.7	4.5	2.8	33.3
Gansu	64.9	3.1	16.9	3.9	9.4	1.8	27.5	9.3	19.1	10.2	10.2	23.7
Ningxia	70.9	0.9	6.4	9.3	12.1	0.3	39.4	7.9	10.5	9.7	12.2	20.1
Qinghai	82.7	1.7	1.9	2.5	11.2	0.0	39.5	0.8	2.4	4.3	13.0	40.1
Xinjiang	37.2	10.0	27.8	4.3	19.2	0.8	21.3	5.8	28.6	6.0	19.5	18.8

The sample proportions of village health clinics in five provinces were from 16.1% to 24.3%. The average distance between villages and the township's administrative center was from 4.28(km) (Qinhai) to 7.06 km (Xinjiang). The average population size of a village in the end of 1998 was 1044.18(Xinjiang) to 1723.25 (Guizhou). The average yearly income per person in 1998 was ¥664.44 (about $95, Qinhai) to 1432.31 (about $205, Xinjiang). The villages in the sample were from poor regions. The average number of doctors per village health clinic was less than two and the age of the chief doctor of village health clinic was over 38 years old (38.55 to 44.78). More detail information about each province is tabulated in Table 6. We noticed from Table 7 that over 60% doctors' education level was secondary school or less, only 2.3% of doctors' education level in Xinjiang graduated from colleges or above, no doctors graduated from colleges and above in Guizhou and Gansu. 88.6% of village doctors in Qinghai were "barefoot doctor," the lowest percentage in Guizhou was 29.5%. The highest percentage (3.4%) of professional training at college level or above of doctors was in Xinjiang.

Table 5. The initial treatment site for childhood illness (%)

Province	Clinic in the same village	Clinic in neighboring village	Township hospital	Hospital of county or above	Maternal and child health center of county or above	Others
Guizhou	69.8	11.5	7.9	1.4	0.5	8.8
Gansu	68.0	9.3	14.1	4.1	0.7	3.8
Ningxia	63.8	5.5	19.4	3.5	0.6	7.2
Qinghai	68.5	17.6	3.4	7.6	1.8	1.2
Xinjiang	46.1	10.6	33.9	2.4	0.9	5.8

Table 6. The information of village

Province	Sample		Distance between village and township (km)		Population of village in 1998		Incoming per person in 1998 (¥)		Number of village doctors		Age of village doctor(year)	
	n	%	Mean	Median	Mean	Median	Mean	Median	Mean	Median	Mean	Median
Guizhou	105	23.8	6.89	5.00	1723.25	1628.00	747.36	700.00	1.81	2.00	38.63	40.00
Gansu	107	24.3	6.08	5.00	1661.01	1350.00	853.89	810.00	1.85	2.00	44.71	46.00
Ningxia	72	16.3	5.14	4.00	1583.26	1356.00	1073.50	602.00	1.25	1.00	44.78	47.00
Qinghai	71	16.1	4.28	3.00	1044.46	1085.00	664.44	589.00	1.17	1.00	43.87	46.50
Xinjiang	86	19.5	7.06	4.00	1299.18	1117.00	1423.31	935.00	1.62	1.00	38.55	40.00

Table 7. Education and professional training of village doctors

Province	Education					Professional Training			
	Less than primary school	primary school	Secondary school	High school	College and above	"barefoot doctor"	County	medical school	Medical college and above
Guizhou	1.9	11.4	48.6	38.1	0.0	29.5	38.4	29.5	2.7
Gansu	4.7	11.2	43.9	40.2	0.0	37.2	51.3	9.7	1.8
Ningxia	5.6	22.2	50.0	20.8	1.4	62.7	17.9	16.4	3.0
Qinghai	1.4	11.3	53.5	32.4	1.4	88.6	2.9	7.1	1.4
Xinjiang	1.2	8.1	51.2	37.2	2.3	69.3	12.5	14.8	3.4

Table 8. The results of evaluation of counties

Province	*D* values								*E* values		E_{2000}- E_{1999}
	Health management		Medical treatment condition		Maternal health care		Child health care				
	1999	2000	1999	2000	1999	2000	1999	2000	1999	2000	
Guizhou	0.291	0.419	0.531	0.441	0.073	0.300	0.372	0.662	0.379	0.443	0.064
Gansu	0.345	0.323	0.294	0.547	0.345	0.589	0.381	0.470	0.327	0.473	0.146
Ningxia	0.406	0.333	0.195	0.395	0.303	0.485	0.191	0.312	0.273	0.376	0.103
Qinghai	0.329	0.651	0.324	0.293	0.062	0.277	0.436	0.508	0.307	0.429	0.122
Xinjiang	0.285	0.573	0.591	0.727	0.887	0.912	0.657	0.805	0.540	0.711	0.171

Comprehensive evaluation

Using AHP, we computed the weighting coefficients of the four aspects, they were 0.311 0.440, 0.124 and 0.124, respectively. According to data of two surveys, we used the TOPSIS to calculate the *D* values of the four aspects of five provinces, we calculated the synthetic indicator of *E* via linear weighting, and the all values are listed in Table 8. The results showed that all *E* values in 2000 were higher than those in 1999. The difference of comprehensive values *E* between these two years was statistically significant ($t = 6.62$, $P = 0.003$) by paired *t* test. However, we found that not all of D values of the four aspects in five provinces in 2000 were higher than those in 1999; the provinces with higher D values in 2000 were Guizhou, Qinghai and Xingjian in health management; Gansu, Ningxia and Xingjian in medical treatment condition; all in maternal health care and in child health care.

Table 9. Indicators of health management in five provinces in two years

Indicators	Guizhou		Gansu		Ningxia		Qinghai		Xinjiang	
	1999	2000	1999	2000	1999	2000	1999	2000	1999	2000
Percentage of having license (%)	80.39	49.07	96.26	90.43	91.67	56.34	98.60	73.91	55.95	44.83
Percentage of having registration of patients (%)	69.52	58.95	64.49	68.47	38.89	33.33	87.14	70.69	40.00	88.89
Percentage of using of prescriptions (%)	39.42	82.18	30.48	94.74	47.22	90.38	30.43	96.61	32.94	98.48
Percentage of having log of drug purchases (%)	57.14	36.11	41.51	52.63	79.17	42.65	94.37	54.41	36.05	36.76
Percentage of having birth certificates (%)	83.81	89.09	62.26	78.57	77.78	88.89	80.28	82.61	90.48	98.88
Percentage of performing health education (%)	48.08	69.64	40.00	71.68	47.76	19.44	38.57	69.57	58.33	96.63
Percentage of attending routine meeting at township hospital (%)	72.38	49.07	81.31	90.43	44.44	56.34	90.14	73.91	75.58	44.83
The total of charge in thirty prescriptions(yuan)	7572.61	8032.34	5966.7	17480.16	6711.68	6606.44	12867.59	6206.5	9371.13	5558.34
The count of antibiotics in thirty prescriptions	929	1909	545	2164	409	931	1032	925	585	776
The count of hormone drugs in thirty prescriptions	302	102	156	167	151	87	327	14	112	22
The count of intravenous injection in thirty prescriptions	125	51	131	283	106	87	214	95	183	113

Table 10. Indicators of medical treatment condition in five provinces in two years

Indicators (%)	Guizhou		Gansu		Ningxia		Qinghai		Xinjiang	
	1999	2000	1999	2000	1999	2000	1999	2000	1999	2000
Percentage of having pressure cooker	65.71	68.47	68.87	90.35	70.83	83.33	46.48	55.07	75.58	55.07
Percentage of using of pressure cooker	66.18	85.53	51.35	69.90	49.02	68.33	93.94	83.78	46.88	83.78
Percentage of having package of delivery	75.24	43.64	42.45	46.09	27.78	22.22	25.35	11.59	67.44	11.59
Percentage of having child weight scale	32.38	10.91	9.43	39.13	23.61	22.22	9.86	18.84	53.49	18.84
Percentage of qualified disinfectant of skin	77.88	85.45	49.04	81.58	31.94	77.46	71.43	82.61	61.18	82.61
Percentage of qualified disinfectant of apparatus	43.81	64.86	35.85	53.10	15.28	52.11	42.86	20.29	38.82	20.29

Table 11. Indicators of maternal health care in five provinces in two years

Indicators (%)	Guizhou		Gansu		Ningxia		Qinghai		Xinjiang	
	1999	2000	1999	2000	1999	2000	1999	2000	1999	2000
Percentage of prenatal care	57.47	72.60	79.56	89.56	72.25	74.21	64.54	72.47	90.65	91.22
Percentage of hospital birth	15.48	21.00	30.19	39.40	27.79	35.71	15.60	27.22	51.17	56.75
Percentage of postnatal visit	53.01	70.64	47.98	64.28	55.28	63.90	46.30	50.94	84.41	76.27

Table 12. Indicators of child health care in five provinces in two years

Indicators	Guizhou		Gansu		Ningxia		Qinghai		Xinjiang	
	1999	2000	1999	2000	1999	2000	1999	2000	1999	2000
Percentage of breast-feeding (%)	97.49	97.05	96.02	94.84	98.42	97.83	93.8	97.19	98.06	94.73
Score of adding grain food	0.64	0.66	0.63	0.63	0.64	0.65	0.59	0.59	0.62	0.64
Score of adding protein food	0.42	0.55	0.37	0.44	0.33	0.42	0.38	0.45	0.44	0.51
Score of adding vegetable food	0.65	0.72	0.58	0.61	0.58	0.6	0.61	0.63	0.65	0.66
Prevalence of common cold in two weeks (%)	38.71	34.26	34.22	35.04	45.91	43.78	28.24	31.81	17.11	18.96
Prevalence of diarrhea in two weeks (%)	28.07	26.59	17.55	24.40	27.00	33.87	15.88	21.09	20.11	22.71

The results of comparative analysis of the indicators of four aspects in two surveys were tabulated in the Table 9 to the Table 12. The differences of some indicators of four aspects were exhibited in the Figure 2 to Figure 5. The bars in all figures illustrated by the differences calculated from the values of indicators in 2000 minus the values in 1999. The symbols "*" in each figure denoted the differences of the indicators were statistically significant Chi-square test ($P < 0.05$).

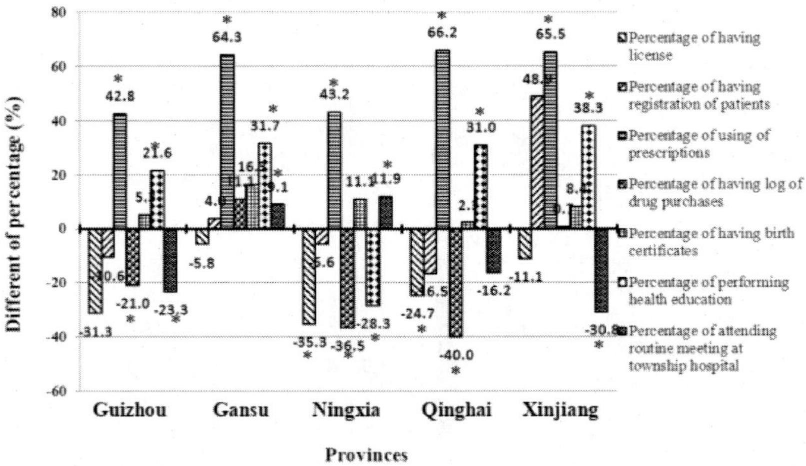

Figure 2. The Differences of Indicators of Health Management in 5 provinces.

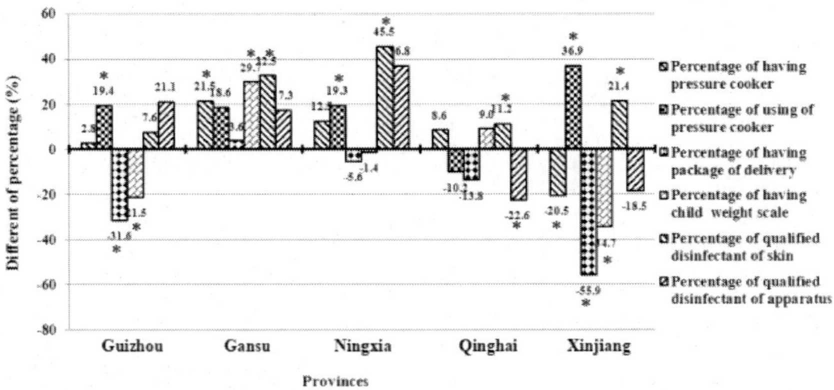

Figure 3. The Differences of Indicators of Medical Treatment Condition in 5 provinces.

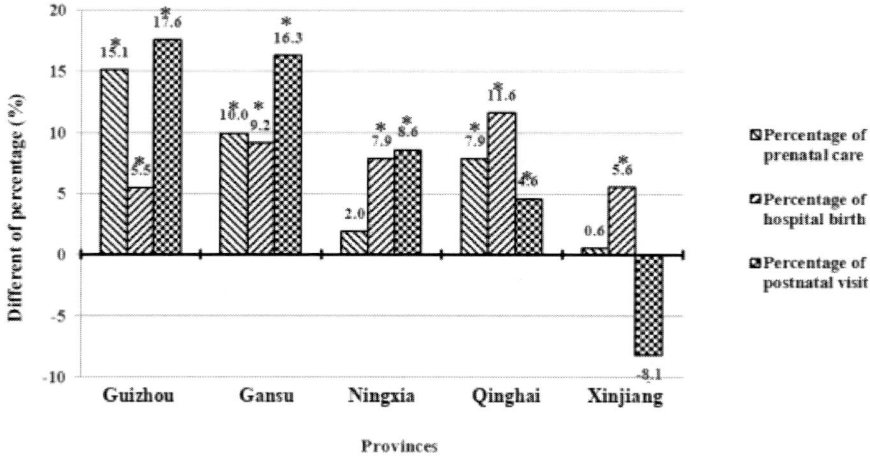

Figure 4. The Differences of Indicators of Maternal Health Care in 5 provinces.

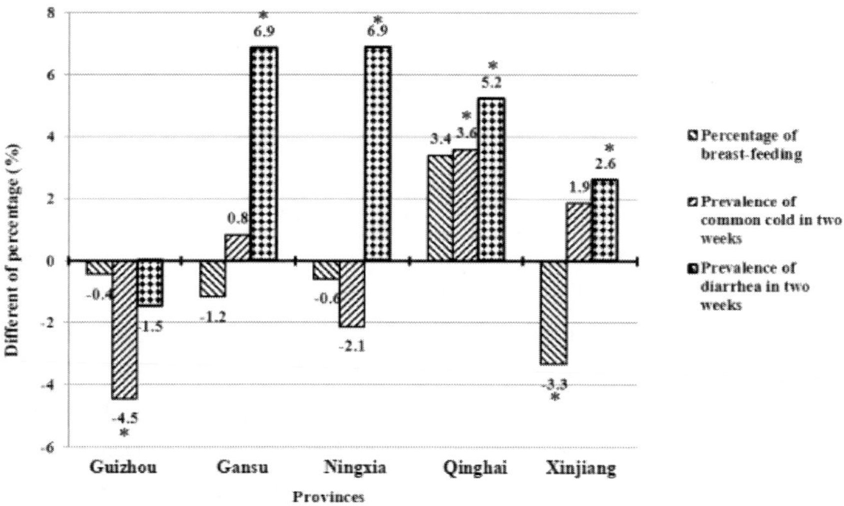

Figure 5. The Differences of Indicators of Child Health Care in 5 provinces.

DISCUSSION

In this article, we use a hybrid procedure of AHP, TOPSIS, linear weighting to evaluate synthetically the interventional effects of the health promotion project by provinces. One of the major findings from this study is that the *E* values of comprehensive evaluation in 2000 were significantly higher than that in 1999 in each of those five provinces (see Table 5). This result indicated that the interventional measures of the project in the five provinces in China were effective. Furthermore, we can see the change from the differences of two-year measurement of *E*. the rank of five provinces from highest to lowest were Xinjiang, Gansu Qinghai, Ningxia and Guizhou. This not only shows us the promotion effects of the project but also revealed the quality of conducting the project. Comparing the D values in 1999 and 2000, we found that maternal health care and child health care in five provinces had been improved, but health management only in Guizhou, Qinghai and Xinjiang had been improved, medical treatment conditions only in Gansu, Ningxia and Xinjiang have been improved. The experiences of the project provided valuable information to help us to form governmental policies on health service promotion in poor rural western region of China. The promotion measures of the project also can be used by other provinces to find an effective health promotion approaches in China. However, our study also found that some disturbing and conflicting results by comparison of the indicators of four aspects in two surveys (see Tables 9-12 and Figures 2-5).

The figures showed us the changes of four aspects in five provinces before and after promotion, the bars over the X-axis in the figures showed the differences between these two years were positive, the promotion had improved the indicators of each province. Otherwise, the promotion had no effect. We can find clearly identify the issues of these four aspects in five provinces, and lead to a better understand the future improvement. Special attention should be paid to the indicators with negative values (below the X-axis).

Figure 2 shows, among the seven indicators of health management, Guizhou, Ningxia and Qinghai had four indicators under the X-axis, namely No.1, 2, 4 and 7, these four indicators. Gansu and Xinjiang was only one indicator, that is 1 and 7 respectively. In fact, it is not difficult to make improvement with strong leadership. From our experience, as long as we assigned the responsibility to the people with proper management, we should be able to have significant improvement for similar projects in the future.

Figure 3 explicits the five indicators of the medical conditions, Xinjiang, Qinghai, Guizhou, and Ningxia had 4, 3, 2 and 2 indicators respectively below the X-axis. A common issue in the five provinces was the lack of child weight scales. Without weight scale, village doctors cannot measure the weight of children and evaluate their growth. How to raise funds to purchase basic health care equipment is a top priority, it is a challenge for developing western five provinces.

Another issue was the disinfection and sterilization, especially Qinghai and Xinjiang. This two provinces need to pay more attention on the disinfectant of skin and apparatus. If disinfection and sterilization of medical devices do not work properly, medical treatment will lead to cross infection and spread disease, especially in the area with high incidence of hepatitis.

It should be noted that in order to increase percentage of hospital delivery, one of the measures of project was to reclaim package of delivery from the village doctors, so the percentage of having package of delivery should be decline. But Gansu is the only province with percentage increasing.

Figure 4 depicted the changes of difference of three indicators in maternal health care, only the Xinjiang had a negative difference of percentage of postnatal visit. Other indicators of 5 provinces had increase at different level. Table 11 showed there were 10-20% of pregnant women had no prenatal care before child delivery. Hospital births in 5 provinces had increased significantly, but highest one was only 56.75% in Xinjiang. There is more work to do next for increase percentage of hospital birth.

Figure 5 described the three indicators of child health care. Although the percentages of breast-feeding had kind of decrease, we are pleased to see that they were still up to or above 94% (see Table 12). A common problem was children diarrhea in five provinces. Therefore, we should focus on the prevention of children diarrhea for further health education to reduce risk factors of diarrhea in children.

CONCLUSION

In summary, although our study has some limitations, data were collected through surveys and therefore subjected to biases in recall, There is no doubt that the comprehensive evaluation results of the projects in this study will play an active role in helping us understand the success experience of the project, and find the problems and defects in the process of project implementation. Provincial health administrative departments are the highest level of local administrative units; they played a major role in the supervision and management of the project and play a direct impact on effect of projects. This study can provide valuable reference for the five provinces to carrying out the project more effectively in future. It will also provide valuable reference for other provinces to implement similar project. Since the re-introduction of Chinese rural health care system at the village level in 1985, many progresses have been achieved. A recent review on the development of village doctors in China is given in (22) with an emphasis on health care finance.

ACKNOWLEDGMENTS

We sincerely thank the Ministry of Health of the People's Republic of China (MOH) and the United Nations Children's Fund (UNICEF) for their great supports and local health bureaus for their strong cooperation. We are very grateful to members of the research teams for their excellent and outstanding work in the surveys. This study was supported by National Natural Science Foundation of China (No. 30771866) and the United Nations Children's Fund (No.YH001). Conflicts of interest: none declared. This chapter is an updated version of an earlier publication in the International Journal of Child Health and Human Development 2019;12 (2) issue with permission.

REFERENCES

[1] Eggleston K, Ling L, Qingyue M, Lindelow M, Wagstaff A.. Health service delivery in China: A literature review. Health Econ 2008;17(2):149-65.

[2] Deng W, Wilkes A, Bloom G. Village health services in rural China. IDS 1997;28(1): 32-8.

[3] Wang Z. Zhu Y. Survey analysis and countermeasures on grass-root hospitals antibacterial drug abuse. Chin J Drug Abuse Prev Treat 1999;2:33-35.

[4] Tang S, Guo Y. Prescribing behaviour in rural health facilities in China. Chin Prim Health Care 1995;8:41-2.

[5] Dong LF, Yan H, Wang DL. Antibiotic prescribing patterns in village health clinics across 10 provinces of Western China. J Antimicrobial Chemother 2008;62(2): 410-5.

[6] Cui WY. China's village doctors take great strides. Bull World Health Organ 2008; 86(12):914-5.

[7] Liu YL. China's public health-care system: facing the challenges. Bull World Health Organ 2004;82(7):532-8.

[8] Jing F. Health sector reform and reproductive health services in poor rural China. Health Policy Plan 2004;19(Suppl 1):140-9.

[9] Tang S, Meng Q, Chen L, Bekedam H, Evans T, Whitehead M. Tackling the challenges to health equity in China. Lancet 2008;372(9648):1493-501.

[10] Zeng L, Dibley MJ, Cheng Y, Dang S, Chang S, Kong L, et al. Impact of micronutrient supplementation during pregnancy on birth weight, duration of gestation, and perinatal mortality in rural western China: Double blind cluster randomised controlled trial. BMJ 2008;337:a2001.

[11] WHO and UNICEF, Low birthweight: Country, regional and global estimates. URL: http://www.who.int/reproductive-health/publications/low_birthweight/low_birthweight_estimates.pdf. 2005.

[12] Liu Y, Lin l. Analysis on the status of supplementary food of Chinese infants in 2000. Chin J Child Health Care 2001;6(3):361-3.

[13] Zheng Q, Lu P, Li Y. The relationship among breastfeeding, supplementary food and growth of children in western China. Chin J Prev Med 2001;35(4):285-6.

[14] Yin S. Supplementary food and nutritional status of infants in developing countries. Chin J Child Health Care 2000;8(6):117-20.

[15] China CDC. China's food and nutrition surveillance in 1999. Beijing: China CDC, 1999: 4-25.

[16] UNICEF. 2000 CHN: An external evaluation report on the Health Management Pilot County Project (1999-2000). URL: https://www.unicef.org/evaldatabase/index_14256.html 2000.

[17] Bi Y, Lai D, Yan H. Synthetic evaluation of the effect of health promotion: Impact of a UNICEF project in 40 poor western counties of China. Public Health 2010;124:376-91.

[18] Saaty TL. Modeling unstructured decision problems: The theory of analytical hierarchies. First Int Conf on Math, 1997;1(1):59-77.

[19] Vargas LG, An overview of the analytic hierarchy process and its applications. J Operat Res Soc 1990;48(1):2-8.

[20] Lai YJ, Liu TY, Hwang CJ. TOPSIS FOR MODM. Eur J Operat Res 1994;76(3):486-500.

[21] Opricovic S, Tzeng GH. Compromise solution by MCDM methods: A comparative analysis of VIKOR and TOPSIS. Eur J Operat Res 2004;156(2): 445-55.

[22] Hu D, Zhu W, Fu Y, Zhang M, Zhao Y, Hanson K, et al. Development of village doctors in China: Financial Compensation and health system support. Int J Equity Health 2017; 16:9.

In: Advances in Chinese Children … ISBN: 978-1-53617-870-8
Editors: Ariel Tenenbaum et al. © 2020 Nova Science Publishers, Inc.

Chapter 4

MATERIALISM IN CHINESE ADOLESCENTS IN HONG KONG: PROFILES AND SOCIO-DEMOGRAPHIC CORRELATES

Daniel TL Shek[1,*], PhD, FHKPS, BBS, SBS, JP, Li Lin[1], PhD, Andrew MH Siu[2], PhD and Britta M Lee[1], MDes

[1]Department of Applied Social Sciences
[2]Department of Rehabilitation Sciences,
The Hong Kong Polytechnic University, Hong Kong, PR China

ABSTRACT

Although youth development models suggest that materialistic beliefs have a negative impact on adolescent development, empirical studies in this area are scarce. Based on a sample of 2,474 high school students in Hong Kong,

[*] Corresponding Author: Daniel TL Shek, PhD, FHKPS, BBS, SBS, JP, Associate Vice President (Undergraduate Programme), Chair Professor of Applied Social Sciences and Li and Fung Professor in Service Leadership Education, Department of Applied Social Sciences, The Hong Kong Polytechnic University, Hung Hom, Hong Kong, PR China.
Email: daniel.shek@polyu.edu.hk.

this study examined the profiles of materialism and socio-demographic correlates of adolescent materialism. Results showed that more than a quarter of the respondents agreed that earning money is more important than other things. Significant proportions of the respondents also agreed that adolescents in Hong Kong were materialistic. However, the respondents perceived themselves to be less materialistic as compared to adolescents in Hong Kong. Regarding socio-demographic correlates of materialism in adolescents, correlation and regression analyses showed that age, gender, parental education, and family intactness were associated with adolescent materialism. Multiple regression analyses further showed that age, gender, and family intactness were significant predictors of adolescent materialism.

INTRODUCTION

The quest for material possession is a feature of the contemporary world with several contributing factors. First, under Capitalism, there is a basic emphasis on material possession. Without material possession, the economy will shrink. In order to push up the GDP, people are persuaded and encouraged to buy commodities which essentially leads to the development of the "consumption" culture. Second, with technological advances, there are many new products such as smartphones, personal computers, and fancy electronic devices. Through aggressive marketing strategies, group pressure, and actual needs, possession of such devices is regarded as trendy and a symbol of identity. Hence, many people, particularly young people "chase" after such new products. Third, with the global issue of poverty (i.e., lack of material possession), people tend to develop the mentality that it is better to have more material possession which can give them a sense of security.

How might materialistic mentality influence adolescent development? In different cultures, over-emphasis on materialism has been regarded as problematic for human development. For example, in the Christian and Catholic traditions, spiritual values are upheld while material values are downplayed. With specific reference to the Chinese culture, materialism is also deemphasized in different social philosophies. In Confucianism, focus is placed on non-material virtues than material possession. In Buddhism, material possession is regarded as illusory and the focus is on transcendence of sensory and material urges. In Taoism, the focus is on harmony and non-material experience such as meditation and harmony with nature.

In different youth developmental models (1), there is also an emphasis on the importance of spiritual values. In the model proposed by the Search Institute, there is an emphasis on positive values which are not materialistic in nature. In particular, the value of "restraint" is the contrary of sensory pleasure and material consumption. In the 5C and 6C models (2,3), character, compassion, and care are developmental ideals which are non-materialistic in nature. In the positive youth development constructs proposed by Catalano et al. (4), spirituality is a PYD construct which can promote the positive development of young people. This construct is in line with the existential approach which focuses on the importance of life meaning and transcendental development in human development. In the "being" approach, spirituality and character are closely related to the process of thriving which represents the healthy and holistic development of adolescents (5, 6).

According to Huta and Ryan (7), there are two motives underlying human happiness. On the one hand, happiness is determined by hedonic motives where a person seeks instant pleasure and comfort through different means, such as physical activities (e.g., shopping and drinking). On the other hand, happiness can be brought forth by eudaimonic motives where happiness is determined by one's intention to achieve development, excellence, authenticity, and meaning (8, 9, 10, 11). Based on this framework, materialism can be regarded as hedonic motive which leads to short term happiness only. Similarly, Peterson and colleagues (12) also differentiated hedonic orientation (i.e., life pleasure) from eudaimonic orientation which includes life of engagement and life of meaning. Again, hedonic motives basically underlie materialistic values and behavior.

Materialism is a hallmark of Capitalism. With particular reference to Hong Kong, it is a melting pot of Western influences and traditional Chinese values. Historically, Hong Kong has also served as an international financial center focusing on business, finance, and trade. Under the Basic Law, the Capitalistic system would continue for 50 years since the handover in 1997. With this backdrop, Shek and Siu (13) argued that materialism is a risk factor for adolescent development in Hong Kong. Developmentally, over-emphasis on materialism would lead to non-holistic development and selective focus on instrumental or utilitarian values.

Although adolescent materialism is an important developmental issue, there are relatively few studies in this area, particularly in the Chinese context (14). One notable exception is the work by Shek, Ma, and Lin (15) who developed the 21-item Chinese Adolescent Materialism Scale based on the data collected from 1,658 Chinese high school students. Confirmatory factor analyses finally suggest a three-factor model with 19 items (e.g., "unless I can make a lot of money, I won't respect myself"; "the most important objective in a woman's life is to marry a rich man"; "possession of money can make people happy"; "no money, no dignity") underlying three dimensions (including "acquisition centrality," "materialistic possessions," and "hedonistic pursuit"). Using five items derived from the Chinese Adolescent Materialism Scale, Shek and Lin (16) examined adolescent development in different domains, including materialism, egocentrism, character strengths, and moral development. The present paper is based on the data collected by this scale.

To understand character and moral development in Chinese high school students in Hong Kong, a series of studies have been conducted by a team of researchers at The Hong Kong Polytechnic University (16-20). This paper utilized the data collected in the study of Shek and Lin (16). There are several research objectives in this paper. First, it attempted to examine the materialistic beliefs in Chinese high school students in Hong Kong. Besides perceived materialistic beliefs in high school students, their perception of the materialistic beliefs in Hong Kong adolescents in general was also explored. Second, we compared high school students' perceptions of their own materialistic attitudes and those of Hong Kong adolescents in general. In the social psychology literature, there are research studies showing that one tends to see oneself as more positive than other people (21). Hence, we examined this hypothesis in the present study. Finally, as there are few studies examining psychosocial correlates of materialism, we examined how materialistic beliefs in adolescents are related to age, gender, family intactness, and economic disadvantage in Chinese high school students in Hong Kong.

OUR STUDY

The data for the present study were derived from a large-scale study examining their character traits, psychosocial competencies, social behavior, family life, and school life of Chinese high school students in Hong Kong (16). A total of 20 local secondary schools participated in the study, with seven schools admitting students with high academic performance (i.e., Band 1 schools), nine schools admitting students with average academic performance (i.e., Band 2 schools) and six schools admitting students with low academic performance (i.e., Band 3 schools). According to the school size, three to five classes of students were randomly selected to join the study. We recruited 2,474 students (Mean age = 14.76, SD = 1.82; 1,271 females and 1,123 males) in this study, with 1,336 junior high school students and 906 senior high school students. Regarding the economic background of the participants, 239 students were on welfare, who could be regarded as experiencing economic disadvantage.

We obtained consent from the school, parents, and students before collecting the data. During data collection, students were requested to complete a questionnaire containing measures of character attributes, psychosocial competencies, social behavior, family life, and school life. Adequate time was provided to the students. A trained research assistant was present throughout the questionnaire administration process.

Instruments

The abridged version of the Chinese Adolescent Materialism Scale (15) was employed in this study to assess the materialistic beliefs of the respondents. Based on theories and research studies on materialism, 21 items assessing adolescent materialism were designed which showed adequate reliability and validity. In this study, five items from the different dimensions of the scale were employed to assess materialistic beliefs in the respondents. These items included: a) "making money is more important than any other things"; b) "I believe that money is everything"; c) "the rich can get respect from others"; d) "I would abandon some principles for the sake of money"; and e) "the amount of money one makes is a fundamental indicator of one's success". A 5-point Likert scale was used, with the response options of "strongly disagree = 1", "disagree = 2", "neither agree nor disagree = 3," "agree = 4," and "strongly agree = 5."

To assess the respondents' perceptions of materialism in adolescents in Hong Kong, these five items were used to capture the related views. The items included: a) "Hong Kong adolescents think that making money is more important than any other things"; b) "Hong Kong adolescents believe that money is everything"; c) "Hong Kong adolescents think that the rich can get respect from others"; d) "Hong Kong adolescents would abandon some principles for the sake of money"; and e) "Hong Kong adolescents believe that the amount of money one makes is a fundamental indicator of one's success". Five response options were used, including "strongly disagree = 1," "disagree = 2," "neither agree nor disagree = 3," "agree = 4," and "strongly agree = 5."

Data analyses

We used Statistical Package for Social Sciences Version 25 (IBM Corp., Somers, NY, USA) to carry out to answer the questions of the study. First, descriptive statistical analyses based on percentages were performed to understand the responses of the participants to the abridged version of the Chinese Adolescent Materialism Scale. Besides, perceptions of the respondents regarding materialistic beliefs amongst adolescents in Hong Kong in general were examined. Second, respondents' views of their own materialistic attitudes and perceptions of the materialistic attitudes of Hong Kong adolescents in general would be compared using matched-sample ANOVAs. For the socio-demographic correlates, Pearson correlation analysis, linear regression, and multiple regression analyses were performed.

FINDINGS

For the first research objective, we conducted descriptive statistical analyses to understand the profiles of materialistic beliefs amongst the respondents via percentage responses. In Table 1 to Table 3, the responses of the students to the items in the 5-item abridged scale in the total, junior form, and senior form samples are presented. There are two observations. First, roughly one-third of the respondents believed that earning money is more important than other things. Second, compared to junior high school students, senior high school students held higher levels of materialistic beliefs than did junior high school students. In Table 4 to Table 6, the respondents' perceptions of the materialistic beliefs in general Hong Kong youth population are outlined. Two observations can be highlighted from the findings. First, high proportions of high school students perceived that adolescents in Hong Kong were materialistic. Second, more senior high school students perceived that young people in Hong Kong were materialistic.

To understand whether there were differences between respondents' perception of their materialistic beliefs and those of general adolescents in Hong Kong, several ANOVAs were carried out (Table 7). Results showed that there were statistically significant differences between perceived materialism in the respondents and perceived materialism in Hong Kong adolescents on materialism, $F(5,4887) = 362.900$, $p < .001$, partial eta squared = 0.27. For univariate effects (ANOVA), results similarly showed statistically significant differences between the two perceptions in the scores of each item ($p < 0.001$) and of the composite score ($p < 0.001$). In short, the respondents saw themselves as less materialistic than did Hong Kong adolescents in general.

Table 1. Perception of materialistic beliefs in the respondents (total sample)

Items	1	2	1+2	3	4	5	4+5	Mean	n
	n (%)	n (%)	n (%)	n (%)	n (%)	n (%)	n (%)		
Making money is more important than any other things.	187 (7.6%)	610 (24.7%)	797 (32.3%)	934 (37.8%)	623 (25.2%)	118 (4.8%)	741 (30.0%)	2.95	2472
I believe that "money is everything".	587 (23.7%)	857 (34.7%)	1444 (58.4%)	590 (23.9%)	362 (14.6%)	76 (3.1%)	438 (17.7%)	2.39	2472
No money, no dignity.	546 (22.2%)	782 (31.8%)	1328 (54.0%)	664 (27.0%)	383 (15.6%)	86 (3.5%)	469 (19.1%)	2.46	2461
I would abandon some principles for the sake of money.	1298 (52.8%)	729 (29.6%)	2027 (82.4%)	288 (11.7%)	101 (4.1%)	43 (1.7%)	144 (5.8%)	1.72	2459
The amount of money one makes is a fundamental indicator of one's "success".	724 (29.3%)	833 (33.8%)	1557 (63.1%)	557 (22.6%)	285 (11.5%)	69 (2.8%)	354 (14.3%)	2.25	2468

Note. 1 = strongly disagree, 2 = disagree, 3 = neither agree nor disagree, 4 = agree, and 5 = strongly agree.

Table 2. Perception of materialistic beliefs in the respondents (junior high school students sample)

Items	1	2	1+2	3	4	5	4+5	Mean	n
	n (%)	n (%)	n (%)	n (%)	n (%)	n (%)	n (%)		
Making money is more important than any other things.	117 (7.9%)	384 (25.9%)	501 (33.7%)	577 (38.9%)	344 (23.2%)	63 (4.2%)	407 (27.4%)	2.90	1485
I believe that "money is everything".	395 (26.6%)	519 (34.9%)	914 (61.5%)	363 (24.4%)	178 (12.0%)	31 (2.1%)	209 (14.9%)	2.28	1486
No money, no dignity.	387 (26.1%)	500 (33.7%)	887 (59.8%)	364 (24.5%)	195 (13.1%)	37 (2.5%)	232 (15.6%)	2.32	1483
I would abandon some principles for the sake of money.	856 (57.9%)	404 (27.3%)	1260 (85.3%)	152 (10.3%)	43 (2.9%)	23 (1.6%)	66 (4.5%)	1.63	1478
The amount of money one makes is a fundamental indicator of one's "success."	497 (33.6%)	505 (34.1%)	1002 (67.7%)	312 (21.1%)	131 (8.8%)	36 (2.4%)	167 (11.3%)	2.12	1481

Note. 1 = strongly disagree, 2 = disagree, 3 = neither agree nor disagree, 4 = agree, and 5 = strongly agree.

Table 3. Perception of materialistic beliefs in the respondents (senior high school students sample)

Items	1	2	1+2	3	4	5	4+5	Mean	n
	n (%)	n (%)	n (%)	n (%)	n (%)	n (%)	n (%)		
Making money is more important than any other things.	70 (7.1%)	226 (22.9%)	296 (30.0%)	357 (36.2%)	279 (28.3%)	55 (5.6%)	334 (33.8%)	3.02	987
I believe that "money is everything."	192 (19.5%)	338 (34.3%)	530 (53.8%)	227 (23.0%)	184 (18.7%)	45 (4.6%)	229 (23.2%)	2.55	986
No money, no dignity.	159 (16.3%)	282 (28.8%)	441 (45.1%)	300 (30.7%)	188 (19.2%)	49 (5.0%)	237 (24.2%)	2.68	978
I would abandon some principles for the sake of money.	442 (45.1%)	325 (33.1%)	767 (78.2%)	136 (13.9)	58 (5.9%)	20 (2.0%)	78 (8.0%)	1.87	981
The amount of money one makes is a fundamental indicator of one's "success."	227 (23.0%)	328 (33.2%)	555 (56.2%)	245 (24.8%)	154 (15.6%)	33 (3.3%)	187 (18.9%)	2.43	987

Note. 1 = strongly disagree, 2 = disagree, 3 = neither agree nor disagree, 4 = agree, and 5 = strongly agree.

Table 4. Perception of materialistic beliefs in Hong Kong adolescents (total sample)

Items	1	2	1+2	3	4	5	4+5	Mean	n
	n (%)	n (%)	n (%)	n (%)	n (%)	n (%)	n (%)		
Adolescents in HK believe making money is more important than any other things.	109 (4.4%)	456 (18.5%)	565 (22.9%)	792 (32.1%)	914 (37.0%)	199 (8.1%)	1113 (45.1%)	3.26	2470
Adolescents in HK believe "Money is everything."	152 (6.2%)	479 (19.4%)	631 (25.6%)	748 (30.3%)	864 (35.0%)	225 (9.1%)	1089 (44.1%)	3.22	2468
Adolescents in HK believe "No money, no dignity."	177 (7.2%)	434 (17.6%)	611 (24.8%)	736 (29.9%)	880 (35.7%)	237 (9.6%)	1117 (45.3%)	3.23	2464
Adolescents in HK believe they would abandon some principles for the sake of money.	332 (13.5%)	566 (23.0%)	898 (36.5%)	756 (30.7%)	645 (26.2%)	166 (6.7%)	811 (32.9%)	2.90	2465
Adolescents in HK believe "The amount of money one makes is a fundamental indicator of one's "success."	193 (7.8%)	486 (19.7%)	679 (27.5%)	715 (29.0%)	798 (32.3%)	275 (11.1%)	1073 (43.4%)	3.19	2467

Note. 1 = strongly disagree, 2 = disagree, 3 = neither agree nor disagree, 4 = agree, and 5 = strongly agree.

Table 5. Perception of materialistic beliefs in Hong Kong adolescents (junior high school students sample)

Items	1	2	1+2	3	4	5	4+5	Mean	n
	n (%)	n (%)	n (%)	n (%)	n (%)	n (%)	n (%)		
Adolescents in HK believe making money is more important than any other things.	78 (5.3%)	291 (19.6%)	369 (24.9%)	485 (32.7%)	519 (35.0%)	111 (7.5%)	630 (42.5%)	3.20	1484
Adolescents in HK believe “Money is everything.”	109 (7.4%)	317 (21.4%)	426 (28.8%)	442 (29.8%)	490 (33.1%)	123 (8.3%)	613 (41.4%)	3.14	1481
Adolescents in HK believe “No money, no dignity.”	128 (8.6%)	288 (19.4)	416 (28.1%)	441 (29.8%)	490 (33.1)	134 (9.0%)	624 (42.1%)	3.14	1481
Adolescents in HK believe they would abandon some principles for the sake of money.	235 (15.9%)	352 (23.8%)	587 (39.7%)	443 (29.9%)	351 (23.7%)	99 (6.7%)	450 (30.4%)	2.82	1480
Adolescents in HK believe “The amount of money one makes is a fundamental indicator of one’s “success.”	146 (9.9%)	320 (21.6%)	466 (31.5%)	422 (28.5%)	455 (30.7%)	137 (9.3%)	592 (40.0%)	3.08	1480

Note. 1 = strongly disagree, 2 = disagree, 3 = neither agree nor disagree, 4 = agree, and 5 = strongly agree.

Table 6. Adolescents' perception of the materialism of their peers in Hong Kong (senior grades)

Items	1	2	1+2	3	4	5	4+5	Mean	n
	n (%)	n (%)	n (%)	n (%)	n (%)	n (%)	n (%)		
Adolescents in HK believe making money is more important than any other things.	31 (3.1%)	165 (16.7%)	196 (19.9%)	307 (31.1%)	395 (40.1%)	88 (8.9%)	483 (49.0%)	3.35	986
Adolescents in HK believe "Money is everything."	43 (4.4%)	162 (16.4%)	205 (20.8%)	306 (31.0%)	374 (37.9%)	102 (10.3%)	476 (48.2%)	3.33	987
Adolescents in HK believe "No money, no dignity."	49 (5.0%)	146 (14.9%)	195 (19.8%)	295 (30.0%)	390 (39.7%)	103 (10.5%)	493 (50.2%)	3.36	983
Adolescents in HK believe they would abandon some principles for the sake of money.	97 (9.8%)	214 (21.7%)	311 (31.6%)	313 (31.8%)	294 (29.8%)	67 (6.8%)	361 (36.6%)	3.02	985
Adolescents in HK believe "The amount of money one makes is a fundamental indicator of one's "success."	47 (4.8%)	166 (16.8%)	213 (21.6%)	293 (29.7%)	343 (34.8%)	138 (14.0%)	481 (48.7%)	3.36	987

Note. 1 = strongly disagree, 2 = disagree, 3 = neither agree nor disagree, 4 = agree, and 5 = strongly agree.

Table 7. Differences in Items and Composite Scores of Materialism between Students and HK Adolescents (N = 2,441 for students, N = 2,452 for Hong Kong adolescents)

	Students	**HK Adolescents**	***F***	**partial η2**
	M (SD)	*M (SD)*	362.900***^	0.27
Making money is more important than any other things	2.95(1.00)	3.26(0.99)	118.798***	0.024
I believe that "money is everything."	2.39(1.09)	3.22(1.05)	734.150***	0.131
No money, no dignity.	2.47(1.10)	3.23(1.07)	604.468***	0.110
I would abandon some principles for the sake of money.	1.73(0.95)	2.90(1.13)	1553.422***	0.241
The amount of money one makes is a fundamental indicator of one's "success."	2.25(1.08)	3.19(1.11)	909.078***	0.157
Composite Score	2.35(0.79)	3.16(0.89)	1125.202***	0.187

Note.****p* <.001; ^Adjusted Bonferroni value = .008.

Table 8. Correlation among variables

Variables	**1**	**2**	**3**	**4**	**5**	**6**
1. Age	-					
2. Gender[b]	0.01	-				
3. Father Education[c]	-0.14***	-0.01	-			
4. Mother Education[c]	-0.13***	-0.00	0.51***	-		
5. Family Intactness[d]	0.10***	0.05*	-0.09***	-0.08[a]	-	
6. Economic Disadvantage[e]	-0.02	-0.14***	0.21***	0.16***	-0.17***	-
7. Materialism	0.18***	-0.09[a]	-0.08**	-0.08[a]	0.10***	-0.03

Note. **p* <.05, ***p* <.01, ****p* <.001, [a]*p* = 0.001;

[b]Male = 1, Female = 2;

[c]The 0-9 values of Father and Mother Education were recoded into three categorical values: Primary and below = 1, Secondary = 2, Above secondary = 3. The value "0" (Do not know) was recoded as missing value (999).

[d]Family Intactness was recoded from variable "Parents' current marital status": First marriage = 1, Non-first marriage = 2.

[e]Economic Disadvantage was recoded from two variables: "Household on CSSA" and "Results of application of Textbook Assistance Scheme": On CSSA and/or receiving textbook allowance = 1, other condition = 2.

Table 9. Results of linear regression independently for each predictor

Predictors	Student Materialism			
	β	*t*	*F*	R^2
Age	0.19	9.25***	85.596***	0.035
Gender[b]	-0.10	-4.91***	24.117***	0.010
Father Education[c]	-0.06	-2.62**	6.847**	0.004
Mother Education[c]	-0.08	-3.25[a]	10.565[a]	0.006
Family Intactness[d]	0.09	4.17***	17.349***	0.007
Economic Disadvantage[e]	-0.01	-0.31	0.098	0.000

Note. *$p < .05$, **$p < .01$, ***$p < .001$, [a]$p = 0.001$;

[b]Male = 1, Female = 2;

[c]The 0-9 values of Father and Mother Education were recoded into three categorical values: Primary and below = 1, Secondary = 2, Above secondary = 3. The value "0" (Do not know) was recoded as missing value (999).

[d]Family Intactness was recoded from variable "Parents' current marital status": First marriage = 1, Non-first marriage = 2.

[e]Economic Disadvantage was recoded from two variables: "Household on CSSA" and "Results of application of Textbook Assistance Scheme": On CSSA and/or receiving textbook allowance = 1, other condition = 2.

Table 10. Results of Multiple Regression

Predictors	Student Materialism			
	β	*t*	*F*	R^2
Age	0.17	6.33***	12.594***	0.052
Gender[b]	-0.09	-3.52***		
Father Education[c]	-0.03	-0.83		
Mother Education[c]	-0.04	-1.33		
Family Intactness[d]	0.08	2.83**		
Economic Disadvantage[e]	-0.01	-0.40		

Note. *$p < .05$, **$p < .01$, ***$p < .001$, [a]$p = 0.001$;

[b]Male = 1, Female = 2;

[c]The 0-9 values of Father and Mother Education were recoded into three categorical values: Primary and below = 1, Secondary = 2, Above secondary = 3. The value "0" (Do not know) was recoded as missing value (999).

[d]Family Intactness was recoded from variable "Parents' current marital status": First marriage = 1, Non-first marriage = 2.

[e]Economic Disadvantage was recoded from two variables: "Household on CSSA" and "Results of application of Textbook Assistance Scheme": On CSSA and/or receiving textbook allowance = 1, other condition = 2.

Table 8 shows the correlations among different variables. While materialistic beliefs in the students were positively correlated with age and family intactness, the related scores were negatively correlated with gender, father education and mother education. However, there was no correlation between student materialism and economic disadvantage. Linear regression analyses were conducted for each predictor separately. As shown in Table 9, except for economic disadvantage, all other variables (age, gender, father education, mother education, and family intactness) significantly predicted student materialism. In short, male students showed higher scores than did female students. Both higher paternal education and higher maternal education predicted lower materialism scores of students. Students from non-intact families (i.e., non-first marriage families) were more materialistic than students from intact families (i.e., first marriage families).

To understand the relative contribution of different predictors to materialistic belief scores, multiple regression analysis was further conducted to predict student materialism from student age, gender, father education, mother education, family intactness, and economic disadvantage (Table 10). Results showed that after controlling other variables, student materialism was positively predicted by age and family intactness and negatively predicted by gender. In other words, older students tended to have higher materialism than did younger students. Male students had higher materialism than did female students. Students from non-intact family had higher materialism than did students from intact family. There was no predicting effect of father and mother education and economic disadvantage on student materialism, when controlling other variables.

DISCUSSION

Despite the importance of the topic of materialism in adolescent development, research studies in this area are surprisingly little. As such, the current study was conducted to understand materialistic beliefs in Chinese high school students in Hong Kong. In particular, we assessed students' perceptions of materialistic beliefs in themselves as compared to adolescents in general. Besides, we also explored the socio-demographic correlates of materialistic beliefs in Chinese high school students in Hong Kong. The current study is pioneering in the field of adolescent materialism as no similar studies have been conducted before.

Based on the responses of the participants to the abridged version of the Chinese Adolescent Materialism Scale, we examined the profiles of materialistic beliefs in high school students in Hong Kong. Several observations can be highlighted from the findings. First, amongst junior secondary school students, roughly one-quarter of them (27.4%) agreed that earning money is more important than other things. The related proportion was higher in senior high school students (33.8%). Besides, roughly one-quarter of the senior high school students agreed that owning money can earn the respect of other people. These observations are disturbing because many students employed money or material possession to be a yardstick to define success and personal achievement. In future, studies should be conducted to examine how materialistic beliefs might contribute to the developmental outcomes in adolescents.

Interestingly, when the participants were asked about materialistic attitudes amongst Hong Kong adolescents in general, the participants saw that quite a high proportion of Hong Kong adolescents showed materialistic attitudes: 40% and 49% of junior and senior high school students agreed that Hong Kong adolescents defined success in terms of richness, respectively; 42.1% and 50.2% of junior and senior high school students agreed that Hong Kong adolescents equated money with respect from others, respectively. ANOVAs results also revealed that the participants saw themselves to be less materialistic than adolescents in Hong Kong in general. In other words, students generally perceived that they were less materialistic as compared to adolescents in general. This observation is generally in line with the social psychology literature that people tend to see themselves as better than others (i.e., social desirability effect).

Regarding sociodemographic correlates of materialistic beliefs in Chinese adolescents, several observations can be highlighted. First, older adolescents showed higher materialism; senior high school students showed stronger endorsement of materialistic beliefs than did junior high school students. There are several factors contributing to this observation. First, when adolescents grow older, their understanding of the importance of money would increase. Second, students in senior forms may actually spend more, hence underscoring the importance of money in the lives of adolescents. Third, older adolescents may be more susceptible to peer influence in material possession which may be used to define their identities.

Regarding gender difference in materialistic beliefs, findings showed that being male was associated with a higher level of materialistic beliefs. There are several possible explanations for this. First, as males are the breadwinners of the family, they would attach higher importance to money and material possession. Second, as males are more instrumental and pragmatic, they would see monetary and material possession to be more important. In future study, we should further examine how such gender differences would be translated into gender differences in other areas, such as psychological well-being and interpersonal relationships.

The present findings also showed that both paternal and maternal education were related to adolescent materialistic beliefs. There are two possible explanations of the findings. First, higher parental education implies higher income for the family, which would reduce the importance of material possession. Second, parents with higher education might nurture their children to develop in a more holistic manner, particularly to look at the world from different angles. Further research is needed to understand how parents would socialize the children, particularly in terms of development of happiness from a hedonic or eudemonic motive.

Finally, materialistic beliefs were higher in high school students in non-intact families than intact families. There are studies showing that parenting and family functioning are less favorable in non-intact families than in intact families. The present study shows that development of materialistic beliefs is adversely affected in non-intact families which is not systematically examined in previous studies. Furthermore, non-intact families might suffer from economic problem which may underscore the importance of material possession. However, as the present findings do not show any relationship between economic disadvantage and materialistic beliefs in adolescents, more research in this area is needed.

Although the present study is a pioneering study in the field, there are several limitations. First, although the sample was large, the students were not randomly selected. Hence, generalizability of the findings should be carefully examined. It is suggested that random samples should be used in future studies. Second, as only five items were used to assess materialistic beliefs, it would be helpful to use more items in future study. Of course, in a survey assessing many constructs, the issue of overloading the respondents should be carefully considered. Finally, regarding the socio-demographics of adolescent materialism, as the effect sizes were not large, there is a need to replicate the findings.

ACKNOWLEDGMENTS

The series of studies on character and moral development in high school students in Hong Kong are financially supported by Wofoo Foundation. This chapter is a re-print with minor revision of an earlier published paper in the *International Journal of Child Health and Human Development* 2019;12(3) issue with permission.

REFERENCES

[1] Shek DTL, Dou D, Zhu X, Chai, W. Positive youth development: Current perspectives. Adolesc Health Med Ther 2019;10:131-41. doi: 10.2147/AHMT.S179946.

[2] Bowers EP, Li Y, Kiely MK, Brittian A, Lerner JV, Lerner RM. The Five Cs model of positive youth development: A longitudinal analysis of confirmatory factor structure and measurement invariance. J Youth Adolesc 2010;39(7):720-35. doi:10.1007/s10964-010- 9530-9.

[3] Lerner RM, Lerner JV, Almerigi JB, Theokas C, Phelps E, Gestsdottir S, et al. Positive youth development, participation in community youth development programs, and community contributions of fifth-grade adolescents: Findings from the first wave of the 4-H study of positive youth development. J Early Adolesc 2005;25(1):17-71. doi:10.1177/0272431604272461.

[4] Catalano RF, Berglund ML, Ryan JAM, Lonczak HS, Hawkins JD. Positive youth development in the United States: Research findings on evaluations of positive youth development programs. Ann Am Acad Pol Soc Sci 2004;591(1):98-124. doi:10.1177/0002716203260102.

[5] Battistich V. Character Education, prevention, and positive youth development. Character Educ Partnership 2005;1-10.

[6] Park N. Building strengths of character: Keys to positive youth development. Reclaiming Child Youth 2009;18(2):42-7.

[7] Huta V, Ryan RM. Pursuing pleasure or virtue: The differential and overlapping well-being benefits of hedonic and eudaimonic motives. J Happiness Stud 2010;11(6):735-62.

[8] Huta V. Linking peoples' pursuit of eudaimonia and hedonia with characteristics of their parents: Parenting styles, verbally endorsed values, and role modeling. J Happiness Stud 2012;13(1):47-61. doi:10.1007/s10902-011-9249-7.

[9] Huta, V. Eudaimonic and hedonic orientations: Theoretical considerations and research findings. In J. Vittersø eds. Handbook of eudaimonic well-being. International handbook of quality of life. Cham, Switzerland: Springer, 2016:215-31.

[10] Huta V, Waterman AS. Eudaimonia and its distinction from hedonia: Developing a classification and terminology for understanding conceptual and operational definitions. J Happiness Stud 2014;15:1425-56. doi:10.1007/s10902-013-9485-0.

[11] Huta V, Pelletier LG, Baxter D, Thompson A. How eudaimonic and hedonic motives relate to the well-being of close others. J Posit Psychol 2012;7(5):399-404.

[12] Peterson C, Park N, Seligman MEP. Orientations to happiness and life satisfaction: The full life versus the empty life. J Happiness Stud 2005;6:25-41. doi:10.1007/s10902-004-1278-z.

[13] Shek DTL, Siu AMH. "UNHAPPY" Environment for adolescent development in Hong Kong. J Adolesc Health 2019;64(6):S1-S4. doi:10.1016/j.jadohealth.2019.01.007.

[14] Shek DTL, Pu E. A review of research on materialism amongst children and adolescents in Hong Kong. Int J Child Adolesc Health 2016;9(4):455-67.

[15] Shek, DTL, Ma CMS, Lin L. The Chinese Adolescent Materialism Scale: Psychometric properties and normative profiles. Int J Disabil Hum Dev 2014;13(2):285-95. doi: 10.1515/ijdhd-2014-0315.

[16] Shek DTL, Lin L. A study on the development of Chinese students (Character, psychosocial competence and behavior): Report No. 1 – Views of students. Hong Kong: Department of Applied Social Sciences, The Hong Kong Polytechnic University, 2017.

[17] Shek DTL, Ma CMS. A study on the development of Chinese students (Character, psychosocial competence and behavior): Report No. 2 – Views of teachers. Hong Kong: Department of Applied Social Sciences, The Hong Kong Polytechnic University, 2017.

[18] Shek DTL, Yu L. A study on the development of Chinese students (Character, psychosocial competence and behavior): Report No. 3 – Views of parents. Hong Kong: Department of Applied Social Sciences, The Hong Kong Polytechnic University, 2018.

[19] Shek, DTL, Leung J. A study on the development of Chinese students (Character, psychosocial competence and behavior): Report No. 4 – Moral education at the crossroad. Hong Kong: Department of Applied Social Sciences, The Hong Kong Polytechnic University, 2018.

[20] Shek DTL, Wu FKY, Leung H. A study on the development of Chinese students (Character, psychosocial competence and behavior): Report No. 5 – A qualitative study of the views of principals and teachers on moral education. Hong Kong: Department of Applied Social Sciences, The Hong Kong Polytechnic University, 2018.

[21] Dunning D. Self-insight: Roadblocks and detours on path to knowing thyself. New York: Psychology Press, 2005.

In: Advances in Chinese Children … ISBN: 978-1-53617-870-8
Editors: Ariel Tenenbaum et al.

Chapter 5

MATERIALISM AND EGOCENTRISM IN CHINESE ADOLESCENTS IN HONG KONG: PERCEPTIONS OF TEACHERS

Daniel TL Shek[1,*], PhD, FHKPS, BBS, SBS, JP, Cecilia Ma[1], PhD, Andrew MH Siu[2], PhD and Britta M Lee[1], MDes

[1]Department of Applied Social Sciences,
The Hong Kong Polytechnic University, Hong Kong, PR China
[2]Department of Rehabilitation Sciences, The Hong Kong Polytechnic University, Hong Kong, PR China

ABSTRACT

While there are studies on materialism and egocentrism based on self-reports of adolescents, there are very few studies focusing on teachers' perceptions of materialism and egocentrism in their students and adolescents in general. In this study, teachers' perceptions (N = 568) of materialism and egocentrism in Chinese adolescents were examined.

* Corresponding Author's E-mail: daniel.shek@polyu.edu.hk.

Findings showed that many teachers perceived that their students and adolescents in Hong Kong showed materialistic beliefs. A significant proportion of teachers also perceived that their students and adolescents in Hong Kong generally showed worrying signs of egocentrism. While background demographic factors (age, gender, religious orientation and teaching grades) were not related to adolescent materialism, teachers' perceptions of their students' egocentrism were related to teaching grades and teachers' perceptions of egocentrism in adolescents in general were related to age, gender, and teaching grades.

INTRODUCTION

Adolescence is an important stage where young people develop beliefs and values about themselves and the world. With cognitive maturation and enlargement of the social circle, adolescents form views about themselves, including their own characteristics and unique features. Besides, adolescents also form views about the world, such as ideological beliefs and philosophies. Amongst the beliefs and values formed by adolescents, there are two important areas to be considered. The first belief is on how adolescents view material possession and money (i.e., materialistic beliefs). With more contact with the world (e.g., buying lunch at school and using money at their own discretion) and peer influence (e.g., it is trendy to possess a pair of limited edition of sports shoes), adolescents begin to form beliefs about material possession and money. Obviously, the development of healthy attitude to material possession is important for adolescent thriving behavior. If adolescents hold unhealthy values, they may engage in delinquency behavior such as theft, shoplifting, and compensated dating to earn quick money in order to get material possession.

Shek, Ma and Lin (1) showed that a high level of materialism was related to a higher level of egocentrism but lower levels of morality, spirituality, and empathy. In different youth development models, particularly in the field of positive youth development (2), it is commonly emphasized that "being" (i.e., non-material values) such as character strengths are important to adolescent development. For example, in the developmental assets proposed by the Search Institute, the developmental assets focus on values and virtues which are non-materialistic in nature (3). In the 5C/6C models on youth development (4, 5), competence, confidence, character, compassion, connection, and contribution are non-materialistic nature. In the existential literature, the theory proposed by Victor Frankl (6) does not focus on "will to sex and aggression" and "will to power"; rather, it focuses on "will to life meaning" which is non-materialistic in nature. In fact, materialism is a by-product of Capitalism which focuses on the importance of material possession and consumption (7).

Another adolescent belief is adolescents' thoughts and experiences when comparing to others. If one always over-estimates one's ability and devaluates others' views, one would develop a "superiority complex". On the other hand, if one always under-estimates one's belief and over-emphasizes others' views, one would develop "inferiority complex". Furthermore, if one looks at things only from his or her own perspective without considering others' views, it is a self-centered orientation. On the other hand, if one looks at things from others' perspectives, it is other-centered orientation. Cognitively speaking, children tend to look at things from one's perspective without making reference to others' perspectives. According to Piaget (8), children's thinking style in late childhood is egocentric. However, with cognitive maturation, adolescents gradually know how to look at the world from one's perceptive as well as others' perspectives, although they initially hold distorted views about oneself and others, such as viewing one's thoughts are superior than others (9-11). According to Shek, Yu and Siu (12), there are two dimensions of egocentrism, including belief that one's thought is better than others (i.e., self-conceit) and not considering the views and experiences of other people (i.e., disregard of others). Developmentally speaking, egocentrism is a normal stage in adolescent development; however, if adolescents cannot grow out of it, it would then be developmental problems to the adolescents.

With widening of the social networks during adolescents, self-centered orientation would impair interpersonal relationships. Besides, adolescent egocentrism would lead to engagement in risky behavior because adolescents believe they are exceptional. Shek, Yu, and Siu (12) showed that adolescent egocentrism was negatively related to spirituality and empathy.

Conceptually, with reference to different youth development models, it is commonly asserted that taking others' perspective and sensitive to others' feelings are important for adolescent healthy development. Positive values and social competences are emphasized in Benson's developmental assets model (3). In the 5C/6C model, it is argued that caring and compassion (i.e., consideration of others) are important. In the social-emotional perspective (e.g., CASEL's model), understanding of others' views is an important competence to be acquired by adolescents. In the character strengths perspective (13-15), social intelligence and modesty are emphasized. In the positive youth development models (16), the importance of considering others' views and experiences is highlighted.

The major drawback of the existing studies on adolescent materialism and egocentrism is that the existing studies are primarily based on self-reports of adolescents. There are several limitations of reliance on the self-report data collected from adolescents. First, it can be argued that adolescents may not have an accurate understanding of themselves because of their emerging cognitive maturity. Second, adolescents may have biases in viewing oneself, particularly because of social desirability effects such as "beauty of beholder side". Third, as self-evaluation of one's weaknesses is painful, self-report of adolescents may not be accurate. Hence, it is methodologically desirable to include the perspectives of other stakeholders (i.e., teachers) to look at the related issues. The engagement of teachers is helpful for several reasons. First, as teachers spend much time with students, they have a better understanding of their students and young people in Hong Kong. Second, through intensive interaction with students, teachers would have a good understanding of the students. Third, with professional teacher training, teachers would have a more informed judgment about the situation of their students and adolescents. With reference to Hong Kong, studies on adolescent materialism are few (7, 17, 18). In the study conducted by Shek and colleagues (7), the finding showed that high school students perceived that adolescents showed worrying signs in materialism and egocentrism. Obviously, it would be illuminating if the views of teachers could be collected.

As there are few studies on the moral character, materialism, egocentrism, and psychosocial development in high school students in Hong Kong, colleagues at The Hong Kong Polytechnic University conducted several studies based on perspectives of adolescents, teachers, and parents (18-22). In this paper, we used the data collected based on teachers' perceptions of materialism and egocentrism of Chinese adolescents (19) with several objectives. First, we examined the perceptions of teachers on materialism and egocentrism of high school students and adolescents in Hong Kong. Second, we examined whether materialism and egocentrism in high school students and adolescents in general are different based on the perspective of teachers. Based on the social psychology literature, it was hypothesized that teachers would see their students to be less materialistic and egocentric as compared to adolescents in the general adolescent population. Third, as there are not many studies on the psychosocial correlates of teachers' perceptions of materialism and egocentrism in their students and adolescents in Hong Kong, we tested several tentative hypotheses: a) as older people tend to be more conservative, older teachers would see their students or adolescents in general to be more materialistic or egocentric; b) as females focus more on affective relationships and they are more empathetic (i.e., less egocentric), female teachers would see their students or adolescents to be more materialistic or egocentric as compared to male teachers; c) compared with those without religion, teachers with religious beliefs would see their students and Hong Kong adolescents to be more materialistic or egocentric; and d) as those who teach both junior and senior high school students would have better understanding of high school students, they would see their students to be more egocentric.

OUR STUDY

To understand the views of teachers on adolescent materialism and egocentrism, teachers from 11 secondary schools in Hong Kong were recruited to participate in this study (N = 568), with 345 female teachers (60.7%) and 216 male teachers (38%). The sample could be categorized into five age groups: 25 years or below (n = 36, 6.3%), 26-35 years (n = 162, 28.5%), 36-45 years (n = 153, 26.9%), 46-55 years (n = 160, 28.2%), and 56 years or above (n = 49, 8.2%). A total of 464 teachers were with teaching experiences of more than six years. Consent from the teachers was obtained before data collection.

Prior to data collection, this study was reviewed and approved by the University Institutional Review Board at a public university in Hong Kong. After getting approval from the school principals, data were collected from the teachers. In each school, we distributed the questionnaires to the school coordinator who helped to collect the completed questionnaires in sealed envelopes without revealing the identity of the respondents.

INSTRUMENTS

Teachers' perception of adolescent materialism

To assess teachers' perceptions of adolescent materialism, we modified the abridged 5-item Chinese Adolescent Materialism Scale (1) which was originally developed to assess materialistic beliefs in Chinese adolescents. These items included: a) "My students believe that making money is more important than any other things"; b) "My students believe that money is everything"; c) "My students believe that the rich can get respect from others"; d) "My students would abandon some principles for the sake of money"; and e) "My students believe that the amount of money one makes is a fundamental indicator of one's success". A five-point Likert scale was used, including "strongly disagree", "somewhat disagree", "neither agree nor disagree", "somewhat agree", and "strongly agree", with higher scores indicating higher levels of materialism.

To understand teachers' perceptions of materialism in Hong Kong adolescents in general, the same five items were used with changing perspectives. The items included: a) "Hong Kong adolescents think that making money is more important than any other things"; b) "Hong Kong adolescents believe that money is everything"; c) "Hong Kong adolescents think that the rich can get respect from others"; d) "Hong Kong adolescents would abandon some principles for the sake of money"; and e) "Hong Kong adolescents believe that the amount of money one makes is a fundamental indicator of one's success". We used a five-point Likert scale in which higher egocentrism was reflected by higher scores.

Teachers' perception of adolescent egocentrism

To assess teachers' perceptions of egocentrism in their students, we modified the abridged 5-item Chinese Adolescent Egocentrism Scale (19) which was originally developed to assess egocentrism in Chinese adolescents based on the perspective of adolescents (12). These items included: a) "My students regard their experiences are more important than those of others"; b) "My students think that their interests are more important than those of others"; c) "My students always find justifications for their behavior"; d) "most of the time, my students think that other people's criticisms about them do not make sense"; e) "even if they make other people unhappy, my students are true to their experience". For each item, there are five response options, including "strongly disagree", "somewhat disagree", "neither agree nor disagree", "somewhat agree", and "strongly agree", with higher scores showing higher levels of egocentrism.

For teachers' perceptions of adolescent egocentrism, we modified the abridged 5-item Chinese Adolescent Egocentrism Scale (19) which was originally developed to assess egocentrism in Chinese adolescents (12). These items included: a) "Hong Kong adolescents regard their experiences are more important than those of others"; b) "Hong Kong adolescents think that their interests are more important than those of others"; c) "Hong Kong adolescents always find justifications for their behavior"; d) "most of the time, Hong Kong adolescents think that other people's criticisms about them do not make sense"; e) "even if they make other people unhappy, Hong Kong adolescents are true to their experience". For each item, there are five response options. A higher total score means a higher level of perceived egocentrism in Hong Kong adolescents in general.

Data analyses

The Statistical Package for Social Sciences Version 25 (IBM Corp., Somers, NY, USA) was used to perform the related analyses. First, we examined percentage findings to look at the profiles of responses of teachers to the modified version of the Chinese Adolescent Materialism Scale as well as the modified Chinese Adolescent Egocentrism Scale. Besides, teachers' perceptions of materialistic beliefs and egocentric beliefs amongst the general adolescent population in Hong Kong were examined.

Table 1. Teacher perception of materialistic beliefs in their own students

Items	1 n (%)	2 n (%)	1+2 n (%)	3 n (%)	4 n (%)	5 n (%)	4+5 n (%)	Mean	n
My students believe making money is more important than any other things.	14 (2.5%)	140 (24.7%)	154 (27.2%)	123 (21.7%)	254 (44.8%)	36 (6.3%)	290 (51.1%)	3.28	567
My students believe "Money is everything".	45 (7.9%)	173 (30.5%)	218 (38.4%)	163 (28.7%)	164 (28.9%)	22 (3.9%)	186 (32.8%)	2.90	567
My students believe that the rich can get respect from others .	15 (2.7%)	144 (25.4%)	159 (28.1%)	153 (27.0%)	221 (39.0%)	33 (5.8%)	254 (44.8%)	3.20	566
My students believe they would abandon some principles for the sake of money.	52 (9.2%)	179 (31.8%)	231 (41.0%)	192 (34.1%)	134 (23.8%)	6 (1.1%)	140 (24.9%)	2.76	563
My students believe "The amount of money one makes is a fundamental indicator of one's success".	17 (3.0%)	128 (22.6%)	145 (25.6%)	169 (29.8%)	222 (39.2%)	31 (5.5%)	253 (44.7%)	3.22	567

Table 2. Teacher perception of materialistic beliefs in HK adolescents

Items	1 n (%)	2 n (%)	1+2 n (%)	3 n (%)	4 n (%)	5 n (%)	4+5 n (%)	Mean	n
Adolescents in HK believe making money is more important than any other things.	4 (0.7%)	58 (10.2%)	62 (10.9%)	109 (19.2%)	336 (59.3%)	60 (10.6%)	396 (69.9%)	3.69	567
Adolescents in HK believe "Money is everything".	13 (2.3%)	74 (13.1%)	87 (15.4%)	160 (28.2%)	272 (48.0%)	48 (8.5%)	320 (56.5%)	3.47	567
Adolescents in HK believe that the rich can get respect from others ".	4 (0.7%)	60 (10.6%)	64 (11.3%)	107 (18.9%)	331 (58.4%)	65 (11.5%)	396 (69.9%)	3.69	567
Adolescents in HK believe they would abandon some principles for the sake of money.	10 (1.8%)	82 (14.5%)	92 (16.3%)	165 (29.1%)	276 (48.7%)	34 (6.0%)	310 (54.7%)	3.43	567
Adolescents in HK believe "The amount of money one makes is a fundamental indicator of one's success".	4 (0.7%)	47 (8.3%)	51 (9.0%)	119 (21.0%)	321 (56.6%)	76 (13.4%)	397 (70.0%)	3.74	567

Table 3. Teacher perception of egocentrism in their own students

Items	1 n (%)	2 n (%)	1+2 n (%)	3 n (%)	4 n (%)	5 n (%)	4+5 n (%)	Mean	n
My students believe their feelings are more important than the feelings of other people.	1 (0.2%)	20 (3.5%)	21 (3.7%)	71 (12.5%)	298 (52.6%)	177 (31.2%)	475 (83.8%)	4.11	567
My students believe their own benefits are more important than the benefits of other people.	4 (0.7%)	19 (3.4%)	23 (4.1%)	107 (18.9%)	335 (59.2%)	101 (17.8%)	436 (77.0%)	3.90	566
My students believe that no matter what happens, they can always justify their behaviors.	3 (0.5%)	19 (3.4%)	22 (3.9%)	83 (14.6%)	291 (51.3%)	171 (30.2%)	462 (81.5%)	4.07	567

My students believe the criticisms on them are usually groundless.	6 (1.1%)	108 (19.1%)	114 (20.2%)	188 (33.2%)	231 (40.8%)	33 (5.8%)	264 (46.6%)	3.31	566
My students are true to their own feelings even if this may upset other people.	1 (0.2%)	52 (9.2%)	53 (9.4%)	178 (31.4%)	270 (47.6%)	66 (11.6%)	336 (59.2%)	3.61	567

Second, teachers' views of the materialistic and egocentric beliefs of their students were compared with their perceptions of the materialistic and egocentric beliefs of Hong Kong adolescents in general, respectively. For the socio-demographic correlates, Pearson correlation analysis and regression analyses were performed.

FINDINGS

The descriptive profiles based on percentage findings on teachers' perceptions of materialism in students, materialism in Hong Kong adolescents, egocentrism in students, and egocentrism in Hong Kong adolescents are presented in Table 1 to Table 4. First, significant proportions of teachers perceived their students and Hong Kong adolescents showed signs of materialism. For example, 51.1% and 69.9% of the teachers regarded their students and Hong Kong adolescents believed that "making money is more important than any other things", respectively. Second, more than half of the teachers perceived their students and Hong Kong adolescents in general showed signs of egocentrism. For example, the teachers believe that "their feelings are more important than the feelings of other people" (83.8% and 89.9%, respectively). Third, teachers generally perceived that materialism in their own students was lower than that in Hong Kong adolescents. Fourth, teacher perceived egocentrism in their own students to be lower than that in Hong Kong adolescents.

MANOVAs and ANOVAs were further performed to look at the third and fourth observations. Results of the one-way MANOVA analyses showed that there were statistically significant differences in materialistic beliefs between students and Hong Kong adolescents perceived by teachers,

$F(5, 1123) = 33.450$, $p < 0.001$, partial eta squared = 0.130. For univariate effects, there were significant differences between teacher perceptions of students and teacher perceptions of Hong Kong adolescents at the item score ($p < 0.001$ in all items) and composite score ($p < 0.001$) levels (see Table 5). Similarly, one-way MANOVA analyses showed that teachers perceived significant difference between egocentrism in their students and Hong Kong adolescents, $F(5, 1124) = 21.379$, $p < 0.001$, partial eta squared = 0.087. For univariate effects, teacher perceptions of students and Hong Kong adolescents were statistically significantly different over Items 2, 4, and 5 ($p < 0.001$) and the composite score ($p < 0.001$) (see Table 6).

Table 4. Teacher perception of egocentrism in HK adolescents

Items	1 n (%)	2 n (%)	1+2 n (%)	3 n (%)	4 n (%)	5 n (%)	4+5 n (%)	Mean	n
Adolescents in HK believe their feelings are more important than the feelings of other people.	2 (0.4%)	10 (1.8%)	12 (2.2%)	45 (8.0%)	351 (62.0%)	158 (27.9%)	509 (89.9%)	4.15	566
Adolescents in HK believe their own benefits are more important than the benefits of other people.	4 (0.7%)	11 (1.9%)	15 (2.6%)	56 (9.9%)	364 (64.3%)	131 (23.1%)	495 (87.4%)	4.07	566
Adolescents in HK believe that no matter what happens, they can always justify their behaviors.	2 (0.4%)	8 (1.4%)	10 (1.8%)	63 (11.2%)	337 (59.6%)	155 (27.4%)	492 (87.0%)	4.12	565
Adolescents in HK believe the criticisms on them are usually groundless.	4 (0.7%)	37 (6.5%)	41 (7.2%)	145 (25.6%)	318 (56.2%)	62 (11.0%)	380 (67.2%)	3.70	566
Adolescents in HK are true to their own feelings even if this may upset other people.	2 (0.4%)	16 (2.8%)	18 (3.2%)	92 (16.3%)	348 (61.5%)	108 (19.1%)	456 (80.6%)	3.96	566

Pearson correlation analyses showed that teachers' perceptions of materialism in students and materialism in Hong Kong adolescents were not correlated with age, gender, religion, and teaching grade of teachers. In contrast, teachers' perception of egocentrism in their students was related to teaching grade whereas perceived egocentrism in Hong Kong adolescents was correlated with age, gender, and teaching grade (see Table 7).

Table 5. Differences in materialistic beliefs between students and HK adolescents perceived by teachers (N = 562 for teacher's perception of students, N = 567 for teacher's perception of Hong Kong adolescents)

	Students	HK Adolescents	*F*	partial η2
My students/HK adolescents believe that…	*M (SD)*	*M (SD)*	33.450***^	0.13
Making money is more important than any other things	3.28(0.99)	3.69(0.82)	57.662***	0.049
Money is everything.	2.91(1.03)	3.47(0.91)	96.525***	0.079
No money, no dignity.	3.20(0.98)	3.69(0.84)	84.224***	0.070
They would abandon some principles for the sake of money.	2.76(0.95)	3.43(0.87)	151.072***	0.118
The amount of money one makes is a fundamental indicator of one's "success".	3.22(0.96)	3.74(0.82)	96.327***	0.079
Composite Score	3.07(0.79)	3.60(0.71)	141.024***	0.111

Note.***p <.001; ^Adjusted Bonferroni value = .008.

Table 6. Differences in egocentrism between students and HK adolescents perceived by teachers (N = 565 for teacher's perception of students, N = 565 for teacher's perception of Hong Kong adolescents)

	Students	HK Adolescents	*F*	partial η2
My students/HK adolescents believe that…	*M (SD)*	*M (SD)*	21.379***^	0.087
Their feelings are more important than the feelings of other people.	4.11(0.77)	4.15(0.66)	0.996	0.001
Their own benefits are more important than the benefits of other people.	3.90(0.75)	4.07(0.68)	15.925***	0.014
Not matter what happens, they can always justify their behaviors.	4.07(0.79)	4.12(0.68)	1.369	0.001
The criticisms on them are usually groundless.	3.31(0.88)	3.70(0.78)	61.380***	0.052
They are loyal to their own feelings even if this may upset other people.	3.61(0.81)	3.96(0.71)	59.122***	0.050
Composite Score	3.80(0.62)	4.00(0.56)	31.988***	0.028

Note.***p <.001; ^Adjusted Bonferroni value = .008.

Table 7. Correlation among variables

Variables	1	2	3	4
Age[a]	-			
Gender[b]	-0.117**	-		
Religion[c]	-0.107**	0.000	-	
Teaching grade[d]	0.031	-0.041	-0.057	-
Materialism in students	-0.023	0.048	0.048	0.020
Materialism in HK adolescents	-0.045	-0.005	0.020	0.066
Egocentrism in students	-0.028	0.062	0.011	0.090*
Egocentrism in HK adolescents	0.125**	0.085*	-0.036	0.147***

Note. *p <.05, **p <.01, ***p <.001.

[a]Aged 25 or below = 1, Aged 26-35 = 2, Aged 36-45 = 3, Aged 46-55 = 4; Aged 56 or above = 5.

[b]Male = 1, Female = 2; [c]Having religion = 1, Having no religion = 2.

[d]Teaching junior forms (S1-S3) = 1, Teaching senior forms (S4-S6) = 2, Teaching both junior and senior forms (S1-S6) = 3.

Table 8. Predicting effects of demographic factors on teacher perceived materialism in their students

Predictors	Materialism in Students			
	β	*t*	*F*	R^2
Age[a]	-0.026	-0.604	0.365	0.001
Gender[b]	0.049	1.149	2.320	0.002
Religion[c]	0.051	1.186	1.407	0.003
Teaching Grade[d]	0.044	0.336	1.113	0.0002

Note. [a]Aged 25 or below = 1, Aged 26-35 = 2, Aged 36-45 = 3, Aged 46-55 = 4; Aged 56 or above = 5.

[b]Male = 1, Female = 2; [c]Having religion = 1, Having no religion = 2.

[d]Teaching junior forms (S1-S3) = 1, Teaching senior forms (S4-S6) = 2, Teaching both junior and senior forms (S1-S6) = 3.

Table 9. Predicting effects of demographic factors on teacher perceived materialism in HK adolescents

Predictors	Materialism in HK Adolescents			
	β	*t*	*F*	R^2
Age[a]	-0.056	-1.318	1.738	0.003
Gender[b]	-0.003	-0.080	0.006	0.000011
Religion[c]	0.012	0.274	0.075	0.000137
Teaching Grade[d]	0.065	1.524	2.323	0.004

Note. [a]Aged 25 or below = 1, Aged 26-35 = 2, Aged 36-45 = 3, Aged 46-55 = 4; Aged 56 or above = 5.

[b]Male = 1, Female = 2; [c]Having religion = 1, Having no religion = 2.

[d]Teaching junior forms (S1-S3) = 1, Teaching senior forms (S4-S6) = 2, Teaching both junior and senior forms (S1-S6) = 3.

Table 10. Predicting effects of demographic factors on teacher perceived egocentrism in their students

Predictors	Egocentrism in Students			
	β	*t*	*F*	R^2
Age[a]	-0.037	-0.869	0.755	0.001
Gender[b]	0.066	1.570	2.466	0.004
Religion[c]	0.012	0.270	0.073	0.00013
Teaching Grade[d]	0.091	2.138*	4.527*	0.008

Note. *p <.05.

[a]Aged 25 or below = 1, Aged 26-35 = 2, Aged 36-45 = 3, Aged 46-55 = 4; Aged 56 or above = 5.

[b]Male = 1, Female = 2; [c]Having religion = 1, Having no religion = 2.

[d]Teaching junior forms (S1-S3) = 1, Teaching senior forms (S4-S6) = 2, Teaching both junior and senior forms (S1-S6) = 3.

Regression analyses were conducted for each predictor separately. Results showed that there were no prediction effects of age, gender, religion, and teaching grade on materialism in students and materialism in Hong Kong adolescents perceived by teachers (Tables 8 and 9). Teachers' perceived egocentrism in students was only predicted by teaching grade ($F(1, 545) = 4.527$, $p < 0.05$) but not by other predictors (Table 10). Teachers' perceived egocentrism in Hong Kong adolescents was predicted by age ($F(1, 558) = 7.039$, $p < 0.01$), gender ($F(1, 559) = 4.482$, $p < 0.05$) and teaching grade ($F(1, 545) = 12.344$, $p < 0.001$) but not religion (Table 11).

Table 11. Predicting effects of demographic factors on teacher perceived egocentrism in Hong Kong adolescents

Predictors	Egocentrism in HK Adolescents			
	β	*t*	*F*	R^2
Age[a]	0.112	2.653**	7.039**	0.012
Gender[b]	0.089	2.117*	4.482*	0.008
Religion[c]	-0.033	-0.768	0.590	0.001
Teaching Grade[d]	0.149	3.513***	12.344***	0.022

Note. *p <.05, **p <.01, ***p <.001.

[a]Aged 25 or below = 1, Aged 26-35 = 2, Aged 36-45 = 3, Aged 46-55 = 4; Aged 56 or above = 5.

[b]Male = 1, Female = 2; [c]Having religion = 1, Having no religion = 2;[d]Teaching junior forms (S1-S3) = 1, Teaching senior forms (S4-S6) = 2, Teaching both junior and senior forms (S1-S6) = 3.

DISCUSSION

Although adolescent materialism and egocentrism are important aspects of adolescent development, few Chinese studies have been conducted. In particular, no study has been conducted to look at the related issues from the perspective of significant-others of adolescents, particularly teachers. Against this background, we conducted this study to examine teachers' perceptions of materialism as well as egocentrism in their students and adolescents in Hong Kong. We also compared the perceived differences between students taught by the respondents and Hong Kong adolescents in general on materialism and egocentrism. Furthermore, as there are very few studies on the socio-demographic correlates of perceptions of materialistic and egocentric beliefs in Hong Kong high school students and adolescents in general, we explored several tentative hypotheses in this study. Because there are very few related studies in the field, this is a pioneer attempt in studying adolescent materialism and egocentrism.

Based on the teachers' responses to the modified version of the Chinese Adolescent Materialism Scale, we observed several phenomena. First, around 45% of the teachers perceived their students believe that "no money, no dignity". Similarly, around 45% of the teachers perceived their students believe that "the amount of money one makes is a fundamental indicator of one's success". Second, more than half of the teachers perceived that adolescents in Hong Kong hold materialistic beliefs: around 70% of the teachers perceived that "adolescents in HK believe making money is more important than any other things"; around 70% of the teachers perceived that Hong Kong adolescents equated money with dignity and regarded money as the criteria of success. These findings are worrying because the over-emphasis on material possession would be detrimental to adolescent development. In future, we should further examine how materialistic beliefs influence adolescent development, particularly on the development of character strengths and virtues.

For adolescent egocentrism, the picture is even more worrying. More than two-third of the teachers perceived that their students are egocentric: around 84% of the teachers perceived that their students regarded their feelings to be more important than those of other people; 77% of the teachers perceived that their students regarded their own benefits are more important than the benefits of other people. Furthermore, most of the teachers perceived that adolescents in Hong Kong were egocentric: around 87% of the teachers perceived that Hong Kong adolescents regarded that their benefits are more important than those of others; around 87% of the respondents perceived that adolescents always have justifications for their behavior. These findings suggest that adolescents should be helped to balance the emphasis on superiority of one's views and feelings while respecting the views and experiences of other people.

Regarding perceptions of teachers regarding materialism and egocentrism in their students and Hong Kong adolescents, the findings showed that teachers generally had relatively positive perceptions of their students as compared to adolescents in general – students were seen as less materialistic and less egocentric as compared to adolescents in Hong Kong. This observation is interesting and it is in line with the previous findings that adolescents saw themselves as less materialistic than did adolescents in general (23).

Several observations can be highlighted from the findings on the socio-demographic correlates of teachers' perceived materialism and egocentrism beliefs in Chinese adolescents. First, socio-demographic correlates were not related to teachers' perceived materialism and egocentrism of their students and Hong Kong adolescents in general. Second, with more teaching exposure (i.e., teaching more grades), teachers tended to perceive that their students were more egocentric. One possible explanation is that teachers might have a more in-depth understanding of their students when they teach junior and senior form students. Third, age, gender, and teaching grades were related to teachers' perceptions of egocentrism of adolescents in Hong Kong. The positive relationship between age and perceived egocentrism is consistent with the conjecture that people with older age are more conservative and they are more critical of young people. Regarding gender, as females attach more emphasis on interpersonal relationship, they would also be more critical of egocentric behavior in adolescents as compared to males. Concerning grade teaching, we can interpret that those with more teaching exposure would understand their students better, hence having a higher level of perceived egocentrism amongst Hong Kong adolescents. However, as the present hypotheses are tentative in nature, there is a need to further refine them in future studies.

Although the present study is a pioneer study in the field, there are several limitations. First, as the sample was not randomly selected, we should be cautious to examine the generalizability of the findings. Further replication of the findings based on random samples is in order. Second, as only abridged scales (i.e., five items) were employed, it would be theoretically and empirically enriching if longer scales could be used. Third, regarding the socio-demographic prediction of teachers' perceived adolescent materialism and egocentrism, the findings are tentative and inconclusive. Hence, there is a need to refine the related hypotheses and theoretical bases. Finally, the origin of materialism and egocentrism in adolescents was not covered in the present study. In the area of materialism, there are studies suggesting that socialization within the family context plays an important role in the development of different motives for happiness in adolescents (24-28). Hence, it would be exciting to explore how family socialization contributes to the development of materialism and egocentrism in adolescents further.

ACKNOWLEDGMENTS

The series of studies on character and moral development in high school students in Hong Kong are financially supported by Wofoo Foundation. This chapter is a re-print with minor revision of an earlier published paper in the *International Journal of Child Health and Human Development* 2019;12(3) issue with permission.

REFERENCES

[1] Shek DTL, Ma CMS, Lin L. The Chinese Adolescent Materialism Scale: Psychometric properties and normative profiles. Int J Disabil Hum Dev 2014;13(2):285-95. doi: 10.1515/ijdhd-2014-0315.

[2] Shek DTL, Dou D, Zhu X, Chai, W. Positive youth development: Current perspectives. Adolesc Health Med Ther 2019;10:131-41. doi: 10.2147/ AHMT.S179946.

[3] Benson PL. All kids are our kids: What communities must do to raise caring and responsible children and adolescents, 2nd edition. San Francisco, CA: Jossey-Bass, 1997. URL: http://psycnet.apa.org/record/2006-13341-000.

[4] Bowers EP, Li Y, Kiely MK, Brittian A, Lerner JV, Lerner RM. The Five Cs model of positive youth development: A longitudinal analysis of confirmatory factor structure and measurement invariance. J Youth Adolesc 2010;39(7):720-35. doi:10.1007/s10964-010- 9530-9.

[5] Lerner RM, Lerner JV, Almerigi JB, Theokas C, Phelps E, Gestsdottir S, et al. Positive youth development, participation in community youth development programs, and community contributions of fifth-grade adolescents: Findings from the first wave of the 4-H study of positive youth development. J Early Adolesc 2005;25(1):17-71. doi:10.1177/0272431604272461.

[6] Frankl V. Man's search for meaning. London: Vintage Publishing, 2004.

[7] Shek DTL, Lin L, Siu AMH, Lee B. Materialism in Chinese adolescents in Hong Kong: Profiles and socio-demographic correlates. Int J Child and Adolesc Dev, in press.

[8] Piaget J. Judgment and reasoning in the child. London: Routledge Kegan Paul, 1972.

[9] Elkind D. Egocentrism in adolescence. Child Dev 1967;38:1025–34.

[10] Elkind D, Bowen R. Imaginary audience behavior in children and adolescents. Dev Psychol 1979;15:38–44.

[11] Enright RD, Lapsley DK, Shukla DG. Adolescent egocentrism in early and late adolescence. Adolescence 1979;14(56):687–95.

[12] Shek DTL, Yu L, Siu AMH. The Chinese Adolescent Egocentrism Scale: Psychometric properties and normative profiles. Int J Disabil Hum Dev 2014;13(2):297-307. doi:10.1515/ijdhd-2014-0315.

[13] Battistich V. Character Education, prevention, and positive youth development. Character Educ Partnership 2005;1-10. URL: https://www.academia.edu/28900720/ Character_Education_Prevention_and_Positive_Youth_Development.

[14] Park N. Building strengths of character: Keys to positive youth development. Reclaiming Child Youth 2009;18(2):42-7.

[15] Park N, Peterson C. Moral competence and character strengths among adolescents: The development and validation of the values in action inventory of strengths for youth. J Adolesc 2006;29:891-909.

[16] Catalano RF, Berglund ML, Ryan JAM, Lonczak HS, Hawkins JD. Positive youth development in the United States: Research findings on evaluations of positive youth development programs. Ann Am Acad Pol Soc Sci 2004;591(1):98-124. doi:10.1177/0002716203260102.

[17] Shek DTL, Siu AMH. "UNHAPPY" Environment for adolescent development in Hong Kong. J Adolesc Health 2019;64(6):S1-4. doi:10.1016/j.jadohealth.2019.01.007.

[18] Shek DTL, Lin L. A study on the development of Chinese students (Character, psychosocial competence and behavior): Report No. 1 – Views of students. Hong Kong: Department of Applied Social Sciences, The Hong Kong Polytechnic University, 2017.

[19] Shek DTL, Ma CMS. A study on the development of Chinese students (Character, psychosocial competence and behavior): Report No. 2 – Views of teachers. Hong Kong: Department of Applied Social Sciences, The Hong Kong Polytechnic University, 2017.

[20] Shek DTL, Yu L. A study on the development of Chinese students (Character, psychosocial competence and behavior): Report No. 3 – Views of parents. Hong Kong: Department of Applied Social Sciences, The Hong Kong Polytechnic University, 2018.

[21] Shek, DTL, Leung J. A study on the development of Chinese students (Character, psychosocial competence and behavior): Report No. 4 – Moral education at the crossroad. Hong Kong: Department of Applied Social Sciences, The Hong Kong Polytechnic University, 2018.

[22] Shek DTL, Wu FKY, Leung H. A study on the development of Chinese students (Character, psychosocial competence and behavior): Report No. 5 – A qualitative study of the views of principals and teachers on moral education. Hong Kong: Department of Applied Social Sciences, The Hong Kong Polytechnic University, 2018.

[23] Dunning D. Self-insight: Roadblocks and detours on path to knowing thyself. New York: Psychology Press, 2005.

[24] Huta V. Linking peoples' pursuit of eudaimonia and hedonia with characteristics of their parents: Parenting styles, verbally endorsed values, and role modeling. J Happiness Stud 2012;13(1):47-61. doi:10.1007/s10902-011-9249-7.

[25] Huta, V. Eudaimonic and hedonic orientations: Theoretical considerations and research findings. In: Vittersø J, eds. Handbook of eudaimonic well-being. International handbook of quality of life. Cham, Switzerland: Springer, 2016:215-31.

[26] Huta V, Ryan RM. Pursuing pleasure or virtue: The differential and overlapping well-being benefits of hedonic and eudaimonic motives. J Happiness Stud 2010;11(6):735-62.

[27] Huta V, Waterman AS. Eudaimonia and its distinction from hedonia: Developing a classification and terminology for understanding conceptual and operational definitions. J Happiness Stud 2014;15:1425-56. doi:10.1007/s10902-013-9485-0.

[28] Huta V, Pelletier LG, Baxter D, Thompson A. How eudaimonic and hedonic motives relate to the well-being of close others. J Posit Psychol 2012;7(5):399-404.

SECTION TWO: FAMILY ENVIRONMENT

In: Advances in Chinese Children … ISBN: 978-1-53617-870-8
Editors: Ariel Tenenbaum et al.

Chapter 6

FAMILY MEALTIME ENVIRONMENT AND CHILD BEHAVIOR OUTCOMES IN CHINESE PRESCHOOL CHILDREN

Cynthia Leung*[*], PhD, Sandra Tsang, PhD, Sing Kai Lo, PhD and Ruth Chan, PhD

Department of Applied Social Sciences, The Hong Kong Polytechnic University, Department of Social Work and Social Administration, The University of Hong Kong, School of Graduate Studies, The Education University of Hong Kong and Department of Medicine and Therapeutics/Centre for Nutritional Studies, The Chinese University of Hong Kong, PR China

[*] Corresponding Author: Professor Cynthia Leung, Department of Applied Social Sciences, The Hong Kong Polytechnic University, Hung Hom, Hong Kong, PR China. E-mail: ssleung@polyu.edu.hk.

Abstract

In this chapter we aimed to examine the influence of family mealtime environment on children's behavior, in addition to styles of parenting and family functioning. This study adopted a two-wave longitudinal design. Data was collected over two rounds, 12 months apart, from 470 parents with children aged three to six. Parents completed measures on their parenting style, family functioning, children's behavior, family meal frequency, family feeding practice and mealtime television. Family feeding practice and parenting style were found to be associated with children's behavior. Family feeding practice mediated between parenting style and children's behavior. Family mealtime environment is important on children's behavior.

Introduction

Young children under parental care are expected to dine at home as part of the general family routine. It is argued that family mealtime behavior is likely to be consistent with other patterns of family social interaction which are associated with child outcomes (1).

There have been a number of cross-sectional studies on the association between family meal frequency and child behavior in preschool and primary school children. For example, higher family meal frequency was associated with reduced externalizing behavior problems and higher prosocial behavior in preschool/primary school children (2, 3). Among adolescents aged 11 to 18 years, a cross-sectional study found a negative association between family meal frequency and substance abuse, after controlling for family connectedness (4). The association between family meal frequency and adolescent problem behavior has also been reported in some longitudinal studies. For example, family meal frequency at baseline was found to be negatively associated with substance use among female adolescents in a 5-year longitudinal study and the mean age of participants was 17.2 at follow-up (5). More recently, a 3-year longitudinal study found that family meal frequency was negatively associated with substance-use, drinking, physical violence and running away among adolescents (6). However, there were few longitudinal studies on the association between family meal frequency and child behavior outcomes among preschool/primary school children.

Many scholars theorized about the association between family meal frequency and child psychosocial outcomes. Family mealtimes offer natural "face-to-face sit-together" chances for parent-child communication, parent monitoring of child activities, and sharing of feelings (1). Parents can be role models for table manners, respect and sharing (5). Family meals within the context of family routine can provide stability, a developmental protective factor (7).

There are some limitations with previous studies. First, most findings on preschool/primary children were based on cross-sectional studies, and it was not possible to establish causal relationship between family meal frequency and behavior outcomes. Second, many studies failed to consider the roles of family functioning or parenting variables. Family functioning involves cohesion (emotional closeness amongst family members) and communication (sharing of ideas and affect among family members) in the family (8). Parenting style can be conceived along two dimensions: demandingness (parent acting as socializing agent) and responsiveness (parent recognition of child individuality) (9). Authoritative parenting is high in demandingness and responsiveness and associated with positive child outcomes. Authoritarian parenting is high in demandingness but low in responsiveness, while permissive parenting is just the opposite (10). Authoritarian parenting and permissive parenting were associated with poorer child outcomes (11). Family meal frequency might be confounded with variables like family functioning or parenting style (12). Third, more frequent family meals might arise from closeness among family members. Family meal frequency might mediate between family relationship and child behavior outcomes, and such role should be examined (12). Fourth, most studies measured family meal frequency as a composite score for all family members. The contribution of individual family members (e.g., father, mother) should be examined.

Other contextual family mealtime environment variables, including mealtime television viewing and family feeding practice, warrant attention in understanding the association between family meal frequency and child outcomes. Sustained television viewing was found to be positively associated with child behavior problems in preschool children (13) though mealtime television viewing was not examined specifically in this study. Mealtime routines were related to children's behavior outcomes. For example, parental rigid demands for the child to finish all food served might lead to child behavior problem and conflict with parents. Disorderly mealtime routine was related to neglect and disregard (1). The impact of these mealtime environment variables on child outcomes should be investigated.

This study addressed the limitations of previous studies. First, it adopted a longitudinal design to provide evidence on causal relationships. Second, it collected data on parenting style and family functioning. The relationship between family mealtime environment variables and family functioning/parenting variables could be investigated. Third, family mealtime environment variables including mealtime television viewing and family feeding practice (type of food served, mealtime behavior management) were investigated. Fourth, to examine the unique contribution of family members, the presence of family members was individually recorded. Finally, to test the cross-cultural applicability of previous findings, the present study targeted Chinese families with preschool children. The results would enable comparison of findings across cultures to map out universal and culture-specific factors.

This study collected two rounds of data from Chinese families with preschool children to examine the influence of family mealtime environment variables (family meal frequency, mealtime television viewing, family feeding practice), parenting style and family functioning on child behavior. Literature review guided this study to examine (i) the direct effect of family mealtime environment variables on child outcomes, in addition to parenting style and family functioning variables; and (ii) family mealtime environment variables as mediators between family functioning/parenting style and child outcomes. The hypotheses were:

1) Family mealtime environment, family functioning and parenting style would be associated with child behavior problems.
2) Family mealtime environment would mediate between family functioning/parenting style and child behavior problems.

OUR STUDY

This was a longitudinal survey. The two rounds of data collection were 12 months apart. The study only included (i) parents who were Cantonese-speaking (Cantonese being the usual language/dialect used at home for 89.5% of the Hong Kong population) (14); and (ii) parents whose children were attending preschools at the time of the study. Parents with children with global developmental delay, physical, severe hearing or visual impairment or Autism Spectrum Disorder were excluded. Since there were two rounds of data collection, parents with children in the final year of their preschools were excluded as their children would have left preschools by the second round of data collection.

Two strategies were used to recruit the participants coming from 24 preschools from 15 of the 18 districts in Hong Kong. First, the investigators used their personal network and contacted organizations providing preschool education. Five organizations nominated preschools within their organizations to participate, and 18 preschools participated. Second, a research assistant made phone calls to invite preschools throughout Hong Kong. Six out of 400 participated. In each participating preschool, the number of participating parents ranged from nine to 141.

The ethics committee of The Hong Kong Polytechnic University approved the study. After getting consent from the preschools and parents, the parent questionnaires were distributed through the preschools. At both rounds of data collection, parents completed the questionnaires at a time and place of their own convenience, and returned the completed questionnaires to the preschools in sealed envelopes.

Measures

Parenting Style and Dimension Questionnaire – Short Form (PSDQ-SF) (15) – Parents completed this 32-item 5-point Likert scale with a validated Chinese version for Hong Kong parents (16) measuring authoritative, authoritarian and permissive parenting styles (e.g., emphasizing the reasons for rules, exploding in anger towards child, spoiling child). A total score was calculated for each style. Higher scores indicated more frequent adoption of that particular parenting style.

Chinese Family Assessment Instrument (C-FAI) (17) – This 33-item measure assessed family functioning (e.g., mutual consideration, harmonious family relationship). It yielded five sub-scales, namely, communication, mutuality, conflict and harmony, parental concern and parental control. The parent version was adapted from the original version for completion by adolescents. Parents rated each statement along a 5-point scale (1: *completely agree*; 5: *completely disagree*). The negatively worded-items were reverse scored. Lower scores represented more harmonious family functioning in all sub-scales.

Hong Kong Parent Feeding Questionnaire (HKPFQ) – This 35-item questionnaire assessed parent knowledge, attitude, cooking and feeding practices with regard to their children (e.g., mealtime regularities, diet profile). Parents rated each item on a 3-point scale. A higher score suggested healthier feeding practices. This scale has been used with Hong Kong parents of preschool children in a recent infant and young child feeding survey (18).

Family meal frequency – Parents had to report the frequency of family members present at family dinner over a week. The number of days within a week that mother ate with the target child was summed up to generate a new variable. A similar variable was created for fathers. Another variable on frequency of grandparents eating with the target child was created by summing up all the meals that grandparents (paternal and maternal) ate with the target child.

Frequency of mealtime television viewing – Parents were requested to report the frequency of dinner time television viewing over a week. The total number of nights the television was on was summed up to form a new variable.

Eyberg Child Behavior Inventory (ECBI) (19) – This was a 36-item measure of parental perception of disruptive behavior (e.g., temper tantrums) in children aged two to 16 years. It included two scales, Intensity scale and Problem scale. ECBI-Intensity measured the frequency of problem behavior on a 7-point rating scale. ECBI-Problem measured the extent to which the parents were concerned about the behavior (1: *yes*; 0: *no*). A validated Chinese version was available (20).

Family background - Parents were asked to supply information on their age, family type, education level, employment, family income and social welfare status. Family income was recoded into a dichotomous variable (at/above versus below median household income).

Data analysis

In this study, the Round 1 and Round 2 variables were measured at the individual level. Owing to the cluster (preschools) nature of the data set, multilevel mediation modelling (21) was used to appropriately model the error structure, treating "preschool" as the random factor. This method allows the testing of mediation effects in clustered datasets. We started by examining the direct effects of Round 1 variables (family mealtime environment, parenting style and family functioning) on Round 2 child behavior outcome. Then, the mediation effect of Round 1 family meal frequency, mealtime television viewing, family feeding practice between Round 1 family functioning/parenting style and Round 2 child behavior outcomes was tested. In the analyses described above, the outcome variables were Round 2 child behavior as measured by ECBI-Intensity and ECBI-Problem. As child gender and family income were found to be associated with child behavior (22, 23), they were controlled for in the analysis.

FINDINGS

The demographic characteristics of the participants and the scale descriptive statistics are shown in Table 1. Table 2 shows the bivariate correlations. As C-FAI mutuality was highly correlated with C-FAI communication ($r = .83$, $p < .001$, $R^2 = .68$) and C-FAI conflict and harmony ($r = .72$, $p < .001$, $R^2 = .52$), C-FAI mutuality was excluded in the following analyses to control for multicollinearity. The direct effects are shown in Table 3.

Table 1. Demographic characteristics of participants and mean and standard deviation scores of scales (*N*= 470)

	Number	Percentage	
Sex of target child - boy	232	49.40%	
Sex of target child - girl	238	50.60%	
Relationship of participant to target child - mother	372	79.15%	
Relationship of participant to target child - father	94	20.00%	
Relationship of participant to target child - grandparents	4	0.85%	
Target child living with both parents	417	88.72%	
Target child living with mother only	21	4.47%	
Target child living with father only	9	1.91%	
Target child not living with parents	22	4.68%	
Mother's education – junior secondary or below	120	25.53%	
Mother's education – senior secondary or above	347	73.83%	
Father's education – junior secondary or below	133	28.30%	
Father's education – senior secondary or above	327	69.57%	
Mother employed	244	51.91%	
Father employed	442	94.04%	
Family income[a] – HK$19,999 or below	196	41.70%	
Family income[a] – HK$20,000 or above	253	53.83%	
	Mean	Standard deviation	Reliability
Age of target child (in years)	4.48	0.64	NA
Age of mother (in years)	34.50	5.27	NA
Age of father (in years)	38.50	6.82	NA
Mother's length of residence in Hong Kong (in years)	20.72	15.37	NA
Father's length of residence in Hong Kong (in years)	31.86	14.45	NA
Number of children	1.74	0.70	NA
Round 2 ECBI-Intensity	108.93	25.63	.94
Round 2 ECBI-Problem	6.09	6.73	.92

	Number	Percentage	
Round 1 authoritative parenting style	58.73	7.51	.89
Round 1 authoritarian parenting style	26.61	5.82	.82
Round 1 permissive parenting style	13.05	2.90	.60
Round 1 C-FAI communication	16.44	6.25	.90
Round 1 C-FAI mutuality	21.56	8.79	.96
Round 1 C-FAI conflict and harmony	11.02	4.23	.73
Round 1 C-FAI parental concern	3.94	1.62	.66
Round 1 C-FAI parental control	6.36	2.36	.67
Round 1 family feeding practice	58.54	7.14	.80
Round 1 frequency of fathers eating with child	4.48	2.67	NA
Round 1 frequency of mothers eating with child	5.79	2.15	NA
Round 1 frequency of grandparents eating with child	5.04	5.09	NA
Round 1 frequency of mealtime television viewing	4.11	2.73	NA

[a] Median household income = HK$20,700.

Table 2. Correlation among variables

	1	2	3	4	5	6	7	8	9	10	11	12	13	14
1														
2	.61**													
3	.30**	.23**												
4	.32**	.21**	.83**											
5	.28**	.22**	.60**	.72**										
6	.17**	.16**	.55**	.52**	.41**									
7	.25**	.20**	.25**	.27**	.34**	.19**								
8	-.29**	-.21**	-.42**	-.35**	-.28**	-.27**	-.24**							
9	.40**	.28**	.24**	.27**	.36**	.17**	.53**	-.33**						
10	.36**	.28**	.24**	.22**	.21**	.09	.24**	-.24**	.40**					
11	-.05**	-.03	-.11*	-.07	-.05	.01	.08	.00	.04	-.06				
12	.02	.02	-.13**	-.05	-.10*	-.04	.06	.05	-.00	-.06	.36**			
13	-.36**	-.27**	-.28**	-.27**	-.25**	-.18**	-.21**	.25**	-.33**	-.43**	.05	.01		
14	.14**	.18**	.18**	.18**	.14**	.08	.03	-.12**	.13**	.23**	-.05	-.11*	-.35**	
15	.03	.07	-.01	-.06	-.04	.00	-.10*	-.06	.00	.08	-.13**	-.14**	-.10*	.10*

* $p \leq .05$ ** $p \leq .01$

Legend:

1: Round 2 ECBI-intensity; 2: Round 2 ECBI-problem; 3: Round 1 C-FAI communication; 4: Round 1 C-FAI mutuality; 5: Round 1 C-FAI conflict and harmony; 6: Round 1 C-FAI parental Concern; 7: Round 1 C-FAI parental control; 8: Round 1 authoritative parenting style; 9: Round 1 authoritarian parenting style; 10: Round 1 permissive parenting style; 11: Round 1 frequency of fathers eating with child; 12: Round 1 frequency of mothers eating with child; 13: Round 1 family feeding practice; 14: Round 1 frequency of mealtime television viewing; 15: Round 1 frequency of grandparents eating with child

Table 3. Direct effect (b and 95% CI) of round 1 family mealtime environment, parenting style, and family functioning on round 2 child behaviour

Round 1 variables	Round 2 ECBI Intensity	Round 2 ECBI Problem
Family income	-.2.61 (-7.02, 1.79), $p = .245$	-0.13 (-1.35, 1.10), $p = .838$
Child gender	-.6.39 (-10.43, -2.35), $p = .002$	-1.44 (-2.59, -0.30), $p = .014$
Authoritative parenting style	-0.29 (-0.61, 0.02), $p = .064$	-0.04 (-0.13, 0.05), $p = .393$
Authoritarian parenting style	0.80 (0.36, 1.24), $p < .001$	0.11 (-0.02, 0.23), $p = .102$
Permissive parenting style	1.59 (0.78, 2.39), $p < .001$	0.39 (0.16, 0.62), $p = .001$
C-FAI Communication	0.28 (-0.20, 0.76), $p = .252$	0.05 (-0.09, 0.19), $p = .490$
C-FAI Conflict and harmony	0.27 (-0.37, 0.91), $p = .408$	0.07 (-0.12, 0.25), $p = .481$
C-FAI Parental concern	-.0.34 (-1.84, 1.17), $p = .661$	0.17 (-0.26, 0.60), $p = .444$
C-FAI Parental control	0.30 (-0.71, 1.32), $p = .557$	0.17 (-0.12, 0.46), $p = .261$
Frequency of fathers eating with child	-0.16 (-0.98, 0.67), $p = .710$	-0.01 (-0.24, 0.23), $p = .942$
Frequency of mothers eating with child	0.43 (-0.60, 1.47), $p = .413$	0.19 (-0.10, 0.49), $p = .199$
Frequency of grandparents eating with child	0.21 (-0.19, 0.62), $p = .300$	0.10 (-0.02, 0.22), $p = .089$
Frequency of mealtime television viewing	-0.02 (-0.80, 0.77), $p = .970$	0.21 (-0.02, 0.43), $p = .076$
Family feeding practice	-0.58 (-0.92, -0.23), $p = .001$	-0.07 (-0.16, 0.03), $p = .168$

The Sample

In Round 1, among 2,492 consent forms distributed, 923 parents consented to participate. Eleven participants were either outside Hong Kong or had changed schools when data was collected. There were 663 sets of complete data out of 912 data sets collected (24). In Round 2, there were 676 parents with complete data. There were 470 parents with complete data in both waves, which provided the basis for the reported analysis.

Participants with complete and incomplete data in both rounds differed. Participants with complete data in both rounds attained lower scores on Round 1 C-FAI conflict and harmony, $t(859) = 2.67$, $p = .008$, and Round 1 authoritarian parenting, $t(847) = 2.07$, $p = .043$. Among those with complete data in both rounds, there was a higher proportion of families with monthly income above HK$20,000, $\chi^2(1) = 8.05$, $p = .005$.

Frequency of Child Behavior Problems (ECBI-Intensity)

Round 2 ECBI-Intensity scores were associated positively with Round 1 authoritarian and permissive parenting and negatively with Round 1 family feeding practice and child gender (Table 3). As Round 1 permissive parenting was negatively associated with Round 1 family feeding practice (b = -0.78, z = -7.01, p < .001), the mediating effect of Round 1 family feeding practice as a mediator between Round 1 permissive parenting and Round 2 ECBI-Intensity scores was tested. The positive indirect (z = 3.00, p = .045) and total (z = 5.12, p < .001) effect of Round 1 permissive parenting on Round 2 ECBI-Intensity scores were significant. Round 1 authoritarian parenting was negatively associated with Round 1 family feeding practice (b = -0.17, z = -2.66, p = .008). The mediating effect of Round 1 family feeding practice as a mediator between Round 1 authoritarian parenting and Round 2 ECBI-Intensity scores was tested. The positive indirect (z = 2.09, p = .037) and total (z = 3.95, p < .001) effect of Round 1 authoritarian parenting on Round 2 ECBI-Intensity scores were significant. In short, higher frequency of child behavior problems was associated with more authoritarian and permissive parenting, less healthy feeding practice, and the child being male. Family feeding practice was a mediator between permissive/authoritarian parenting and frequency of child behavior problems.

Parent Concern over Child Behavior Problems (ECBI-Problem)

Round 2 ECBI-Problem scores were negatively associated with child gender and positively associated with Round 1 permissive parenting (Table 3). More parent concern over child behavior problems was associated with the child being male and more permissive parenting.

DISCUSSION

In terms of Hypothesis 1, the results indicated that family mealtime environment variables had direct contributions to child behavior, after controlling for family functioning, parenting style, and family income. Specifically, healthier feeding practices were associated with lower frequency of child behavior problems. The longitudinal design of the present study provided further support for the causal relationship between family feeding practices and child behavior outcomes. The emphasis on healthy food (rather than the often more appealing unhealthy food) and regular meal routines implies a sense of self-regulation which is conducive to positive behavior outcomes. The results confirmed that mealtime routines were related to children's mental health (1). The results also concurred with literature and provided support for the negative effect of authoritarian and permissive parenting on child behavior (11).

With regard to Hypothesis 2, the results provided evidence of family mealtime environment variables as mediators of parenting style on child behavior outcomes. Permissive parenting styles negatively influenced child behavior outcomes through family feeding practices. Parents with permissive styles were more likely to allow unhealthy feeding practices (e.g., unhealthy food, lax meal routines), which then predicted more child behavior problems. Authoritarian parenting rigidly demanding the child to finish all food served might lead to parent-child conflict and child problem behavior (1).

The present study illuminated on parenting practices for Hong Kong Chinese families with preschool children. The findings generally concurred with the international literature on the impact of parenting style and family mealtime environment on children's outcomes. Family mealtime environment variables reflected actual parenting practices such as type of food eaten, arrangement of meal routines, and management of mealtime behavior. The results indicated that actual parenting practices and parenting styles were both influential on child developmental outcomes.

Limitations

First, the family and parenting measures were only based on parent reports. Second, the reporting parents were mostly mothers, while views from both parents should be useful to identify possible couple differences in parenting styles or practices, as well as their impact on child and family outcomes. Third, the sample did not include preschools in all administrative districts of Hong Kong, and is not adequately representative of the Hong Kong population. Fourth, participants with incomplete data were more disadvantaged and less positive in parenting practices than those with complete data. These should be fully considered in the interpretation of the data.

CONCLUSION

This study underscores the importance of considering family mealtime environment in understanding family influence on child development. Family mealtime environment variables and parenting style variables contributed directly to child behavior. Family feeding practice was associated with parenting style, and family feeding practice mediated the effect of parenting style on child outcome. This study reinforces the efforts to conduct longitudinal studies in families. Such attempts in this study successfully generated meaningful causative information that can directly enrich health education and the practice of professionals working with young children. The findings allow for evidence-based assertions that parenting styles are associated with child outcomes. It will be helpful for parents to learn to be responsive to their children, harbor realistic expectations on their children and be reasonably demanding on their age-appropriate performance. Parents should try to create more opportunities to cultivate healthy and pleasant family atmosphere. Parents should set limits and rules for appropriate mealtime behavior, provide a variety of food, and let the child decide how much to eat and what to eat (18).

Acknowledgment

This project was supported by the Research Grants Council General Research Fund (PolyU 5422/13H). This chapter is an adapted version of a re-print with minor revision of an earlier paper published in the *International Journal of Child Health and Human Development* 2018;11(3) issue with permission.

References

[1] Fiese BH, Foley KP, Spagnola M. Routine and ritual elements in family mealtimes: Contexts for child well-being and family identity. New Direct Child Adolesc Dev 2006;111:67-89.

[2] Hofferth SL, Sandberg JF. How American children spend their time. J Marriage Fam 2001;63:295-308.

[3] Lora KR, Sisson SB, DeGrace BW, Morris AS. Frequency of family meals and 6-11-year-old children's social behaviors. J Fam Psychol 2014;28:577-82.

[4] Eisenberg M, Olson R, Neumark-Sztainer D, Story M, Bearinger L. Correlations between family meals and psychosocial well-being among adolescents. Arch Pediatr Adolesc Med 2004;158:792-6.

[5] Eisenberg ME, Neumark-Sztainer D, Fulkerson JA, Story M. Family meals and substance use: Is there a long-term protective association? J Adolesc Health 2008;43:151-6.

[6] Sen B. The relationship between frequency of family dinner and adolescent problem behaviors after adjusting for other family characteristics. J Adolesc 2010;33:187–96.

[7] Munoz DJ, Israel AC, Anderson DA. The relationship of family stability and family mealtime frequency with bulimia symptomatology. Eat Disord 2007;15:261–71.

[8] Olson DH, DeFrain J. Marriages and families: Intimacy, strengths, and diversity, 4th ed. New York: McGraw-Hill, 2003.

[9] Darling N, Steinberg L. Parenting style as context: An integrative model. Psychol Bull 1993;113 (3):487-96.

[10] Maccoby E, Martin J. Socialization in the context of the family: Parent-child interaction. In: Hetherington EM, Mussen PH, eds. Handbook of child psychology, vol 4. Socialization, personality, and social development. New York: Wiley, 1983:1-101.

[11] Williams LR, Degnan KA, Perez-Edgar KE, Henderson HA, Rubin KH, Pine DS, et al. Impact of behavioral inhibition and parenting style on internalizing and

externalizing problems from early childhood through adolescence. J Abnorm Child Psychol 2009;37:1063-75.

[12] Miller DP, Waldfogel J, Han WJ. Family meals and child academic and behavioral outcomes. Child Dev 2012;83(6):2104-20.

[13] Mistry KB, Minkovitz CS, Strobino DM, Borzekowski DLG. Children's television exposure and behavioral and social outcomes at 5.5 years: Does timing of exposure matter? Pediatrics 2007;120:762-9.

[14] Census and Statistics Department. 2011 population by-census main report, volume 1. Hong Kong: Government Publications Unit, 2012.

[15] Robinson C, Mandleco B, Olsen SF, Hart CH. The Parenting Styles and Dimension Questionnaire (PSDQ). In: Perlmutter BF, Touliatos J, Holden GM, eds. Handbook of family measurement techniques, volume. 3. Instruments and index. Thousand Oaks, CA: Sage, 2001:319-32.

[16] Tse H. Translation and Validation of Parenting Styles and Dimensions Questionnaire – Short Form (PSDQ-SF). Dissertation. Hong Kong: The Hong Kong Polytechnic University, 2011.

[17] Shek DTL, Ma CMS. The Chinese Family Assessment Instrument (C-FAI): Hierarchical confirmatory factor analyses and factorial invariance. Res Social Work Prac 2010;20:112-23.

[18] Leung S, Leung C, Luk WY. A survey of infant and young child feeding in Hong Kong: Parental perceptions and practices, 2012. URL: http://www.fhs.gov.hk/english/archive/files/reports/Survey_IYCF_parents%20perception.pdf.

[19] Eyberg SM, Ross AW. Assessment of child behaviour problems: The validation of a new inventory. J Clin Psychol 1978;16:113-6.

[20] Leung CM, Chan SCM, Pang RCY, Cheng WKC. Validation of the Chinese version of the Eyberg Child Behaviour Inventory for use in Hong Kong. Hong Kong: Education Bureau, Hong Kong SAR Government, 2003.

[21] Krull JL, MacKinnon DP. Multilevel modeling of individual and group level mediated effects. Multivariate Behav Res 2001;36(2):249-77.

[22] Flouri E, Midouhas E, Joshi HJ. Family poverty and trajectories of children's emotional and behavioural problems: The moderating roles of self-regulation and verbal cognitive ability. J Abnorm Child Psychol 2014;42:1043.

[23] Leung C, Leung S, Chan R, Tso K, Ip F. Child behaviour and parenting stress in Hong Kong families with young children. Hong Kong Med J 2005;11(5):373-80.

[24] Leung C, Lo SK, Tsang S, Chan R, Kung E. The relationship between family dining practices, parenting style and family functioning and child learning. Int J Disabil Hum Dev 2015. Doi: 10.1515/ijdhd-2015-0013.

In: Advances in Chinese Children … ISBN: 978-1-53617-870-8
Editors: Ariel Tenenbaum et al.

Chapter 7

FAMILIES IN TRANSITION IN HONG KONG: IMPLICATIONS TO FAMILY RESEARCH AND PRACTICE

Janet TY Leung*[1,*], *PhD
and Daniel TL Shek*[1-6], *PhD, FHKPS, BBS, SBS, JP
[1]Department of Applied Social Sciences, The Hong Kong Polytechnic University, Hong Kong, PR China
[2]Centre for Innovative Programmes for Adolescents and Families, The Hong Kong Polytechnic University, Hong Kong, PR China
[3]Department of Social Work, East China Normal University, Shanghai, PR China
[4]Kiang Wu Nursing College of Macau, Macau, PR China
[5]Hong Kong Institute of Service Leadership and Management Limited, Hong Kong, PR China
[6]Division of Adolescent Medicine, Department of Pediatrics, Kentucky Children's Hospital, University of Kentucky School of Medicine, Lexington, Kentucky, United States of America

[*] Corresponding Author's E-mail: janet.leung@polyu.edu.hk.

ABSTRACT

Utilizing the life course perspective, historical time and events that have influenced family development, delay of social timing of family development, linked lives that supported families and emergence of different modes of the families in Hong Kong were examined. The analyses showed several changes in the structures and functions of families in Hong Kong during the past few decades, which include: 1) reduced birth rate due to the success of the "birth control" campaign, the change of the conception of childbearing and the rising burden associated with child rearing; 2) delay of social timing of marriage and parenthood as more females participated in the labor force; 3) increased involvement of grandparents and foreign domestic helpers in taking care of children; 4) parents are heavily affected by the educational opportunities and achievement of their children, resulting in the mushrooming of "monster parents" (helicopter parents) who "hover" over their children's lives; 5) emergence of "DINK" (Double Income, No Kids) families; 6) an increase in cross-border marriages; 7) an increasing trend of marital disruption in families; and 8) a growing demand for the recognition of non-traditional forms of families. The implications of these family developments to family research and practice were discussed.

INTRODUCTION

Family is regarded as the "vital component of the society" (1). It is the basic unit of production, reproduction and perpetuation, protection of members from external forces, socialization, nurturing for the next generations, mutual support and emotional security (2, 3). However, the socio-economic and cultural transformations in Hong Kong in the past few decades have brought about dramatic changes to families. The reduction of family size, an increasing number of mothers entering into the labour force, the rise of divorce rate, an emergence of "DINK" (double income with no kids) families, the blossoming of "monster parents" (helicopter parents) who "hover" over their children's lives (4) are examples illustrating the inevitable structural and functional changes that have happened in the families in Hong Kong. While some changes are the result of global transformation of families, some changes are unique to the social, political and economic conditions in Hong Kong. Against such macro social changes, several questions should be asked - What have happened to the cohorts who are now the main actors of the families? What were the historical, social and cultural transformations that have influenced the family structures and functions? What were the changes of the families during this transition?

The generation theorists have offered special labels to different cohorts born after the World War II, namely the "Baby Boomers" (1943-1960), "Generation X" (1961-1981), and "Generation Y" or "The Millennial" (1982-2000) (5, 6). According to such views, each cohort showed very special characteristics due to the social changes that happened during those eras. The cohort studies provided an insightful lens for scholars and policy makers to understand how social changes affected these generations, and how one generation affected the other generations. However, they did not specifically employ the family as the basic unit of study, and they paid inadequate attention to the changes of the family structures and functions. Moreover, the studies took US as the backstage and the observations might not be applicable to non-American cultures, as culture is an important determinant of the development of families (7). To understand the changes of families during the transition in Hong Kong, the life course perspective (8, 9) provides a useful angle to examine the historical and social transformations that have influenced Hong Kong family development in the past few decades.

The Life Course Perspective

As suggested by Bengtson and Allen (10), the life course perspective is a "contextual, processual, and dynamic approach to the study of change in the lives of individual family members over time, and of families as social units as they change over historical periods" (10). Elder (8) concretely gave a definition to the life course as "age-graded life patterns embedded in social structures and cultures that are subject to historical change" (8). Three basic components are intrinsic to this definition: age-graded life patterns, social structure and culture, and historical change. Regarding the age-graded life patterns, they are formulated by the ontogenetic development of individuals as well as the stages of family life cycle. Life span theories, such as Erikson's (11) psychosocial stages of development, give an account of the ontogenetic development of individuals. A family life cycle portrays the stages of family development by examining different family developmental tasks in response to the development of its members (12). Concerning the social structure and culture, there are four dimensions: social structural context, social construction of meaning, cultural context and the interplay of macro-micro levels of analysis (10). Finally, historical time is the "events, periods, or eras dominated by watershed geopolitical or economic events" (10). In summary, the life course perspective emphasizes the interplay of life span development, historical time and events, as well as the social context. White and Klein (13) regarded the life course perspective to focus on the "sociological meaning of development" (13). Hence, the evolvement of the life course perspective put the two lines of inquiries, including life span development (i.e., the intra-individual changes) and social development (i.e., the extra-individual changes), together.

PARADIGMATIC THEMES OF THE LIFE COURSE PERSPECTIVE

Elder and his colleagues (8, 9, 14) suggested four paradigmatic themes that are central to the life course perspective, including a) human lives in historical time and place, b) the timing of lives, c) linked or interdependent lives, and d) human agency in the choice making and social constraints. These themes do not only constitute the essential elements of the life course perspective; they also identify important mechanisms through which the history and social contexts influence human development.

Human lives are influenced by the historical events and social contexts. In the life course, people of different ages are exposed to different historical worlds and may have different impacts in their lives. Thus, history brings the "cohort effect" to a particular birth cohort when there are social changes that affect and differentiate their life patterns from other cohorts (8).

The timing of lives emphasizes the concept of "social timing" that defines the start and the termination of social roles, their duration and sequence in respect to the relevant age expectations and beliefs (8). The social timing of lives is essential as it gives the structure to the life course where age norms, sequences, durations of life events and trajectories are embodied.

Linked or interdependent lives are the social relationships with kin, friends and the significant others across the life span (8). It is expected that one's life course would knit with those of the others sharing the significant relationships (9). Finally, as differentiated from social determinism that human agency is determined by the social environment, the life course theory respects the choices of individuals in determining their live course. However, there are social constraints and age-graded norms that may create restrictions. Individuals may need to make their own choices with the interpretations of the opportunities and constraints [8].

HONG KONG FAMILIES IN TRANSITION

Hong Kong has undergone rapid demographic and social changes that have strong impacts on the family development during the past few decades. Furthermore, the Government policies also provided structural opportunities and constraints to individuals that may affect their marital and parental trajectories (15). Thus, identifying the historical development as well as the policies implemented during the past decades would be important for understanding the families in transition.

The birth control campaign in the 1970s: "Two is enough"

The baby boom in the post-war period as well as the influx of immigrants from mainland China resulted in a rapid increase of the population from

1950s to 1970s in the last century in Hong Kong. There was a need for the Government to control the population growth. Against this background, the Family Planning Association of Hong Kong launched the "Two is enough" campaign to arouse public concern on birth control in 1975. The Association used a series of propaganda and educational means to encourage families to have two children at most, accompanied with other birth control services such as the use of contraceptives, sterilization and pregnancy termination operation. The campaign not only resulted in a sharp decrease in the fertility rate (from 3,459 children per 1,000 women in 1971 to 2,047 in 1980) in Hong Kong; it also altered the Chinese beliefs of "child-bearing" in the Hong Kong society. In the traditional Chinese culture, childbearing was considered as a natural biological imperative in the Chinese families. The Chinese cultural focus of "*chuan zong jie dai*" (continuation of posterity) and "*ji hou xiang deng*" (to have descendents for lighting the joss stick and lantern) was considered as the primary function of the family. Thus, contraception and termination of pregnancy were considered as anti-natural, immoral and anti-familial concepts that were not generally embraced by the Chinese values. The consequences of "*sha sheng*" (killing lives) and "*jue hou*" (prohibiting posterity) were social taboos in the traditional Chinese culture.

However, the "Two is enough" campaign constructed a new conception of childbearing that birth could be "controlled". Birth control was no longer considered as an anti-natural and anti-familial concept that resulted in "*sha sheng*" or "*jue hou*", but a new connotation of "family planning". With the advancement and popularity of contraceptive methods, people are more acceptable to use these methods to "control birth". The frequent use of contraceptive practice (almost every time of sexual intercourse) was 86%, 79.5% and 74.8% in 2002, 2007 and 2012 respectively. The rate of induced abortion was 26.3%, 20.6% and 14.1% in 2002, 2007 and 2012 respectively (16). Though there were decreasing trends of frequent use of contraceptive practice and induced abortion during the past decade (probably due to the use of other means of contraception), the figures were still striking. The campaign not only helped to legitimatize the use of contraception and termination of pregnancy, but also altered the Chinese cultural value of "continuation of posterity". In a survey on understanding the change of family values, it was found that the young generation showed less agreement on "having descendants to carry on the family name is very important" than did their parents (17).

The attitudinal changes on childbearing as well as common practice of contraceptive methods have facilitated the couples to have fewer kids, or even have no kids. From the statistics of the Census and Statistics Department (18, 19), it was found that the average domestic household size has gradually decreased from 4.3 in 1981 to 2.9 in 2014. The total fertility rates also dropped rapidly over the past three decades. There were only 927 children per 1,000 women in 2001, which were far below the replacement level of 2,100 children per 1,000 women (20). "The small family culture" (21) characterized by very few kids and child-centered family practice was evolving.

Compulsory and free education

In 1971, the Government launched the policy of "six-year compulsory and free education" in Hong Kong. The policy was expanded to nine years in 1978 and free education was further expanded to twelve years in 2008. The policies provided dramatic changes on the educational attainment of citizens in Hong Kong. Before that, it was not easy for children to receive education to the secondary level, especially for females. With the traditional cultural discourse of "man is superior to woman" (*nan zun nu bei*) in the Chinese society, the chance for females to receive education was less. However, the implementation of "compulsory and free education" policy became a turning point for educational attainment of women, where women were treated the same as men in receiving free and compulsory education. The policy has three important impacts: higher educational attainment of women, increased women's participation in the labor force, and rising aspirations for career prospect for women. It was found that female students studying in the programs funded by the University Grants Committee (sub-degrees, undergraduates, postgraduates) had been increased from 15,609 (32.9%) in

1986/1987 to 52,598 (53.9%) in 2014/2015 (22). The related percentages of females had surpassed the percentages of males from 1996/1997 onwards (19). In particular, the percentage share of female students enrolled in postgraduate and undergraduate programs were 60.6% and 54.7% respectively, which further exceeded the percentages of males enrolled in these programs (19). When considering women's participation into the labor force, there was a steady increase of females entering into the labor force. In the past three decades, the female to male ratio in labor force has increased from 0.58 in 1986 to 0.95 in 2014 (19). The gap between the labor force participation between males and females was narrowing. Furthermore, there were increasing numbers of women occupying higher positions in the labor market. The numbers of females occupying the posts of managers/ administrators and professionals have increased from 403,000 and 377,000 respectively in 1993 to 1,065,000 and 861,000 respectively in 2010 (19). Women in Hong Kong have been gaining better career prospects.

Open-door economic policy of mainland China since 1978

The open-door economic policy of mainland China is an important milestone of the changes of the economic structure in Hong Kong. Before that, Hong Kong was dominated by the manufacturing industries which required unskilled or semi-skilled labor. Women were commonly engaged in low-wage factory work which required a low educational standard and skills. With the open-door economic policy of mainland China since 1978, there was a great expansion of tertiary industries such as banking, finance, legal advice and consultation, information technology, etc. A high level of knowledge and professional skills were required. Managerial and professional positions increased and required employees with higher educational attainment and career commitment. As mentioned, this attracted more females to fill the managerial and professional positions (19).

The open-door economic policy of mainland China has also facilitated the emergence of cross-border marriages, extra-marital affairs across the border, and educational problems of children across the border (23).

Engagement of foreign domestic helpers

In the face of the labor policy of the Philippines to encourage and promote export of labor in the form of overseas Filipino workers, the Hong Kong Government has opened up the legal immigration channels for the families to hire foreign domestic helpers (FDH) since 1974. The employer families need to sign up a two-year standard employment contract with the foreign domestic helpers and apply for a visa from the Immigration Department.

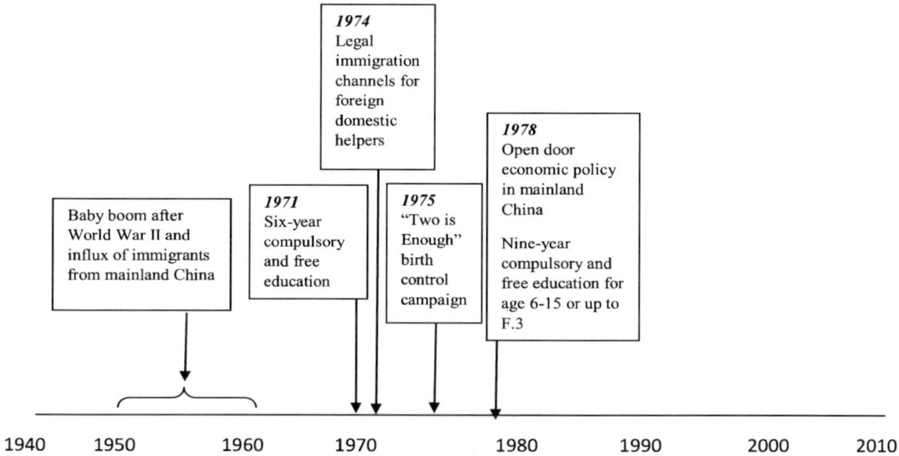

Figure 1. The occurrence of historical events during 1961-1980 in Hong Kong that influenced family development.

With the economic prosperity of Hong Kong in the 1980s and 1990s, the employment of foreign domestic helpers was becoming very popular in Hong Kong. The number of foreign domestic helpers increased from 172,119 in 1998 to 330,650 in 2014. Among them, Philippino and Indonesian maids accounted for 52.3% and 45.3% of the number of foreign domestic helpers, respectively (19).

In summary, Figure 1 illustrates the occurrence of the historical events during 1961-1980 in Hong Kong that influenced family development.

The delay of timing in different stages of family development

The popularity of education resulted in the delay of school completion age of adults. A crucial effect is that there was a time delay for a person to enter the work force. The labor force participation rate of males and females aged 15-24 dropped significantly from 65.5% and 61.7% respectively in 1986 to 8.0% and 8.6% respectively in 2014 (19). Obviously, the delay of timing of school completion implies prolonged dependency of adult children to their families.

Besides, women nowadays have a higher chance to hold jobs with better career prospect. To sustain the requirement of their jobs, they need to invest longer working hours, more work commitment, educational advancement and on-job training. According to the human capital theory (24), increased economic opportunities may influence the marriage pattern and decision of women. The career commitment and human capital investment happened early in the life course of adulthood may delay the decision of women to engage in marriage. Wong (25) provided support for this view which showed the relationship between the rising educational attainment and employment opportunities of women and the postponement of timing of marriage in Hong Kong.

During the past three decades, it was found that the median ages of first marriage of males and females have risen from 27.0 and 23.9 respectively in 1981 to 31.2 and 29.1 respectively in 2014 (22). With the normative sequence that marriage precedes parenthood, the delay of timing of marriage definitely delays the timing of parenthood.

To understand the timing of parenthood, it is important to differentiate the concepts of the biological timing from the social timing. Biological timing of parenthood refers to biological capability of individuals to remain reproductive. Biological capability sets a non-negotiable deadline to parenthood, with the loss of fecundity of women [15]. Normally, the childbearing ages of women are between 15 and 49 years of age (22). Social timing of parenthood takes into account of the readiness of an individual to enter into the parental role. Marital status, life transition, social expectations and constraints would propose a relative "social timing" (15). In the past three decades, there was a disparity between biological timing and social timing in marriage and parenthood in Hong Kong. The couples were biologically "fit" to enter marriage and parenthood, but the social timing to enter into the social roles of being married and as parents lagged behind. There are three consequences of the delay of timing of parenthood. First, women gave birth to a child at an older age. The median age of women at the first birth rose from 25.1 in 1981 to 31.3 in 2014 (19). Second, the couple did not have many children. The changes of cultural beliefs on "child-bearing" resulted from the "birth control" campaign also fascinated the delay of timing of child-bearing. Third, some parents might consider having no children due to the high risk of dystocia and anxiety for bearing an abnormal child in late pregnancy, as well as the anticipated difficulties in finance and effort to rear a child. Interestingly, there has been a social discourse generated by the mass media that rearing a child lifelong requires HK$4,000,000 (roughly US$500,000).

"Linked lives" --- The support but indulgent care of grandparents and foreign domestic helpers

In the life course perspective, linked lives are essential for a family to establish significant relationships with others across the life span (9). Among all, two significant relationships are critical for the Hong Kong families: the family of origin as well as foreign domestic helpers.

The families of origin are important supportive systems of the nuclear families. Grandparents played an important role of taking care of their grandchildren and were often regarded as "substitute parents" (21). Although grandparents might not live together with their adult children due to the limited space in Hong Kong, the non-cohabitation did not restrict the genuine needs of the adult children as well as the grandparents' enthusiasm to take care of their grandchildren. In a household survey commissioned by the Family Council in 2013, it was found that 58.3% of the respondents agreed on the high values of roles played by grandparents in family life, and

65.3% agreed that grandparent's involvement was appreciated by the adult parents (26).

The opening-up of legal immigration channels for foreign domestic helpers from the Asian countries by the Hong Kong Government has facilitated more women to enter into the labor force, while foreign domestic helpers manage the family housework as well as take care of the elderly and the children at home. Though employing foreign domestic helpers in childcare was regarded as the reluctant choice of the working parents, it became an actual reality of many families in Hong Kong (27).

As there was an increasing trend of mothers participating in the labor force, grandparents were more involved in taking care of their grandchildren. However, the parenting style of grandparents might be different from that of the parents (28) and this might result in intergenerational conflicts and disputes (29). Moreover, the involvement of grandparents might intrude into the family life of the adult child's family and create power dynamics between the grandparents and adult parents. Intergenerational discrepancies in parenting styles might generate opportunities for the children to manipulate the family members in order to get the most benefits (28).

As a consequence, there was a creation of "4-2-1 indulgence" culture (i.e., four grandparents and two parents spoiling one child) (30). In addition to the popularity of employing foreign domestic helpers to do housework and take care of the children, there were totally seven adults serving one child. The child becomes the "little emperor" of whom the family adults give superior attention, human and material resources (31). The adolescents today are labeled as the "spoilt generation" who show signs of narcissist traits (32). They are also regarded as "Hong Kong Kids" who are "unable to look after themselves, have low emotional quotient and even lower adversity quotient." (33). This would make them grow up in a "greenhouse" and become more egocentric (34).

Due to the very few children in the family as well as the "*wang zi cheng long*" (expecting the son to become a dragon) beliefs embedded in the Chinese culture, the parents have high expectation about their children's future (3). They were heavily affected by the educational opportunities and achievement of their children, hoping that their children could be competitive in their future. The parents paid great effort and plenty of resources to nurture their children, with the expectation that they could win "at the starting line". As a consequence, they were highly involved and intervened frequently in their children's lives. Different terminologies of "helicopter parenting" (35), "monster parenting", "lawnmower parenting" (36) have been used to describe the over-parenting or over-nurturing phenomenon. The parents have faced much stress in nurturing their children and may further affect the parent-child relationship. In a household survey commissioned by the Family Council in 2013, it was found that 72.0% of the parents felt more tired than before, 63.2% expressed that their large part of life was controlled by the child's needs, and 60.4% suffered from the severe lack of personal time (26).

Choices of the couples – Emergence of different forms of families

Though there were historical events and social constraints shaping the life course trajectories of the families, the couples could still make their own choice in constructing their families. There were three types of families that are prevalent in Hong Kong: the "DINK" families, cross-border marriages and the divorced families.

"DINK" means "Double income with no kids". "DINK" families are childless or childfree families with the couples participating in the labor force. In the past, the phenomenon was considered as "deviant" and "abnormal", especially in the Chinese culture that continuation of posterity is emphasized. Childlessness was considered as "*jue hou*" (prohibiting posterity) in the traditional Chinese culture which was regarded as a taboo. It was up to 1970s and 1980s that "child-free" was considered as an "alternative lifestyle" that families could have outside the traditional norms of a nuclear family (37). According to the Family Planning Knowledge, Attitude and Practice in Hong Kong Survey in 2012, it was found that there were 23.4% of the respondent families reported childless (excluding those families with involuntary infertility or sub-fecundity). There were also 7.1% of females and 5.3% of males who preferred to be "child-free" (16).

Besides personal choices, there are social constraints that might affect the couples to choose childlessness. Work is one of the barriers for married couples to have children. Career advancement, employment opportunities, long-hour work culture are considerations of the married couples to remain "childless" (38). Age is another important factor that the couple would prefer childfree, especially those entering middle adulthood. Rowland [39] highlighted two components for the age-related fertility decline: a reducing probability of conceiving and an increasing risk of spontaneous abortion. Furthermore, the high risk of dystocia as well as anxiety for bearing an abnormal child in late pregnancy would forbid the couples to consider childbearing. In addition, rearing a child requires huge responsibilities and financial costs that have become a social constraint of childbearing. Jones (40) suggested the ideology of having "quality" child and financial costs of childbearing were factors that lower the desire of childbearing among the married couples in Pacific Asia. Among the respondent couples who did not want to have children in the Family Planning Knowledge, Attitude and Practice in Hong Kong Survey in 2012, 43.3% of females and 42.0% of males suggested that the financial constraint was the main reason for childlessness.

The open-door economic policy of mainland China has facilitated the emergence of the cross-border marriages in Hong Kong. In 2014, there were 26,330 cases of cross-border marriages in Hong Kong, of which 20,698 marriages registered in Hong Kong, occupying 36.7% of the total marriages registered that year (19). There were some unique features arising from the cross-border marriages, which include the marriages between a young wife and an old husband, split families and pseudo single parent (either children live with father in Hong Kong while mother stays in China, or the children stay with mother in China while father resides in Hong Kong), and cross-border education of children (41, 42). Though the cross-border marriage has been a common form of marriage in recent years, concerns and problems such as adjustment difficulties of migrant mothers and children, increased risk for marital stability and harmony, accommodation problems in Hong

Kong with limited living space, parenting difficulties, problems in children's education, poorer care, nurture and modeling of the children, social isolation and higher risk of spousal violence (23, 42, 43) are emerging.

When looking at the divorce rate figures, the crude divorce rate has been increasing steadily from 0.76 in 1984 to 3.1 in 2013, with the first time of decrease to 2.8 in 2014 (19,44,45). It is worth noting that divorce as a percentage of marriage remained high (33% to 35%) during the past five years. One reason accounting for the change was the direct influence of the Western romantic conception of marriage that has eroded the Chinese cultural values of familism (46). The conception of marriage in Hong Kong has been moving away from a traditional and patriarchal mode to a modern and egalitarian one (47). Instead of preserving a long-lasting conjugal relationship based on the Confucian virtues of familism, the couples would consider divorce when they experienced marital dissatisfaction. The temptation of extramarital affairs also constituted the increase of divorce rate (46, 48). Moreover, the general acceptance of divorce by the public makes divorce become a "means" to solve marital dissatisfaction. In a household survey commissioned by the Family Council, 63.2% of the respondents agreed that if a married couple did not have children, divorce was the best solution for them when they could not live harmoniously. Even if the couple has children, 32.3% still agreed that divorce was the best choice if they could not live together agreeably [26].

Table 1. Summary of family changes in Hong Kong under the paradigmatic themes of the life course perspective

Paradigmatic themes		Family changes
• Humans live in historical time and place	• The birth control campaign in 1975: "Two is Enough" • Compulsory and free education • Open door economic policy in mainland China	• Reduced birth rate • Change of the conception of childbearing and less emphasis on the Chinese value of "continuation of posterity" • Delay of social timing of marriage and parenthood • More mothers participated in the labor force • The employment of foreign domestic helpers for childcare and family housework

	• Legal immigration channels for foreign domestic helpers

Table 1. (Continued)

Paradigmatic themes	Family changes
• The timing of lives	• Delay of social timing of marriage and parenthood • Reduced birth rate • Emergence of "DINK" (Double Income, No Kids) families
• Linked or interdependent lives	• Increased involvement of grandparents and foreign domestic helpers in taking care of the child • Indulgence parenting with seven adults (four grandparents, two parents and one foreign domestic helper) in nurturing one child in a family • Parental stress due to high expectation on education and achievement of their children • The mushrooming of "monster parents" (helicopter parents) who "hover" over their children's lives
• Human agency in choice making and social constraints	• Emergence of "DINK" (Double Income, No Kids) families • Increase in cross-border marriages involving young wives and old husbands • Increasing trend of marital disruption in families • A growing demand for the recognition of non-traditional forms of families

Apart from the increase of DINK families, popularity of cross-border marriages and high divorce rate, there is a growing demand for the recognition of non-traditional forms of families. Similar to the Western world, the voice of LGBT (lesbian, gay, bisexual and transgender) communities to recognize their rights for marriage, adoption of children and formation of family was blooming. In 2013, the court ruling on transgender marriage has raised the hopes for sexual minorities to pursue their rights in marriage and family formation (49). At the same time, it has brought great challenges to the traditional values of marriage and family. As mentioned by the dissenting judge of the court case, to consider a transsexual's marriage a right implies "a radical change to the traditional concept of marriage" (50). The traditional forms of marriages are confronted with strong pressure, which may bring revolutionary changes to the family forms, values and systems. Table 1 summarizes the family changes in the transition under the paradigmatic themes of the life course perspective.

IMPLICATIONS TO FAMILY RESEARCH AND PRACTICE

With reference to the analyses based on the life course perspective, the families in Hong Kong are exhibiting several changes. These included: 1) reduced birth rate due to the success of the "birth control" campaign, the change of the conception of childbearing and the rising burden associated with child rearing; 2) delay of social timing of marriage and parenthood as more females participated in the labor force; 3) increased involvement of grandparents and foreign domestic helpers in taking care of the children; 4) parents are intensely affected by the educational opportunities and achievement of their children, resulting in the mushrooming of "monster parents" (helicopter parents) who "hover" over their children's lives; 5) emergence of "DINK" (Double Income, No Kids) families; 6) an increase in cross-border marriages involving young wives and old husbands; 7) an increasing trend of marital disruption in families; and 8) a growing demand for the recognition of non-traditional forms of families. The changing family trends draw attention of social scientists, researchers and clinical practitioners on family research and practice.

The life course perspective provides thoughtful ideas in understanding how the historical and social contexts influence the development of family life patterns. This is especially meaningful in the Chinese families, as familism is central in the Chinese culture (51, 52). It is insightful and important if longitudinal panel studies across cohorts were conducted to examine how different historical and social contexts influence family beliefs and life patterns in the life course trajectories.

As suggested by Elder and Shanahan (9), the temporal location of reproductive cycle greatly influenced the family life cycle. Early childbearing would hasten the cycle and shorten the distance between generations. In contrast, late childbearing may decelerate the cycle and reduce the age similarities across generations. In Hong Kong, the delay of social timing of marriage and parenthood is salient and affects the family life patterns across adjacent generations. Thus, it is important to examine the influence of temporal location and timing of family life cycle on human development and life patterns.

The life course perspective not only sketches the temporal changes in the patterns of family life cycle, it also portrays the changes of roles within the family. The social contexts have influenced greatly on the roles and division of labor in the family. With more mothers participating in the labor force and grandparents and foreign domestic helpers offer support in childcare and housework, their roles within the family are changing. It is interesting and important to examine the changes in roles and functions of different members in families, as well as the family dynamics such as family boundary, rules, power and interactions, etc. The importance of linked lives across the life span and generations should catch more research attention. Furthermore, timing also matters to the role and identity change of the family members. The implications of marriage and parenthood may vary in accordance with the social timetable, age norms and age-graded sanctions (9). Ebaugh (53) used the term "role exit" to describe an identity change in response to the transformation of roles in the life span. Indeed, temporality of family roles may be an emerging area that needs to be explored.

The prevalence of divorce and child-free couples has strong impact on the family life development across generations. However, it is criticized that the life cycle which only focuses on reproduction and parenting has "limited value as a way of viewing the lives and developmental trajectories of children and adults because it does not apply to never married, non-parent, or divorced persons, all of whom have become increasingly common" (9). In fact, divorce may imply multiple families in a person's life which may lead to interwoven roles and complex kin relationship. Regarding the child-free families, there is a concern about the changes of the family life patterns as well as the developmental life tasks of the couples. "Parenthood" has been expected as an important developmental task in one's life span, which may result in generativity in the middle age (54). Thus, the absence of parenthood in the family life cycle may have great impact on their members. The effects of the divorce and DINK to the family members may need to be further researched.

From a macro perspective, the changes of forms and patterns of the families may have significant impact on the social values, structure and functions. For instance, the delay of marriage and parenthood would result in a reduced birth rate of Hong Kong, which may further bring the future risk of the aging population. The cross-border marriages may bring the demographic, cultural and social concerns to the society, as the education, value systems and lifestyles in China may be different from those in Hong Kong. Social scientists need to be sensitive to the changes and explore the impact on the society as a whole. In fact, family research in Hong Kong with respect to these areas is grossly inadequate (55).

Regarding family practice, the "small family culture" characterized by very few kids and child-centered family practice is evolving in Hong Kong. The "seven adults serving one kid" phenomenon (four grandparents, two parents and one foreign domestic helper) has happened in the Hong Kong families, with more resources being allocated for the child development, but at the same time the children are over-parented and over-protected. Further research to examine the impact of over-parenting on child development in Hong Kong is urged. Besides, it is important for family practitioners to understand the new forms of parenting in the Chinese families and to provide parenting education to the family members. In particular, grand-parenting is becoming more and more popular in Hong Kong when both parents enter the labor force in the recent decades. However, grandparent education programs are not well developed in Hong Kong. Thus, it is important to develop effective training strategies on grandparent education.

Furthermore, the life course perspective suggests that historical events, age-graded experiences and role identity may influence individual's life span and family life development across generations. In the swiftly changing world, grandparents, parents and children may share different cultures and experiences. These may influence the family values, dynamics and interaction among the family members. The discrepancies of perceived roles and expectation among the family members, as well as the differences in parenting styles and practices between the two generations may result in family conflicts (28). Thus, family practitioners should be sensitive to the intergenerational conflicts that may generate between the grandparents and adult parents, and resolve the conflicts when these arise. It is necessary to explore the collaborative roles between grandparents and adult children of which complementary parenting as well as respectful participation could be nurtured (56).

In view of the prevalence of the cross-border marriages in Hong Kong, there are concerns to the adjustment of the families, educational needs of the children as well as the high risks of family instability. Supportive and counseling services are definitely essential. However, the differences in social welfare policies across the border make the service difficult to be delivered to the cross-border families. Negotiation with the Chinese Government is necessary so that more resources and services can be provided to help the cross-border families. Again, we need more research in this area to illuminate the issues involved.

The rising trend of divorce has set an alarm to the family development in Hong Kong. Family breakdown and dysfunctions has detrimental effects to parental distress and adolescent development. Marital counseling and post-divorced parenting education programs are necessary. Besides, family mediation services are important.

Last but not least, new family forms and patterns challenge the conventional values of the Chinese culture and social expectation to the families. Family practitioners should be sensitive to the cultural changes and work against the social disharmony and stigmatization that may arise. Obviously, we need more research to understand how the public look at these “non-conventional” families and examine the needs, problems and resilience facing by such families. Besides, training family practitioners need to be sensitive to the “macro” social conditions instead of just focusing on the “micro” dyadic or family issues.

CONCLUSION

Hong Kong families have undergone dramatic changes in these few decades. The life course perspective provides a sociocultural lens for social scientists to explore the family life cycle and patterns of the Hong Kong families. The success of birth control campaign, free and compulsory education, increased work opportunities for women in the labor market have brought forward the delay of social timing of marriage and parenthood. Linked with the support of grandparents and foreign domestic helpers in childcare and family management, the indulgence culture of rearing the children and over-parenting was created. The increase of divorced families, cross-border marriages, DINK families and emergence of non-traditional forms of families also became one of the concerns of family development in Hong Kong. The social account of family life course in Hong Kong is just the beginning of the long journey to explore the family life development in the Chinese communities. More scientific research should be conducted to explore how historical time and socio-cultural contexts influence family life course across generations. With the belief that people can "work out their life course in relation to established, institutionalized pathways and their regulatory constraints" [9, p.706], the studies of family life course in the Chinese communities may open a door for scholars and social scientists to have a better understanding of the Chinese families in the transition.

ACKNOWLEDGMENTS

This chapter is a revised and adapted version of an earlier published paper in the International Public Health Journal 2018;10(2) issue with permission.

REFERENCES

[1] Social Welfare Department, Hong Kong Special Administrative Region. Social welfare into the 1990's and beyond. Hong Kong: Social Welfare Department, 1989.
[2] Chu P. Promoting family well-being: Future direction on family and child welfare services. Hong Kong J Paediatr 2001;6:9-13.
[3] Leung JTY, Shek DTL. Parental beliefs and parenting characteristics of Chinese parents experiencing economic disadvantage in Hong Kong. Int J Disabil Hum Dev 2013;12(2):139-49.

[4] Nelson MK. Parenting out of control: Anxious parents in uncertain times. New York: New York University Press, 2010.
[5] Howe N, Strauss W. Millennials go to College. Great Falls, VA: LifeCourse Associates, 2007.
[6] Twenge JM. Generation ME: Why today's young Americans are more confident, assertive, entitled – and more miserable than ever before. New York: Free Press, 2006.
[7] Shweder RA, Goodnow JJ, Hatano G, LeVine RA, Markus HR, Miller PJ. The cultural psychology of development: One mind, many mentalities. In: Damon W, Lerner RM, eds. Handbook of child psychology: Theoretical models of human development. Vol 1. New York: Wiley, 1998:865-937.
[8] Elder GH Jr. Human lives in changing societies: Life course and developmental insights. In: Cairns RB, Elder GH Jr, Costello EJ, eds. Developmental science. New York: Cambridge University Press, 1996:31-62.
[9] Elder GH Jr, Shanahan MJ. The life course and human development. In: Damon W, Lerner RM, eds. Handbook of child psychology: Theoretical models of human development. 6th ed. Vol 1. New York: Wiley, 2006:665-715.
[10] Bengtson VL, Allen KR. The life course perspective applied to families over time. In: Boss PG, Doherty WJ, LaRossa R, Schumm WR, Steinmetz SK. Sourcebook of family theories and methods: A contextual approach. New York: Plenum Press, 1993:469-99.
[11] Erikson EH. Identity and the life cycle. New York: International Universities Press, 1959.
[12] Hill R, Rodgers RH. The developmental approach. In: Christensen HT, ed. Handbook of marriage and the family. Chicago, IL: Rand McNally, 1964:171-211.
[13] White JM, Klein DM. Family Theories. 3rd ed. Los Angeles, CA: Sage, 2008.
[14] Elder GH Jr. Time, human agency, and social change: Perspectives on the life course. Soc Psychol Q 1994;57:4-15.
[15] Hagestad GO, Call VRA. Pathways to childlessness: A life course perspective. J Fam Issues 2007;28(10):1338-61.
[16] The Family Planning Association of Hong Kong. Family Planning Knowledge, Attitude and Practice (KAP) in Hong Kong survey 2012. Hong Kong: Family Planning Association of Hong Kong, 2013. [PowerPoint available in Chinese only]. URL: http://www.famplan.org.hk/fpahk/zh/press/press/20130521-press-chi.pptx.
[17] Hong Kong Women Foundation Limited, Department of Social Work and Social Administration, The University of Hong Kong. Contemporary Hong Kong families in transition. Hong Kong: Department of Social Work and Social Administration, HKU, 1995.
[18] Census and Statistics Department, Hong Kong Special Administrative Region. Hong Kong 2011 population census. Hong Kong: The Government of the Hong Kong Special Administrative Region, 2011.

[19] Census and Statistics Department, Hong Kong Special Administrative Region. Hong Kong annual digest of statistics 2015 edition. Hong Kong: The Government of the Hong Kong Special Administrative Region, 2015.

[20] The Task Force on Population Policy, Hong Kong Special Administrative Region. Report of the Task Force on population policy. Hong Kong: The Government of the Hong Kong Special Administrative Region, 2003. URL: http://www.info.gov.hk/info/population/eng/index.htm.

[21] Settles BH, Zhao J, Mancini KD, Rich A, Pierre S, Oduor A. Grandparents caring for their grandchildren: Emerging roles and exchanges in global perspectives. J Comp Fam Stud 2009;40(5):827-48.

[22] Census and Statistics Department, Hong Kong Special Administrative Region. Women and men in Hong Kong: Key statistics 2015 edition. Hong Kong: The Government of the Hong Kong Special Administrative Region, 2015.

[23] So AY. Cross-border families in Hong Kong: The role of social class and politics. Crit Asian Stud 2003;35(4):515-34.

[24] Becker GS. Human capital: A theoretical and empirical analysis, with special reference to education. Chicago, IL: University of Chicago Press, 2009.

[25] Wong OMH. Postponement or abandonment of marriage? Evidence from Hong Kong. J Comp Fam Stud 2003;34(4):531-54.

[26] Policy 21 Limited. Family survey 2013 [Internet]. Hong Kong: The University of Hong Kong, 2014. URL: http://www.familycouncil.gov.hk/tc_chi/files/research/Family_Survey_2013_Report.pdf.

[27] Tam VC. A family ecological analysis of child care use in Hong Kong. Child Soc 2001;15(3):181-92.

[28] Goh ECL, Kuczynski L. "Only children" and their collation of parents: Considering grandparents and parents as joint caregivers in urban Xiamen, China. Asian J Soc Psychol 2010;29(4):499-525.

[29] Goh ECL. Raising the precious single child in urban China: An intergenerational joint mission between parents and grandparents. J Intergener Relatsh 2006;4(3):7-28.

[30] Cutler B. China's little emperors. Am Demogr 1988;10:58.

[31] Settles BH, Sheng X, Zang Y, Zhao J. The one-child policy and its impact on Chinese families. In: Chan KB, ed. International handbook of Chinese families. New York: Springer, 2013;627-46.

[32] Chong D. Hong Kong's parents raising 'spoiled brats', warns study. South China Morning Post [Internet]. 2013 Apr 24. URL: http://www.scmp.com/news/hong-kong/article/1221770/hong-kong-raising-spoilt-generation-only-out-themselves-academic.

[33] Ho CP. Kong kids phenomenon. China Daily [Internet]. 2011 Jan 11. URL: http://www.cpho.hk/a/44565-cht.

[34] Leung JTY, Busiol D. Adolescents growing up in a "Greenhouse": A literature review. Int J Child Adolesc Health 2016;9(4):413-22.

[35] Hunt J. Make room for daddy… and mommy: Helicopter parents are here. J Acad Adm High Educ 2008;4(1):9-11.

[36] Locke JY, Campbell MA, Kavanagh D. Can a parent do too much for their child? An examination by parenting professionals of the concept of overparenting. Aust J Guid Couns 2012;22(2):249-65.

[37] Bulcroft R, Teachman J. Ambiguous constructions: Development of a childless or child-free life course. In: Coleman M, Ganong LH, eds. Handbook of contemporary families. Thousand Oaks, CA: Sage, 2004:116-35.

[38] Wood GJ, Newton J. Childlessness and women managers: 'Choice', context and discourses. Gend Work Organ 2006;13(4):338-58.

[39] Rowland DT. Historical trends in childlessness. J Fam Issues 2007;28(10):1311-37.

[40] Jones GW. Delayed marriage and very low fertility in Pacific Asia. Popul Dev Rev 2007;33(3):453-78.

[41] Hui DL. The changes of cross-border families between China and Hong Kong: Overview of Hong Kong future population. Cross-Border Fam Forum 2013;1:4-15. [Chinese]. URL: http://webcontent.hkcss.org.hk/FAMILY_wellness/download/Cross-border_Families_Forum_Issue1_Final.pdf.

[42] Choi SYP, Yeung WY, Chiu SY. Cross-border families in Shenzhen situations and challenges. Cross-Border Fam Forum 2013;1:41-50. [Chinese]. URL: http://webcontent.hkcss.org.hk/FAMILY_wellness/download/Cross-border_Families_Forum_Issue1_Final.pdf.

[43] Choi SYP, Cheung YW, Cheung AKL. Social isolation and spousal violence: Comparing female marriage migrants with local women. J Marriage Fam 2012;74(3):444-61.

[44] Census and Statistics Department, Hong Kong Special Administrative Region. Hong Kong annual digest of statistics 1995 edition. Hong Kong: The Government of the Hong Kong Special Administrative Region, 1995.

[45] Census and Statistics Department, Hong Kong Special Administrative Region. Hong Kong annual digest of statistics 2005 edition. Hong Kong: The Government of the Hong Kong Special Administrative Region, 2005.

[46] Kung WW, Hung SL, Chan CL. How the socio-cultural context shapes women's divorce experience in Hong Kong. J Comp Fam Stud 2004;35:33-50.

[47] Young KPH. Understanding marriage: A Hong Kong case study. Hong Kong: Hong Kong University Press, 1995.

[48] Fan CS, Lui HK. Extramarital affairs, marital satisfaction, and divorce: Evidence from Hong Kong. Contemp Econ Policy 2004;22(4):442-52.

[49] Chan C. Court ruling on transgender marriage raises hopes for other minorities. South China Morning Post [Internet]. 2013 May 21. URL: http://www.scmp.com/comment/insight-opinion/article/1242095/court-ruling-transgender-marriage-raises-hopes-other.

[50] Fedrigotti LM, Lam PF. Concerned about court's decision. South China Morning Post [Internet]. 2013 May 22. URL: http://www.scmp.com/comment/letters/article/ 1242943/ concerned-about-courts-decision.
[51] Yang CF. Familism and development: An examination of the role of family in contemporary China mainland, Hong Kong, and Taiwan. In: Sinha D, Kao HSR, eds. Social values and development: Asian perspectives. New Delhi: Sage, 1988.
[52] Yeh MH, Yang KS. Chinese familism: Conceptual analysis and empirical assessment. Bulletin of the Institute of Ethnology, Academia Sinica (Taiwan) 1997;83:169-225. [Chinese].
[53] Ebaugh HRF. Becoming an ex: The process of role exit. Chicago, IL: University of Chicago Press, 1988.
[54] Erikson EH. Generativity & ego integrity. In: Neugarten B, ed. Middle age and aging. Chicago, IL: University of Chicago Press, 1968.
[55] Shek DTL. Chinese family research: Puzzles, progress, paradigms, and policy implications. J Fam Issues 2006;27(3):275-84.
[56] Thang LL, Mehta K, Usui T, Tsuruwaka M. Being a good grandparent: Roles and expectations in intergenerational relationships in Japan and Singapore. Marriage Fam Rev 2011;47(8):548-70.

In: Advances in Chinese Children … ISBN: 978-1-53617-870-8
Editors: Ariel Tenenbaum et al.

Chapter 8

SUBJECTIVE OUTCOME EVALUATION OF THE TIN KA PING P.A.T.H.S. PROJECT IN CHINA: VIEW OF THE STUDENTS

Daniel TL Shek[1,*], PhD, FHKPS, BBS, SBS, JP, Tak Yan Lee[2], PhD, Xiaoqin Zhu[1], PhD and Lawrence K Ma[1], PhD

[1]Department of Applied Social Sciences, The Hong Kong Polytechnic University, Hong Kong, PR China

[2]Department of Applied Social Sciences, City University of Hong Kong, Hong Kong, PR China

ABSTRACT

Utilizing the client satisfaction approach, the present paper reports the program participants' perceptions of a positive youth development program (Tin Ka Ping P.A.T.H.S. Project) in China. Upon the completion of the program, altogether 7,289 Secondary 1 and 2 students completed a valid and reliable questionnaire (Form A) to rate on different aspects

* Corresponding Author's E-mail: daniel.shek@polyu.edu.hk.

including program content, program implementer, and program effectiveness. As anticipated, most students evaluated all the three aspects positively. Grade differences were observed, with Secondary 1 students reporting higher satisfaction on program content, program implementer, and overall satisfaction than did their Secondary 2 counterparts. Furthermore, perceived program content and implementer quality predicted perceived program effectiveness. In short, the findings underscore the effectiveness of the Tin Ka Ping P.A.T.H.S. Project launched in the academic year 2015-2016.

INTRODUCTION

Since the beginning of the "open-door policy" in the early 1980s, China has developed rapidly. China has become the world's second largest economy and is forecasted to surpass the United States by 2030 (1). Such an economic growth goes hand in hand with the urbanization of the contemporary Chinese youth communities. Accordingly, how such an economic transition in China has shaped the psychological development of Chinese adolescents attracts growing interest in the research community. For instance, utilizing the cross-temporal meta-analytic data from thousands of Chinese youth, Xin and associates (2, 3) revealed that urbanization level was a significant positive correlate of adolescents' anxiety level, depressive symptoms, and mental illness across cohorts, and the mental health of young people in China had deteriorated throughout time.

In view of such a backdrop, the Ministry of Education (4) published "The Outline of Education Guide for Pupil's Mental Health". One key strategy entails the permission for primary and secondary schools to hire mental health teachers to implement mental health education and offer counseling service to the students. There is, nonetheless, still a lack of systematic teaching resources for these mental health teachers regarding how psychosocial competencies of the students can be strengthened. As such, there is an urgent need to develop related curriculum materials based on the positive youth development (PYD) approach. According to Damon (5), problem prevention alone is not enough to promote healthy youth development and it is important to discover and nurture adolescents' strengths, talents, and potentials.

With reference to Hong Kong, adolescents also display problems such as substance abuse, materialism, and bullying (6). Nonetheless, Shek and Yu (7) highlighted the paucity of robustly evaluated, multi-year PYD programs in Hong Kong. Against such a backdrop, a multi-year project entitled "Positive Adolescent Training through Holistic Social Programs" (Project P.A.T.H.S.), funded by The Hong Kong Jockey Club Charities Trust, was launched in 2005. The Project P.A.T.H.S. which comprises two tiers is a comprehensive PYD program tailored for junior secondary-schoolers in Hong Kong. While the Tier 1 Program represents a curriculum-based intervention targeting the general junior secondary-schooler population, the Tier 2 Program was catered to adolescents with greater psychosocial needs. Results from a multitude of evaluation studies (8) corroborate the effectiveness of the Project P.A.T.H.S. over the years in promoting the holistic youth development alongside eradicating risk behavior in junior secondary students in Hong Kong.

Despite the remarkable achievement of the Project P.A.T.H.S., we have to ask whether the related programs can be successfully applied in other Chinese communities (9). Funded by the Tin Ka Ping Foundation, the first phase of the program entitled "Tin Ka Ping Positive Adolescent Training through Holistic Social Program" (Tin Ka Ping P.A.T.H.S. Project) was embarked on in four schools in East China (Shanghai, Suzhou, Changzhou, and Yangzhou) since 2011. This pioneer project in China was well-received as evidenced by findings derived from both subjective outcome evaluation (10) and objective outcome evaluation studies (11). Accordingly, started from the academic year 2015-2016, the second phase of the Tin Ka Ping P.A.T.H.S. Project targeting both junior and senior secondary schoolers was launched in 30 secondary schools in mainland China. Given the geographical socioeconomic differences across provinces, it is necessary to examine if the second phase, which involves schools from both inside and outside East China, would be similarly effective.

Resembling other PYD programs, the Tin Ka Ping P.A.T.H.S. Project emphasizes program evaluation. Shek and Sun (12) outlined five key elements to a successful PYD program, including program, process, policy, people, and place (i.e., the 5Ps). Particularly, the element "people" which encompasses program participants and implementers was identified as one of the most decisive factors of all (12). Thus, utilizing the client satisfaction approach, the present paper is primarily concerned with the program participants' subjective evaluation of the Tin Ka Ping P.A.T.H.S. Project. The client satisfaction approach, which has been adopted cross-culturally in the field of human services (13, 14), permits researchers to examine the participants' perceptions of program effectiveness in a cost-effective manner. For instance, Walsh and Lord (15) adopted the Client Satisfaction Questionnaire (16) to gather participants' views on a social work intervention program. Likewise, utilizing the subjective outcome evaluation approach, Shek and Sun (17) assessed students' perceived effectiveness of a university subject designed to nurture their leadership skills and intrapersonal development.

Nonetheless, Larson and colleagues (18) noted that students, despite being the target recipients of a program, often had their views overlooked when implementers attempted to evaluate program effectiveness. Such a negligence may stem from the stereotype that adolescents are incapable of expressing dissatisfaction in meaningful ways or that they seldom do so because of early dropout (19). While findings from subjective outcome evaluation studies regarding the Project P.A.T.H.S in Hong Kong are well-documented (e.g., 20, 21), we could hardly say the same about the Tin Ka Ping P.A.T.H.S. Project in China. Therefore, it is imperative that we scrutinize the views of the participants on the different aspects of the program such as program content and implementers of the project and how these aspects would interrelate with each another.

In short, utilizing the client satisfaction approach, this study examined the following research questions and hypotheses with reference to the Tin Ka Ping P.A.T.H.S. Project launched in the academic year 2015-2016:

- How do the program participants evaluate the curricula-based program (i.e., Tier 1 Program)? Based on the findings from previous evaluation studies (10), we hypothesized that a high proportion of the program participants would be satisfied with the program (Hypothesis 1). Specifically, with reference to the previous Hong Kong findings that around four-fifths of the respondents were positive about Tier 1 Program, we expected that at least four-fifths of the current respondents would show positive responses.

- How do perceived program content, implementer quality, and program effectiveness inter-relate with one another? Results from the evaluation studies of the Project P.A.T.H.S. in Hong Kong (20, 21) suggested a significant inter-correlation among these three program facets (Hypotheses 2a, 2b, and 2c).
- Are satisfaction ratings different across grades? Based on previous studies (22), it was predicted that the three aspects of client satisfaction would be inter-related (Hypotheses 3a, 3b, and 3c)?
- Are perceived program content and perceived implementer quality predictive of perceived program effectiveness? Based on previous findings (21, 22), we hypothesized that these two factors would predict perceived program effectiveness (Hypotheses 4a and 4b).

OUR STUDY

In the academic year 2015-2016, the curricula-based Tin Ka Ping P.A.T.H.S. Project was implemented in 30 secondary schools in mainland China. Amongst them, eighteen junior secondary schools participated in the current evaluation study. Of these schools, all implemented the program at Secondary 1 (S1 hereafter, equivalent to Grade 7), with three implementing the program also at Secondary 2 (S2 hereafter, equivalent to Grade 8).

To examine the effectiveness of the Tin Ka Ping P.A.T.H.S. Project, students were invited to complete the Subjective Outcome Evaluation Form (the Form A) upon the completion of the program. The program implementers who had attended training workshops over evaluation topics were responsible for data collection. An evaluation manual with standardized instructions on data collection was also distributed to each of the schools concerned. The principles of confidentiality, anonymity and voluntary participation were reiterated upon the administration of the survey. All students provided their consent prior to participation. Altogether 7,289 questionnaires were returned to Research Team. Amongst them, 6,222 were S1 students and 1,067 were S2 students.

Instruments

A well-validated and extensively used (20, 22) instrument (Form A) was adopted to solicit participants' feedback on the program. The Form A contains four parts. Part 1 examined students' overall appraisal of Program content, such as program objectives, design, and interaction among classmates (10 items). Part 2 assessed students' perception of qualities exhibited by the program implementers via ten items measuring aspects like preparation for lessons, degree of involvement, and professionalism. Items of Parts 1 and 2 were rated on a six-point Likert scale with 1 representing "strongly disagree" while 6 representing "strongly agree". The sixteen-item Part 3 assessed students' perceived program effectiveness via a five-point Likert scale (1 = unhelpful; 5 = very helpful). Part 4 contains three additional items measuring the likelihood of the respondents recommending the program to others, participating in a similar program in future, and their overall satisfaction with the program. Additionally, Form A consists of four open-ended questions on students' experience of the program (e.g., aspects of the program worthy of their appreciation). The focus of the present paper is on the quantitative data collected from the program participants.

Data analyses

The individual data of students were adopted as the units of analysis. Reliability analyses were conducted for the present three subscales (i.e., program content, program implementers, and program effectiveness). Descriptive statistical analyses using the percentage of positive responses to each item were conducted to reveal students' perceptions of the various facets of the program (i.e., Hypothesis 1). To test Hypothesis 2, we examined the associations among the three subscales using the Pearson's correlation tests. Additionally, multivariate analysis of variance (MANOVA) was adopted to test whether there were differences in students' subjective program evaluation across grades (i.e., Hypothesis 3). Finally, Hypothesis 4 was examined via several multiple regression analyses.

FINDINGS

Results on the reliability of Form A are detailed in Table 1. All three parts each recorded excellent internal consistency as evidenced by the high alpha values (ranged from 0.93 to 0.96). The Cronbach's alpha for all three parts combined (i.e., 36 items) was 0.97.

Table 1. Mean, standard deviations, Cronbach's alphas, and mean of inter-item correlations

	Secondary 1		Secondary 2		Overall	
	M (SD)	α (Mean#)	M (SD)	α (Mean#)	M (SD)	α (Mean#)
Program content (10 items)	5.04 (.83)	.92 (.55)	4.99 (.97)	.95 (.66)	5.03 (.85)	.93 (.57)
Program implementers (10 items)	5.26 (.81)	.95 (.66)	5.08 (1.05)	.97 (.77)	5.23 (.85)	.96 (.69)
Program effectiveness (16 items)	4.05 (.81)	.96 (.59)	4.07 (.92)	.98 (.72)	4.06 (.83)	.96 (.61)
Total effectiveness (36 items)	4.67 (.70)	.97 (.46)	4.61 (.67)	.95 (.34)	4.66 (.70)	.97 (.44)

Note. # Mean inter-item correlations.

Tables 2 to 5 show the numbers and percentages of students having a positive evaluation on the program. As most of the respondents showed positive evaluation of all facets of the program, there was support for Hypothesis 1. Table 2 shows the descriptive statistics on students' evaluation of the program content. Results showed that an overwhelming proportion of the sample responded positively. For instance, 93.1% thought highly of the curriculum design, 93.8% appreciated the clarity of the curriculum objectives, and 92.7% reported that they generally "liked the curriculum very much".

Table 2. Descriptive statistics of the participants' evaluations on the program content

	Respondents with positive responses (Options 4-6)					
	Secondary 1		Secondary 2		Overall	
	n	%	*n*	%	*n*	%
The objectives of the curriculum are very clear.	5834	94.2	969	91.2	6803	93.8
The design of the curriculum is very good.	5782	93.5	964	90.7	6746	93.1
The activities were carefully planned.	5695	92.3	951	89.5	6646	91.9
The classroom atmosphere was very pleasant.	5526	89.5	966	90.9	6492	89.7
There was much peer interaction amongst the students.	5581	90.5	947	89.2	6528	90.3
I participated actively during lessons (including discussions, sharing, games, etc.).	5596	90.6	967	91.1	6563	90.7
I was encouraged to do my best.	5575	90.2	921	86.7	6496	89.7
The learning experience I encountered enhanced my interest towards the lessons.	5659	91.6	944	88.8	6603	91.2
Overall speaking, I have a very positive evaluation of the program.	5583	90.4	940	88.4	6523	90.1
On the whole, I like this curriculum very much.	5756	93.2	955	89.8	6711	92.7

Note. All items were rated on a 6-point Likert scale with 1 = strongly disagree, 2 = disagree, 3 = slightly disagree, 4 = slightly agree, 5 = agree, 6 = strongly agree. Only the positive responses (Options 4-6) are shown.

Regarding participants' evaluation of the program implementers, over 92% of the respondents rated positively on all the ten items. Some examples included perceived mastery of the curriculum (93.8%), professionalism exhibited (94.0%), preparation for the lessons (94.9%), and overall satisfaction with the implementers (94.9%).

Table 3. Descriptive statistics of the participants' evaluations of the program implementers

	Respondents with positive responses (Options 4-6)					
	Secondary 1		Secondary 2		Overall	
	n	%	*n*	%	*N*	%
The instructor(s) had a good mastery of the curriculum.	5839	94.4	951	90.1	6790	93.8
The instructor(s) was well prepared for the lessons.	5894	95.4	967	91.7	6861	94.9
The instructor(s)' teaching skills were good.	5861	94.9	947	89.8	6808	94.2
The instructor(s) showed good professional attitudes.	5830	94.5	961	91.2	6791	94.0
The instructor(s) was very involved.	5864	95.0	962	91.2	6826	94.5
The instructor(s) encouraged students to participate in the activities.	5880	95.4	983	93.3	6863	95.1
The instructor(s) cared for the students.	5851	94.9	942	89.4	6793	94.1
The instructor(s) was ready to offer help to students when needed.	5902	95.7	960	91.1	6862	95.0
The instructor(s) had much interaction with the students.	5792	93.6	936	88.7	6728	92.9
Overall speaking, I have a very positive evaluation of the instructors.	5901	95.5	966	91.6	6867	94.9

Note. All items are rated on a 6-point Likert scale with 1 = strongly disagree, 2 = disagree, 3 = slightly disagree, 4 = slightly agree, 5 = agree, 6 = strongly agree. Only the positive responses (Options 4-6) are shown.

Table 4 details the descriptive statistics on students' ratings regarding perceived program effectiveness. Over 85% of the respondents showed positive ratings on all the 16 items. For instance, 91.8%, 93.1%, and 92.4% of the students felt that the program had raised their self-confidence, self-awareness, and social competence, respectively. There were 94.4% of them indicating that the program had "enriched my overall development". Table 5 presents students' ratings on the three additional items. Over 90% indicated that they would recommend the program to others (94.5%) and participate in a future similar program (93.2%). Furthermore, 94.3% expressed satisfaction with the program. In short, Hypothesis 1 was supported.

Table 4. Descriptive statistics of the participants' evaluations of the program effectiveness

The extent to which the course (i.e., the program that all students have joined) has helped you:	Respondents with positive responses (Options 3-5)					
	Secondary 1		Secondary 2		Overall	
	n	%	*n*	%	*N*	%
It has strengthened my bonding with teachers, classmates and my family.	5496	88.8	933	87.5	6429	88.7
It has strengthened my resilience in adverse conditions.	5610	90.9	984	92.3	6594	91.1
It has enhanced my social competence.	5707	92.5	984	92.3	6691	92.4
It has improved my ability in handling and expressing my emotions.	5675	92.0	978	91.7	6653	92.0
It has enhanced my cognitive competence.	5584	90.6	975	91.5	6559	90.8
My ability to resist harmful influences has been improved.	5778	93.8	971	91.1	6749	93.4
It has strengthened my ability to distinguish between the good and the bad.	5830	94.5	969	90.9	6799	93.9
It has increased my competence in making sensible and wise choices.	5715	92.6	976	91.6	6691	92.4
It has helped me to have life reflections.	5549	89.9	941	88.3	6490	89.7
It has reinforced my self-confidence.	5676	91.9	969	90.9	6645	91.8
It has increased my self- awareness.	5745	93.1	995	93.3	6740	93.1
It has helped me to face the future with a positive attitude.	5715	92.7	993	93.2	6708	92.7
It has helped me to cultivate compassion and care about others.	5647	91.6	970	91.0	6617	91.5
It has encouraged me to care about the community.	5253	85.1	916	85.9	6169	85.2
It has promoted my sense of responsibility in serving the society.	5646	91.4	952	89.3	6598	91.1
It has enriched my overall development.	5846	94.6	995	93.3	6841	94.4

Note. All items are rated on a 5-point Likert scale with 1 = unhelpful, 2 = not very helpful, 3 = slightly helpful, 4 = helpful, 5 = very helpful. Only the positive responses (Options 3-5) are shown.

Table 5. Summary of the participants' positive perceptions toward other aspects

Items	Secondary 1		Secondary 2		Overall	
	n	%	*n*	%	*n*	%
Willingness to suggest other students to participate in the program*	5856	95.1	974	91.3	6830	94.5
Willingness to participate similar programs in future*	5795	94.1	942	88.3	6737	93.2
The extent to which the participants satisfied with the program^	5853	95.5	943	88.5	6796	94.4

Note. *A 4-point Likert scale was used (1 = definitely will not, 2 = will not, 3 = will, 4 = definitely will). Only the positive responses (Options 3–4) are shown in this table.

^A 6-point Likert scale was used (1 = very dissatisfied, 2 = moderately dissatisfied, 3 = slightly dissatisfied, 4 = satisfied, 5 = moderately satisfied, 6 = very satisfied). Only the positive responses (Options 4–6) are shown.

Table 6. Comparison of participants' subjective evaluation of the program by grade levels

	S1 (N = 5,719)		S2 (N = 1,047)		MANOVA	
	Mean	***SD***	***Mean***	***SD***	***F-value***	$p\eta^2$
1) Program content (10 items)	5.05	0.83	4.99	0.97	4.54*^	.001
2) Program implementers (10 items)	5.27	0.80	5.08	1.05	48.12***^	.007
3) Program effectiveness (16 items)	4.06	0.81	4.07	0.92	0.29^	.000
4) Overall score (i.e., total of 1 to 3, 36 items)	4.67	0.70	4.61	0.67	7.70**^	.001

Note. * $p < .05$; ** $p < .01$; *** $p < .001$; ^ Adjusted Bonferroni value = .0125; $p\eta^2$ = partial eta-squared.

Results of the Pearson correlation analyses showed that the three subscales were significantly and positively correlated with one other. Both program content (r (6,869) = 0.55, $p < .001$) and program implementer (r (6,881) = 0.45, $p < .001$) were correlated with program effectiveness. The relationship between subscales program content and program implementer was the strongest (r (6,954) = 0.59, $p < .001$). Hence, Hypotheses 2a to 2c were supported.

Table 6 illustrates the findings of the MANOVA. As expected, results showed that Secondary 1 students had significantly more positive evaluation than did their S2 counterparts on program content (F = 4.54, p = .033, $p\eta^2$ = .001), program implementers (F = 48.12, p < .001, $p\eta^2$ = .007), and the overall score (F = 7.70, p = .006, $p\eta^2$ = .001). However, differences across grade levels were not observed in students' evaluation of program effectiveness (p > .05). As such, Hypothesis 3c was not supported.

Lastly, results of the multiple regression analyses (see Table 7) demonstrated that students' evaluations of program content (S1: β = 0.42, p < .001; S2: β = 0.32, p < .001; overall: β = 0.43, p < .001) and program implementers (S1: β = 0.25, p < .001; S2: β = 0.07, p = .021; overall: β = 0.20, p < .001) were significant predictors of their perceived program effectiveness. The overall model explained 32.67% of the variance of perceived program effectiveness. In a nutshell, Hypothesis 4 was confirmed at every grade level and for the entire sample.

Table 7. Multiple regression analyses predicting program effectiveness by program content and implementers

	β^a			
	Program content	Program implementers	***F***	R^2
Secondary 1	0.42***	0.25***	1837.94***	0.39
Secondary 2	0.32***	0.07*	67.91***	0.12
Overall	0.43***	0.20***	1642.14***	0.33

Note. [a] Standardized Beta coefficients. * p < .05(two-tailed). ** p < .01(two-tailed). *** p < .001(two-tailed).

Discussion

Utilizing the subjective outcome evaluation approach, the present study examined the views of students on the Tin Ka Ping P.A.T.H.S. Project in mainland China. Consistent with the previous findings, results showed that the program was well-received by the majority of program participants. This was evidenced by their positive evaluation of the program content, program implementer, program effectiveness, and their eagerness to recommend this program to others and to participate in a similar program in future. The overwhelmingly positive client satisfaction findings strongly supported Hypothesis 1. The findings also replicated those of Shek et al.'s (10) study covering the first phase of the project launched in East China, thus corroborating the evidence which supports the success of the Tin Ka Ping P.A.T.H.S. Project across China.

Echoing previous research findings from both East China and Hong Kong, significant inter-correlations among the three major program dimensions were observed, giving support to Hypotheses 2a to 2c. While no significant difference in program effectiveness was found across grade levels, Secondary 1 participants had a more positive evaluation of program content, program implementers and they also generally felt more satisfied. Nonetheless, judging by the small effect sizes ($p\eta^2 < 0.01$ for all cases) associated with all the significant grade effects (see Table 6) and taking into account the overall high satisfaction of the entire sample (see Table 1), one could legitimately conclude that both Secondary 1 and 2 participants were indeed very satisfied with the program in terms of its content, implementers, and effectiveness.

Regarding Hypothesis 4, results of multiple regression analyses indicated that both perceptions of program content and implementers were significant predictors of perceived program effectiveness. This finding resonates with Shek and Sun's (12) argument that "people" and "process" are vital to successful PYD programs. Nonetheless, the fact that the present model could only explain 32.67% of the variance implies that additional factors such as "policy" or "place" might be worthy areas of investigation in future evaluation studies.

There are several strengths of the present paper. Supplementing Shek et al.'s (10) pioneer subjective evaluation study of the first phase of the Tin Ka Ping P.A.T.H.S. Project, the present study adds to the scanty empirical work utilizing the client satisfaction approach in the mainland China context. Additionally, a valid and reliable subjective outcome evaluation instrument (i.e., the Form A) was presently adopted to comprehensively examine the different facets of the program. Lastly, via scrutinizing various prospective predictors of perceived program effectiveness and satisfaction, this paper could help researchers build models regarding subjective outcome evaluation in the mainland China context. Particularly, our results suggested that the promotion of perceived effectiveness would hinge on the improvement of the quality of both the program content and its implementers.

There are several limitations of this study. First, as the current analyses were predominantly quantitative, it may be insightful to also examine the open-ended responses to gain an understanding of the feelings of the participants. Second, the present findings may not be representative of the entire school sample (N = 30) of the Tin Ka Ping P.A.T.H.S. Project as only eighteen of them took part in the current study. Third, impression management (23) may underlie the present overwhelmingly supportive findings. Students may give desirable ratings as to avoid appearing ungrateful for the implementers' hard work. Nevertheless, this possibility can be conveniently ruled out because of the anonymous nature of the present survey (24). Finally, although subjective outcome evaluation has been widely used in the human services domain, it is methodologically superior to incorporate other evaluation methods such as the objective outcome and process evaluation as to reinforce the robustness of the findings. Despite these limitations, the present findings suggest that the Tin Ka Ping P.A.T.H.S. Project launched in the academic year 2015-2016 could be regarded as a success.

ACKNOWLEDGMENTS

The preparation for this paper and the Tin Ka Ping P.A.T.H.S. Project were financially supported by the Tin Ka Ping Foundation. This chapter is a reprint with minor revisions of an earlier published paper in the *International Public Health Journal* 2018;10(1) issue with permission.

REFERENCES

[1] PriceWaterhouseCoopers. The long view: How will the global economic order change by 2050? Aberdeen, UK: PricewaterhouseCoopers LLP, 2017.

[2] Xin Z, Zhang L, Liu D. Birth cohort changes of Chinese adolescents' anxiety: A cross-temporal meta-analysis, 1992-2005. Pers Individ Dif 2010;48(2):208-12.

[3] Xin Z, Zhang M. Changes in Chinese middle school students' mental health (1992~2005): A cross-temporal meta-analysis. Xin Li Xue Bao 2009;41(1):69-78. [Chinese]

[4] Ministry of Education. The outline of education guide for pupil's mental health Rev. ed. The People's Republic of China: Ministry of Education, 2012. [Chinese]

[5] Damon W. What is positive youth development? Ann Am Acad Pol Soc Sci 2004;591(1):13-24.

[6] Shek DTL, Ma HK, Sun RCF. A brief overview of adolescent developmental problems in Hong Kong. ScientificWorldJournal 2011;11:Article ID 896835. doi: 10.1100/2011/896835

[7] Shek DTL, Yu L. A review of validated youth prevention and positive youth development programs in Asia. Int J Disabil Hum Dev 2011;23(4):317-24.

[8] Shek DTL, Sun RCF, eds. Evaluation of the Project P.A.T.H.S. in Hong Kong: Findings based on multiple methods. Hong Kong: Department of Applied Social Sciences, The Hong Kong Polytechnic University, 2012.

[9] Shek DTL, Han XY. The relationship between subjective outcome evaluation and objective outcome evaluation findings: Evidence from China. Int J Disabil Hum Dev 2014;13(4):497-503.

[10] Shek DTL, Han XY, Lee TY, Yu L. Subjective outcome evaluation of a positive youth development program in China. Int J Disabil Hum Dev 2014;13(2):275-83.

[11] Shek DTL, Yu L, Sun RCF, Lee TY, Han X, Yan, Li XX, et al. Objective outcome evaluation of a positive youth development program in China. Int J Disabil Hum Dev 2014;13(2):255-65.

[12] Shek DTL, Sun RCF. The Project P.A.T.H.S. in Hong Kong—Lessons learned and implications for positive youth development programs. ScientificWorldJournal 2012;2012(3):Article ID 687536. doi: 10.1100/2012/687536

[13] Shek DTL, Siu AMH, Lee TY. The Chinese Positive Youth Development Scale: A validation study. Res Soc Work Pract 2007;17(3):380-91.

[14] Shek DTL, Tang VMY, Lo CY. Evaluation of an internet addiction treatment program for Chinese adolescents in Hong Kong. Adolescence 2009;44(174):359-73.

[15] Walsh T, Lord B. Client satisfaction and empowerment through social work intervention. Soc Work Health Care 2004;38(4):37-56.

[16] Larsen DL, Attkisson CC, Hargreaves WA, Nguyen TD. Assessment of client/patient satisfaction: Development of a general scale. Eval Program Plann 1979;2(3):197-207.

[17] Shek DTL, Sun RCF. Post-lecture evaluation of a university course on leadership and intrapersonal development. Int J Disabil Hum Dev 2013;12(2):185-91.

[18] Larson R, Walker K, Pearce N. A comparison of youth-driven and adult-driven youth programs: Balancing inputs from youth and adults. J Community Psychol 2005;33(1):57-74.

[19] Collins ME, Lemon C, Street E. A consumer view of teen living programs: Teen parents' satisfaction with program components and services. Fam Soc 2000;81(3):284-93.

[20] Shek DTL, Law MYM. Evaluation of the Project P.A.T.H.S. based on the client satisfaction approach: View of the students. J Pediatr Adolesc Gynecol 2014;27 Suppl:S2-9.

[21] Shek DTL, Leung JTY, Law MYM, Chan KSY. Perceived effectiveness and satisfaction of a community-based positive youth development program: findings based on high school students. Int J Disabil Hum Dev 2016. Epub ahead of print 03 Dec 2016. doi: 10.1515/ijdhd-2017-7005

[22] Shek DTL, Sun RCF. Effectiveness of the Tier 1 program of Project P.A.T.H.S.: Findings based on three years of program implementation. ScientificWorldJournal 2010;10:1509-19.

[23] Paulhus DL. Measurement and control of response bias. In: Robinson JP, Shaver PR, Wrightsman LS, eds. Measures of personality and social psychological attitudes. San Diego, CA: Academic Press, 1991: 17-59.

[24] Paulhus DL. Self-Deception and impression management in test responses. In: Angleitner A, Wiggins JS, eds. Personality assessment via questionnaires: Current issues in theory and measurement. Berlin: Springer, 1986:143-65.

In: Advances in Chinese Children … ISBN: 978-1-53617-870-8
Editors: Ariel Tenenbaum et al.

Chapter 9

EVALUATION OF THE PROJECT P.A.T.H.S. IN MAINLAND CHINA: VIEWS OF THE PROGRAM IMPLEMENTERS IN SENIOR HIGH SCHOOLS

Daniel TL Shek[1,*], PhD, FHKPS, BBS, SBS, JP, Florence KY Wu[2], EdD, Rachel CF Sun[2] and Mengtong Chen[3], PhD

[1]Department of Applied Social Sciences,
The Hong Kong Polytechnic University, Hong Kong, PR China
[2]Faculty of Education, The University of Hong Kong,
Hong Kong, PR China
[3]Hong Kong Baptist University, Hong Kong, PR China

---

* Corresponding Author: Daniel TL Shek, PhD, FHKPS, BBS, SBS, JP, Associate Vice President (Undergraduate Programme) and Chair Professor of Applied Social Sciences, Department of Applied Social Sciences, The Hong Kong Polytechnic University, Hunghom, Hong Kong, PR China. E-mail: daniel.shek@polyu.edu.hk.

Abstract

In this chapter we investigated program implementers' views on the Tin Ka Ping Project P.A.T.H.S. in its first year of implementation in senior high schools in mainland China. After completion of the program, 33 program implementers completed the Subjective Outcome Evaluation Form (Form B). Results showed that over 90% of the implementers had positive views of program content, their self-performance and program effectiveness. In line with previous evaluation studies, perceived worker performance was found to predict perceived program effectiveness. Nevertheless, program content did not predict program effectiveness. Findings of the present study underscore the benefits of implementing the Project P.A.T.H.S. in senior high schools in mainland China.

Introduction

While adolescence is often regarded as a period with rapid physical development, it is also a transitional period during which adolescents have to go through many challenges (1). According to World Health Organization (WHO), adolescents may engage in a range of risk behaviors and health issues, including violent behaviors, alcohol and drug abuse, tobacco use, self-harm, and mental health issues (2). These health compromising behaviors often have negative impacts on the current and future health of adolescents (3). Based on the statistics of WHO (2), health compromising behaviors among adolescents are prevalent throughout the world.

The problem of health comprising behaviors among adolescents have also drawn public attention in China. In the study of Hesketh, Ding, and Tomkins (4), it was found that nearly 16% of the junior and senior school students responding to the survey were ever smokers. Alcohol use among Chinese adolescents is another serious problem that more attention should be paid. A meta-analytic study of Feng and Newman (5) indicated that over 35% of male students and over 20% of female students in senior high schools had used alcohol in the last 30 days. Regarding illicit drug use, the prevalence rate was about 4% based on a survey of 15 secondary schools in Wuhan (6). A large-scale study (7) investigated self-harm behaviors among secondary school students in China, and the findings suggested that 17% of the students had injured themselves deliberately in the past 12 months, which was higher that Western countries (7, 8).

Mental health issue is another leading cause of health problem among adolescents (9). According to a large-scale survey in China, approximately 10% of Chinese school children had suffered from one or more types of psychiatric disorders (10). Correspondingly, it was estimated that every trained child psychiatrist has to serve more than 40,000 children with behavioral and emotional problems in mainland China (11). Thus, prevention of health compromising behaviors and mental health problems among children and adolescents is an urgent and important job in mainland China. Unfortunately, there is a lack of prevention programs designed for Chinese adolescents.

Both individual and contextual factors affect adolescent behavior and shape their development (12). Turbin et al. (13) suggested that adolescent involvement in health-promoting behaviors were more likely to be affected by protective and risk factors in social context (e.g., family and peers), rather than by their individual-level factors. Therefore, providing prevention in the social context would be effective to reduce the risk of adolescent behavior problems and psychiatric disorders. As school is an important place for adolescents to learn knowledge, develop social skills and build social support (1), it would be appropriate to implement prevention programs in school setting, since Chinese adolescents spend more than 8 hours at school each day (14). Therefore, school-based positive youth development (PYD) programs for the general adolescent population is a promising approach to promote holistic development in adolescents.

With respect to the above-mentioned issues, a PYD program entitled "P.A.T.H.S. to Adulthood: A Jockey Club Youth Enhancement Scheme" was initiated in Hong Kong in the 2005-2006 academic year and then piloted in mainland China from 2007-2008 academic year to 2009-2010 academic year (15, 16). The initial version of the Project P.A.T.H.S. was designed by the first author and his collaborators from five universities in Hong Kong and funded by The Hong Kong Jockey Club Charities Trust. Two tiers of programs were included in the project to help adolescents with different levels of need. The Tier 1 Program provides a series of curricula-based training programs to the general adolescent population in junior secondary schools that students participate in 10 to 20 hours of training on 15 PYD constructs in each school year, whereas the Tier 2 Program is designed for one-fifth of the students who have greater psychosocial needs (17).

Because of the prominent success in the implementation of the project in Hong Kong, a pilot project was funded by Tin Ka Ping Foundation and implemented in four schools in mainland China (including Shanghai, Suzhou, Changzhou and Yangzhou) in 2011-2014. As a transplant of the Project P.A.T.H.S. (i.e., Tin Ka Ping P.A.T.H.S. Project), the pilot project had very good performance. Thus, a second phase of the project was funded to fully implement the project from 2014-2015 academic year (18, 19). In the academic year of 2015-2016, a total of 30 secondary schools joined the project and the curriculum for senior high schools was also developed. To facilitate program implementation, a series of in-service training programs were provided to school teachers and social workers from participating schools.

Subjective outcome evaluation is a useful approach to gather feedback from stakeholders of programs (e.g., program participants and implementers) and assess their satisfaction. The views of the stakeholders can provide ideas to improve program content and process, which have implications to the application of the program in the general population. Previous evaluation studies using subjective outcome evaluation approach showed that both students and school teachers held very positive views toward the project, which echoes the results of qualitative evaluation and objective outcome evaluation of the project (18-21). However, the perceptions of program implementers from senior schools are still unknown.

As implementers are an indispensable part of a program, the feedback from these well trained professionals in the field of positive adolescent development could be very helpful to improve program content. Moreover, their first-hand experience of delivering program to students would provide practical data to review the program, as they would not adapt materials which are not fit in their situation (22). Implementers could review their own practice when they are doing evaluation, and such evaluation could provide them with a sense of respect and fairness (23).

The purpose of the present study was to examine program implementers' perceptions toward the project implemented in senior high schools in China. Subjective outcome evaluation approach was used to collect feedback of implementers who delivered the senior curriculum. As there are very few programs focusing on promoting holistic and positive development for students of senior high schools in mainland China, the evaluation study can provide good insight into the efficacy of the Project P.A.T.H.S. and the factors associated with program success. Three sets of research questions and hypotheses were examined in the present study:

- What are program implementers' perceptions of the project implemented in senior high school? Would the findings be consistent with the findings of previous evaluation studies of programs conducted in junior secondary school? Based on previous studies, it was expected that a majority of the respondents (at least 80%) would have positive view of the program (Hypothesis 1).
- Are there any significant inter-relationships among the three aspects of subjective outcome evaluation? Based on the results of previous findings, we hypothesized that perceived program effectiveness would be significantly associated with program content (Hypothesis 2a) and perceived worker performance (Hypothesis 2b).
- What are the predictors of perceived effectiveness of the program? Based on the findings of previous study, we hypothesized that program content and perceived worker performance would predict the effectiveness of the project (Hypothesis 3a and 3b, respectively).

OUR STUDY

In the academic year of 2015-2016, the Tin Ka Ping P.A.T.H.S. Project was implemented in 30 junior and/or senior high schools in mainland China. To explore program implementers' viewpoints toward the program and their self-performance, and to evaluate program effectiveness, school teachers who taught the senior school programs were invited to complete the

Subjective Outcome Evaluation Form for Instructors (Form B) after program curriculum was finished.

A total of 33 implementers from four senior secondary schools in mainland China, with a range from five to twelve teachers in each school, have submitted the Form B after the completion of program. To ensure survey response quality, an evaluation manual with a clear guideline on the completion of Form B was provided to the teachers before they started to fill in the evaluation form. Relevant training on evaluation was also included in different training workshops.

Instruments

The Subjective Outcome Evaluation Form for Instructors (Form B) has been widely applied over the past decade and evaluation studies of the project demonstrate that Form B is a valid and reliable measure gathering feedback from program implementers of the project (24). Form B consists of both open-ended questions that provide qualitative data and quantitative scales. As shown in Table 1, the three subscales used in Form B have demonstrated very good internal consistency with Cronbach's αs above .90. Due to space limitation, the present study focused on the quantitative data collected from the following items/subscales:

- A 6-point Likert scale assessing implementers' perceptions of program content (10 items);
- A 6-point Likert scale assessing implementers' perceptions of self-performance (10 items);
- A 5-point Likert scale assessing implementers' perceptions of program effectiveness (16 items);
- One item assessing the degree to which implementers would recommend other students to join the program;
- One item assessing the degree to which teachers would teach similar curriculum in the future;

- One item assessing implementers' view toward their professional growth through the program.

Table 1. Mean, standard deviations, Cronbach's alphas, and mean of inter-item correlations

	M	SD	*α*	Mean#
Program content (10 items)	5.17	0.87	.97	.75
Program implementers (10 items)	5.08	0.89	.97	.78
Program effectiveness (16 items)	4.10	0.77	.98	.72
Total effectiveness (36 items)	4.66	0.78	.99	.66

Note: # Mean inter-item correlations.

Data analyses

First, reliability analyses were conducted to examine the internal consistency of the three subscales in Form B and the inter-item correlations among them. Second, descriptive analyses were performed to compute the percentage of positive responses of implementers' perception of program components (program content and implementers' self-performance) and program effectiveness. Third, to examine the correlations between program content, implementers' self-performance and program effectiveness, Pearson correlation analysis was performed. Finally, multiple regression analysis was conducted to test the potential predictors of perceived program effectiveness, including program content and implementers' perceived self-performance. All statistical analysis was performed using SPSS 23.0.

FINDINGS

Program implementers' perceptions of program content, self-performance and program effectiveness are shown in Tables 2-4, respectively. Generally speaking, their views toward the aspects measured in Form B were very positive. Over 96% of the respondents had positive responses on eight out of ten items regarding program content, such as design of the program, program activities, atmosphere in the classroom, student classroom participation, theoretical support and teacher's interest toward the curriculum. Over 90% of the respondents agreed that "the objectives of the curriculum are very clear," and "there was much peer interaction amongst the students." Overall speaking, the respondents perceived positive features of program content (see Table 2). Similarly, the majority of the respondents also had positive perceptions toward their own performance. Seven out of ten questions regarding implementers' perceived self-performance received positive responses from over 96% of the respondents (see Table 3).

Table 2. Summary of the program implementers' perceptions toward the program content

		N	Mean	SD	Respondents with positive responses (Options 4-6)	
					n	%
1.	The objectives of the curriculum are very clear.	32	5.22	1.04	30	93.8
2.	The design of the curriculum is very good.	32	5.06	0.91	31	96.9
3.	The activities were carefully planned.	32	5.19	0.93	31	96.9
4.	The classroom atmosphere was very pleasant.	32	5.19	1.00	31	96.9
5.	There was much peer interaction amongst the students.	32	5.19	1.12	30	93.8
6.	Students participated actively during lessons (including discussions, sharing, games, etc.)	32	5.16	0.95	31	96.9
7.	The program has a strong and sound theoretical support.	32	4.88	0.98	31	96.9
8.	The teaching experience I encountered enhanced my interest towards the lessons.	32	5.16	0.99	31	96.9
9.	Overall speaking, I have very positive evaluation of the program.	32	5.25	1.02	31	96.9
10.	On the whole, students like this curriculum very much.	32	5.41	0.98	31	96.9

Note: All items are on a 6-point Likert scale with 1 = strongly disagree, 2 = disagree, 3 = slightly disagree, 4 = slightly agree, 5 = agree, 6 = strongly agree. Only respondents with positive responses (Options 4-6) are shown in the table.

Table 3. Summary of the program implementers' perceptions toward their own performance

		N	Mean	SD	Respondents with positive responses (Options 4-6)	
					n	%
1.	I have a good mastery of the curriculum	32	4.88	1.07	29	90.6
2.	I prepared well for the lessons.	32	4.94	1.05	30	93.8
3.	My teaching skills were good.	32	4.75	0.98	30	93.8
4.	I have good professional attitudes.	32	5.00	1.02	31	96.9
5.	I was very involved.	32	5.06	0.95	31	96.9
6.	I gained a lot during the course of instruction.	32	5.09	1.00	31	96.9
7.	I cared for the students.	32	5.28	0.99	31	96.9
8.	I was ready to offer help to students when needed.	32	5.41	0.98	31	96.9
9.	I had much interaction with the students.	32	5.19	0.97	31	96.9
10.	Overall speaking, I have very positive evaluation of myself as an instructor.	32	5.19	0.93	31	96.9

Note: All items are on a 6-point Likert scale with 1 = strongly disagree, 2 = disagree, 3 = slightly disagree, 4 = slightly agree, 5 = agree, 6 = strongly agree. Only respondents with positive responses (Options 4-6) are shown in the table.

Table 4. Summary of the program implementers' perceptions toward the program effectiveness

The extent to which the Tier 1 Program (i.e., the program in which all students have joined) has helped your students:		N	Mean	SD	Respondents with positive responses (Options 3-5)	
					n	%
1.	It has strengthened students' bonding with teachers, classmates and their families.	33	4.18	0.88	32	97.0
2.	It has strengthened students' resilience in adverse conditions.	33	4.03	0.85	32	97.0
3.	It has enhanced students' social competence.	33	4.30	0.85	32	97.0
4.	It has improved students' ability in handling and expressing emotions.	33	4.39	0.83	32	97.0
5.	It has enhanced students' cognitive competence.	33	3.97	0.88	32	97.0

Table 4. (Continued)

The extent to which the Tier 1 Program (i.e., the program in which all students have joined) has helped your students:		N	Mean	SD	Respondents with positive responses (Options 3-5)	
					n	%
6.	Students' ability to resist harmful influences has been improved.	33	4.03	0.95	31	93.9
7.	It has strengthened students' ability to distinguish between the good and the bad.	33	4.09	0.95	31	93.9
8.	It has increased students' competence in making sensible and wise choices.	33	3.91	0.91	31	93.9
9.	It has helped students to have life reflections.	33	3.94	0.90	32	97.0
10.	It has reinforced students' self-confidence.	32	4.19	0.78	31	96.9
11.	It has increased students' self-awareness.	32	4.31	0.86	31	96.9
12.	It has helped students to face the future with a positive attitude.	33	4.30	0.81	32	97.0
13.	It has helped students to cultivate compassion and care about others.	33	4.06	0.90	32	97.0
14.	It has encouraged students to care about the community.	33	3.55	1.00	30	90.9
15.	It has promoted students' sense of responsibility in serving the society.	33	3.94	1.06	30	90.9
16.	It has enriched the overall development of the students.	33	4.30	0.85	32	97.0

Note: All items are on a 5-point Likert scale with 1 = unhelpful, 2 = not very helpful, 3 = slightly helpful, 4 = helpful, 5 = very helpful. Only respondents with positive responses (Options 3-5) are shown in the table.

Results in Table 4 indicated that there were a number of perceived benefits of the project. Over 96% of the respondents agreed that the program could strength students' bonding with their families, teachers and classmates, enhance students' resilience and their competence in regard to social skills, emotion capital and cognitive functioning, and increase students' self-awareness and self-confidence, etc. The great majority (97%) of the respondents agreed that the program enriched students' overall development. From the program implementers' subjective views toward other aspects of the program, all of them (100%) would suggest the students who have similar needs join the program. In addition, 97% of the respondents had intention to teach similar programs again in the future, and over 93% of respondents perceived the program as helpful in their professional growth (Table 5). In short, the findings supported Hypothesis 1.

Table 5. Other aspects of subjective outcome evaluation based on the program implementers' perceptions

		N	Mean	SD	Respondents with positive responses	
					n	%
Q3.	If you have a student/client whose needs and conditions are similar to those of your students who have joined the program, will you suggest him/her to participate in this program?	33	3.58	0.50	33	100
Q4.	If there is a chance, will you teach similar programs again in the future?	33	3.58	0.56	32	97.0
Q5.	Do you think the implementation of the program has helped you in your professional growth (e.g., enhancement of your skills)?	32	4.28	0.89	30	93.8

Note: For Q3 & Q4, the item is on a 4-point Likert scale with 1 = definitely will not teach, 2 = will not teach, 3 = will teach, 4 = definitely will teach. Only respondents with positive responses (Options 3-4) are shown in the table. For Q5, the item is on a 5-point Likert scale with 1 = unhelpful, 2 = not very helpful, 3 = slightly helpful, 4 = helpful, 5 = very helpful. Only respondents with positive responses (Options 3-5) are shown in the table.

The results of correlation analyses showed that program content, program implementers' perceived worker performance and program effectiveness were significantly associated with each other (*r*s ranged from .73 to .92, *p*s < .01; see Table 6). The findings gave support to Hypotheses 2a and 2b. Table 7 presents the results of multiple regression analysis. Consistent with Hypothesis 3b, the overall perception of program implementers' self-performance predicted program effectiveness ($\beta = .65$, $p < .05$). However, Hypothesis 3a was rejected, as program content was not a significant predictor of the benefits of the program based on the data of the present study. This model explained 59% of the variance of program effectiveness.

Table 6. Correlation coefficients on the relationship between program components and program effectiveness

Variable	1	2	3
1. Program content (10 items)	–	–	–
2. Program implementers (10 items)	.92**	–	–
3. Program effectiveness	.73**	.77**	–

** p < .01.

Table 7. Multiple regression analyses predicting program effectiveness

	Predictors			
	Program content	Program implementers	Model	
	β^a	β^a	R	R^2
Program effectiveness	.12	.65*	.77	.59

Note: Missing values were replaced with mean ; [a] Standardized coefficients ; * $p < .05$.

Discussion

To promote students' whole person development in senior high schools, innovative units and topics based on PYD constructs were developed and incorporated into the senior curriculum of P.A.T.H.S. programs in mainland China. This initiative is groundbreaking in different Chinese communities. Utilizing the subjective outcome evaluation approach, this study examined stakeholder satisfaction of program components (quality of content and implementers) and program effectiveness based on the perceptions of program implementers who taught the senior curriculum of Tier 1 Program in the academic year of 2015-2016. Generally speaking, the great majority of the implementers who responded to the survey were satisfied with the project and recognized its positive influences on adolescent development. The present study replicated the previous evaluation findings in junior secondary schools (24, 25).

As the first subjective evaluation regarding implementers' views of senior school program, several observations can be highlighted. First, approximately 97% of the respondents held positive views toward program content, self-performance and benefits of the program. Second, relatively fewer teachers (90.9%) agreed that the program promoted students' sense of social responsibility and encouraged them to care more about community development, which was consistent with previous evaluation findings (25, 26). One explanation is that community involvement is more difficult to observe, as activities in the project are mainly conducted within school settings. However, the findings can still be regarded as very positive. Third, this study replicated the relationships among the three aspects of subjective outcome evaluation that both program content and implementers' self-performance had strong and positive relationships with program effectiveness. Fourth, the performance of program implementers was identified as a significant predictor of positive effects of the program. However, in contrast to previous studies based on student participants, program effectiveness was not statistically significant.

There are several reasons why the project was successful and positive feedbacks were received. First, the remarkable success of the junior school programs in Hong Kong and mainland China provides experience and materials for implementing similar programs in senior secondary schools. Second, as implementers in the present study were school teachers who aspired to pass on their knowledge and positive attitude toward life to students, they would have a higher motivation to deliver the program. Third, teaching and learning behavior expected in PYD programs is different from traditional way of education in China. Because different teaching and learning methods are used in the programs, including group discussion, role play, self-reflections, and multimedia teaching, students can be more actively involved (17). Fourth, in-service training programs for teachers can help strengthen their understanding of PYD constructs and program content (15). Implementers would be more likely to evaluate their performance and the program positively if they observe that students have positive changes after attending the program (27).

The findings in the present study would be a good reference for similar research and programs in the future, which provide a synthesis of stakeholder satisfaction on program implementation and effectiveness. It is important to collect the views of program implementers, since they play the role of a medium between program participants and program operation. As an indispensable factor contributing to an effective program in the 5P model (i.e., policy, program, place, process and people), program implementers have crucial influence on program effectiveness (28). In future studies, researchers may investigate if implementers' perceptions are consistent with students' subjective and objective evaluation of the program.

The present study has several limitations. First, because this is an initial evaluation study of the senior school program of Project P.A.T.H.S., the sample size is relatively small. Hence, the findings could only represent the views of teachers in a few project schools. Second, as few schools joined the evaluation, it is unclear if implementers teaching different grades have different views on the program. Third, only quantitative data were reported in this study. Obviously, a more comprehensive picture of implementers' feedback on the program requires both quantitative and qualitative evaluation. Therefore, it is helpful to include more teachers using different evaluation methods in future evaluation studies.

Despite these limitations, the results of this study demonstrated that the Tier 1 Program of the Tin Ka Ping P.A.T.H.S. Project in mainland senior high schools was positively evaluated by program implementers and they had positive effects on adolescent development, which is pioneer in the Chinese contexts. In view of the limited international and local research on positive youth development programs in China, the present study provides an insight into the initial application of Tin Ka Ping P.A.T.H.S. Project among senior high school students and teachers.

ACKNOWLEDGMENTS

The preparation for this paper and the Tin Ka Ping P.A.T.H.S. Project are financially supported by Tin Ka Ping Foundation. This chapter is a re-print with minor revisions of an earlier published paper in the *International Public Health Journal* 2018;10(1) issue with permission.

REFERENCES

[1] Tang SKC, Wong WC, Leung PM, Chen WQ, Lee A, Ling DC. Health compromising behaviors among Chinese adolescents: Role of physical abuse, school experience, and social support. J Health Psychol 2011;16(3):457-66. DOI: 10.1177/13591 05310384297.

[2] World Health Organization. Health for the world's adolescents: A second chance in the second decade. Accessed 2017 Feb 27. URL: http://www.who.int/maternal _child_adolescent/documents/second-decade/en/.

[3] McDonald CC, Sommers MS, Fargo JD. Risky driving, mental health, and health-compromising behaviours: Risk clustering in late adolescents and adults. Inj Prev 2014;20(6):365-72. DOI: 10.1136/injuryprev-2014-041150.

[4] Hesketh T, Ding QJ, Tomkins A. Smoking among youths in China. Am J Public Health 2001;91(10):1653-5. DOI: 10.2105/AJPH.91.10.1653.

[5] Feng Y, Newman IM. Estimate of adolescent alcohol use in China: A meta-analysis. Arch Public Health 2016;74:45. DOI: 10.1186/s13690-016-0157-5.

[6] Gong J, Chen X, Zeng J, Li F, Zhou D, Wang Z. Adolescent addictive internet use and drug abuse in Wuhan, China. Addict Res Theory 2009;17(3):291-305. DOI: 10.1080/16066350802435152.

[7] Wan YH, Hu CL, Hao JH, Sun Y, Tao FB. Deliberate self-harm behaviors in Chinese adolescents and young adults. Eur Child Adolesc Psychiatry 2011;20(10):517-25. DOI: 10.1007/s00787-011-0213-1.

[8] Morey C, Corcoran P, Arensman E, Perry IJ. The prevalence of self-reported deliberate self harm in Irish adolescents. BMC Public Health 2008;8:79. DOI: 10.1186/1471-2458-8-79.

[9] Kieling C, Baker-Henningham H, Belfer M, Conti G, Ertem I, Omigbodun O, et al. Child and adolescent mental health worldwide: Evidence for action. Lancet 2011;378(9801):1515-25. DOI: 10.1016/S0140-6736(11)60827-1.

[10] Yang X, Jiang C, Pan W, Xu W, Liang F, Li N, et al. Prevalence of psychiatric disorders among children and adolescents in Northeast China. PLoS One 2014;9(10):e111223. DOI: 10.1371/journal.pone.0111223.

[11] Zheng Y, Zheng X. Current state and recent developments of child psychiatry in China. Child Adolesc Psychiatry Ment Health 2015;9:10. DOI: 10.1186/s13034-015-0040-0.

[12] Shek DTL. The role of positive youth development and family functioning in Chinese adolescent well-being: Theoretical considerations and empirical evidence. In:

Maggino F, ed. A life devoted to quality of life. Cham, Switzerland: Springer International Publishing, 2016:43-58.

[13] Turbin MS, Jessor R, Costa FM, Dong Q, Zhang H, Wang C. Protective and risk factors in health-enhancing behavior among adolescents in China and the United States: Does social context matter?. Health Psychol 2006;25(4):445-54. DOI: 10.1037/0278-6133.25.4.445.

[14] Xu H, Minca E. How Chinese children spend their time. In: Murdock SH, Swanson DA, eds. Applied demography in the 21st century. Dordrecht: Springer Netherlands, 2008:299-334.

[15] Shek DTL, Liang RLY, Lee TY. Evaluation of a training program of Tin Ka Ping P.A.T.H.S. Project in China. Int J Child Adolesc health, in press.

[16] Shek DTL, Sun RCF. The Project P.A.T.H.S. in Hong Kong: Development, training, implementation, and evaluation. J Pediatr Adolesc Gynecol 2013;26(3 Suppl):S2-9. DOI: 10.1016/j.jpag.2013.03.009.

[17] Shek DTL, Wu FKY. The Project P.A.T.H.S. in Hong Kong: Work done and lessons learned in a decade. J Pediatr Adolesc Gynecol 2016;29(1 Suppl):S3-11. DOI: 10.1016/j.jpag.2015.10.003.

[18] Shek DTL, Han XY, Lee TY, Yu L. Subjective outcome evaluation of a positive youth development program in China. Int J Disabil Hum Dev 2014;13(2):275-83. DOI: 10.1515/ijdhd-2014-0313.

[19] Shek DTL, Yu L, Sun RCF, Lee TY, Han XY, Li XX, et al. Objective outcome evaluation of a positive youth development program in China. Int J Disabil Hum Dev 2014;13(2):255-65. DOI: 10.1515/ijdhd-2014-0311.

[20] 20 Shek DTL, Ma CMS. Impact of the Project P.A.T.H.S. in the junior secondary school years: Objective outcome evaluation based on eight waves of longitudinal data. ScientificWorldJournal 2012;2012:Article ID 170345. DOI: 10.1100/2012/170345.

[21] Shek DTL, Sun RCF. Qualitative evaluation of Project P.A.T.H.S.: An integration of findings based on program participants. ScientificWorldJournal 2012;2012:Article ID 591816. DOI: 10.1100/2012/528483.

[22] Flannery DJ, Torquati J. An elementary school substance abuse prevention program: Teacher and administrator perspectives. J Drug Educ 1993;23(4):387-97. DOI: 10.2190/3N63-D19V-CJ0G-VLUJ.

[23] Sun RCF, Shek DTL. Perceived program qualities and outcomes of a youth program in Hong Kong based on the views of the workers. J Pediatr Adolesc Gynecol 2014;27 Suppl:S10-
6. DOI: 10.1016/j.jpag.2014.02.007.

[24] Shek DTL, Yu L. Subjective outcome evaluation of the Project P.A.T.H.S. (extension phase) based on the perspective of program implementer. ScientificWorldJournal 2012;2012:Article ID 589257. DOI: 10.1100/2012/589257.

[25] Shek DTL, Ma CMS. Program implementers' evaluation of the Project P.A.T.H.S.: Findings based on different datasets over time. ScientificWorldJournal 2012;2012:Article ID 918437. DOI: 10.1100/2012/918437.

[26] Shek DTL, Ma CMS, Zhu X. Evaluation of a community-based positive youth development program in Hong Kong: Views of program implementers. Int J Disabil Hum Dev, in press.

[27] Judge TA, Thorese CJ, Bono JE, Patton GK. The job satisfaction-job performance relationship: A qualitative and quantitative review. Psychol Bull 2001;127(3):376-407. DOI: 10.1037/0033-2909.127.3.376.

[28] Shek DTL, Sun RCF. Implementation of a positive youth development program in a Chinese context: The role of policy, program, people, process, and place. ScientificWorldJournal 2008;8:980-96. DOI: 10.1100/tsw.2008.120.

In: Advances in Chinese Children … ISBN: 978-1-53617-870-8
Editors: Ariel Tenenbaum et al.

Chapter 10

EVALUATION OF THE TRAINING PROGRAM OF A POSITIVE YOUTH DEVELOPMENT PROGRAM: TIN KA PING P.A.T.H.S. PROJECT IN CHINA

Daniel TL Shek[1,*], PhD, FHKPS, BBS, SBS, JP, Janet TY Leung[1], PhD, Rachel CF Sun[2], Mengtong Chen[3], PhD and Chi Kin Chung[1], MA

[1]Department of Applied Social Sciences,
The Hong Kong Polytechnic University, Hong Kong, PR China
[2]Faculty of Education, The University of Hong Kong,
Hong Kong, PR China
[3]Hong Kong Baptist University, Hong Kong, PR China

---

* Corresponding Author: Daniel TL Shek, PhD, FHKPS, BBS, SBS, JP, Associate Vice President (Undergraduate Programme) and Chair Professor of Applied Social Sciences, Department of Applied Social Sciences, The Hong Kong Polytechnic University, Hunghom, Hong Kong, PR China. Email: daniel.shek@polyu.edu.hk.

ABSTRACT

In this chapter we investigated the participants' perceptions of a training program conducted in Tin Ka Ping P.A.T.H.S. Project in China using the subjective outcome evaluation approach. The participants (N = 151) completed an evaluation form at the end of the training program. Results showed that a very high proportion of the participants were satisfied with the training program in terms of program content, instructors, administrative arrangements, and their own performance. Several significant predictors of effectiveness of the training program were identified, including program quality, instructor quality, administrative arrangement, and participants' perceived self-performance. Perceived program quality also predicted overall satisfaction of the participants. Together with previous evaluation findings, the present study suggests that the Tin Ka Ping P.A.T.H.S. Project training program was effective and well received by colleagues in mainland China.

INTRODUCTION

With the implementation of one-child policy from 1978 to 2015 and the expanding urban-rural gap in China, adolescent developmental problems have been a critical issue for psychologists, educators, scholars, and the Government in China. Research on the mental health condition of only-child expanded at a remarkable rate in past 10 years. For instance, Hesketh and his colleagues (1) estimated that the suicide rate of adolescents in China was around three times the global average. Xing et al. (2) reported that Chinese adolescents with suicide attempts usually have family problems, such as improper parental rearing behavior, parental divorce, and parental gambling problem. Moreover, it is estimated that over 24 million (14.1%) adolescents in urban cities displayed symptoms of internet addiction (3). In addition, it also revealed that the adolescents from less developed areas in China have higher prevalence rates of youth internet addiction problem (14.8%) than those from high developed cities (8.4%) (3).

In view of the above observations, it is advocated that effective positive youth development (PYD) programs to strengthen the psychosocial competencies of adolescents are in urgent need in China. The PYD approach emphasizes that "problem-free is not fully prepared" and utilizes the ecological (person-in-environment) and strengths-based principles (4). It focuses on preventing a wide range of adolescent developmental problems and needs, instead of merely preventing a single adolescent problem.

With particular reference to Hong Kong, adolescents are also facing different types of risk behavior such as substance abuse, materialism, suicide, and bullying (5). As such, a PYD program entitled "P.A.T.H.S. to Adulthood: A Jockey Club Youth Enhancement Scheme" funded by Hong Kong Jockey Club Charities Trust was launched in 2004. The project comprised of two tiers programs. While the Tier 1 Program was a universal curriculum-based program based on 15 PYD elements identified in the effective programs, such as bonding, social competence, cognitive competence, and behavioral competence (6), the Tier 2 Program was developed for participants who were identified with greater psychosocial needs and tailor-made special programs were constructed. Multiple evaluation studies revealed that project in Hong Kong has received notable success in promoting holistic youth development and preventing problem behavior among junior secondary school students (7-10).

Given the overwhelming success of project in Hong Kong, it is important to ask whether the program can promote the holistic development of adolescents in other Chinese communities. With the financial support from Tin Ka Ping Foundation, a project entitled "Tin Ka Ping P.A.T.H.S. Project" was implemented in four schools in East China, including Shanghai, Suzhou, Changzhou, and Yangzhou from 2011 to 2014, with good outcomes based on subjective and objective outcome evaluation (11, 12).

Despite the encouraging evaluation findings reported in four East China secondary schools (11, 12), we need to further understand the applicability of the program in other parts of China. Hence, a second phase of the Project P.A.T.H.S. designed for the junior secondary school students was implemented in more than 30 secondary schools in mainland China from the 2014-2015 academic year, with the first year as the preparatory year of a full-implementation stage.

Unlike other traditional youth prevention programs, this project emphasizes systematic training through experiential and reflective learning approaches. With respect to the training programs for the potential implementers of the project in Hong Kong, all potential implementers were expected to actively participate in the training process as students (13). Participants were given opportunities to reflect on their own values, teaching methods, and attitude towards adolescent development (14). Such an emphasis was also adopted in the training programs in mainland China. Specifically, four junior form training sessions were offered in Shanghai, Suzhou, and Chongqing in the preparatory year (2014-2015 academic year).

From 2015-2016 to 2016-2017 academic year, the program was launched in over 30 secondary schools in China. In the 2015-2016 academic year, three training workshops targeting potential implementers of the junior and senior secondary programs were held in Zhaoqing, Shaoguan (in Guangdong province), and Changchun (in Jilin province), respectively. The evaluation findings of the training held in Zhaoqing and Shaoguan have been documented (15, 16).

In this chapter, perceptions of the participants joining the training conducted in Changchun were examined. As the training was conducted during the summer holiday, the research team extended the training period from 3 days to 4 days. Therefore, more lesson demonstrations and in-depth sharing sessions from project schools were included. The contents of the third training workshop in Changchun are shown in the Appendix. There were several objectives of this training program: (a) to understand the concepts and rationale of PYD; (b) to understand the features of adolescent development and to develop positive attitudes towards adolescents; (c) to comprehend the rationales, design, implementation, and evaluation of the project; (d) to understand the contents and activities developed for the project; (e) to encourage participants to review and obtain appropriate attitude, knowledge, and teaching skills to facilitate program implementation; and (f) to develop a self-help network among the participants.

Although the importance of prevention programs and PYD programs for adolescents have been highlighted in previous studies, the significance of training programs for implementers tends to be overlooked. Clarke (17) believed that training program should be treated as a key strategy to help trainees familiarize with the program philosophy and content, and strengthen their enthusiasm and support for the program. Fullan (18) also pointed out that the impact of shared meaning and collaboration from the implementers would determine the effectiveness of educational program. Shek and Sun (19) listed five key factors contributing to the success of the PYD program, including program, process, policy, people, and place (i.e., 5 P's). Amongst these factors, "people," which included both program participants and implementers, was identified as the most influential factor affecting the effectiveness of the project (19). As such, providing systematic and on-site training for the potential program implementers should be taken into account in program delivery. Moreover, since there are very few PYD programs in China, it is important to provide comprehensive support and resources to the project schools and implementers through all-rounded in-service training.

In addition, it is advocated that training evaluation is necessary in every training program. Training evaluation refers to "the process of determining the merit, worth, and value of things, or the product of that process" (20). In other words, it is a methodological approach for measuring a training program's achievement with regard to program design and content, and changes in trainees. Kirkpatrick's (21) four dimensional training evaluation model (i.e., reactions, learning, behavior, and results) is widely used for understanding the purpose of in-service training evaluation. Training evaluation results can give scientific evidence to explain how the objectives of training program, content, and methods achieve the expected outcomes or benefits in the training (22). Furthermore, program developer can identify successful factors through evaluation and then improve program design and implementation in the future.

To date, several training evaluation studies of the project based on subjective outcome evaluation strategy have been conducted in Hong Kong (23-26). Comparatively speaking, there are still very few training evaluations conducted in Chinese communities. As reviewed by Yang and Guo (27), there were only 86 Chinese studies related to teacher training evaluations published in the last decade in 11 major Chinese or international databases. Besides, most of these studies simply focused on conceptual issues rather than investigating the efficacy of training programs. Most importantly, as the Project P.A.T.H.S. has moved to a full implementation stage, it is worth exploring the influence of its training program on potential implementers and collecting their feedbacks for further improvement.

The current study attempted to examine the effectiveness of the Project P.A.T.H.S. training program conducted in Changchun in August 2016. Similar to other training evaluation studies reported previously (15, 16), there are three research objectives of this paper: 1) to explore potential implementers' viewpoints towards the training program in the areas of training content, instructors' quality, self-performance, and administrative arrangements; 2) to examine the predictors of perceived benefits through the training program from the perspective of the participants; 3) to investigate the predictors of overall satisfaction with the training program amongst the participants.

OUR STUDY

In the academic year of 2015/2016, the third training workshop of the Tin Ka Ping P.A.T.H.S. Project was held in Changchun, China. There were altogether 208 teachers from 35 junior and/or senior secondary schools registering to attend this 4-day workshop.

During the last session of the workshop in Day 4, the participants reflected on their gains through the training, and they were invited to complete an anonymous questionnaire regarding their evaluation on this training workshop. Because of transportation constraints, some participants had to leave earlier upon the completion of the training. Finally, a total of 151 questionnaires were collected, including 70 (46.4%) questionnaires completed by junior secondary school teachers and 81 (53.6%) completed by senior secondary school teachers. Overall speaking, there were more female teachers (N = 103, 68.2%) than male teachers (N = 48, 31.8%) completing the evaluation after the training. Among all the respondents, 62.9% (N = 95) had over 10 years of teaching experience. In addition, the mean years of working experience of the respondents was 12.6 (SD = 8.42).

Instruments

The participants' perceptions of the training workshop were measured utilizing the Subjective Outcome Evaluation Questionnaire developed by Shek and his colleagues (24). The evaluation questionnaire consists of 33 items, including four subscales measured by 31 closed-ended questions and two open-ended questions.

Regarding the four subscales, each respondent is asked to rate the items on a 5-point Likert scale with responses ranging from "strongly disagree" to "strongly agree." The first subscale, comprising 16 items, measures participants' overall view of the program training content, including the perceived benefits of the program (9 items), perceived program quality (5 items) and satisfaction degree of participants (2 items). The second subscale investigates participants' perceptions of the instructors with 5 items. The third subscale, consisting of 4 items, assesses participants' reflections on their own performance. The fourth subscale focuses on participants' evaluations of the administrative arrangements of the training. The two open-ended questions examine participants' most appreciated part of the training and their suggestion for the workshop.

The quantitative part of the questionnaire has demonstrated excellent internal consistency (Cronbach's $\alpha > .9$) in previous studies evaluating the training programs in Hong Kong (25, 26). The current study focused on the participants' perceptions by analyzing the data from the four subscales.

FINDINGS

Table 1 shows that the reliability measures for the total scale (Cronbach's $\alpha = .95$) and subscales of the Subjective Outcome Evaluation Questionnaire (Cronbach's alpha ranged from .66 to .93) had good reliability status. Although the alpha value for the overall satisfaction subscale was not high (Cronbach's $\alpha = .66$), it can be regarded as reasonable because there are only two items in this subscale.

Participants' perceptions of the program content, program instructors, their own performance and the administrative arrangements of the training are shown in Tables 2-5 respectively. The numbers and percentages of positive responses (scores equal to or above 4) to each item and subscale are presented. In general, the majority (over 80%) of the participants held a positive view regarding program benefits, program quality, program instructors and the administrative arrangements. And taken as a whole, nearly 90% of the participants were satisfied with the workshop. However, relatively fewer participants (74.7%) expressed positive views about their self-performance, although the value was respectable.

Table 1. Means, standard deviations, Cronbach's alphas, and mean of inter-item correlations

Subjective Outcome Evaluation Scales	*M*	*SD*	Cronbach's *α*	Mean Inter-item correlation
Perception of the training program (16 items)	4.42	0.43	.93	.47
Perceived benefits (9 items)	4.44	0.44	.89	.49
Program quality (5 items)	4.39	0.48	.81	.47
Overall satisfaction (2 items)	4.33	0.54	.66	.49
Perception of program instructor (5 items)	4.49	0.46	.85	.54
Perception of self-performance (4 items)	4.15	0.53	.81	.52
Perception of administrative arrangements (6 items)	4.44	0.49	.91	.65
Total scale (31 items)	4.41	0.39	.95	.40

Table 2. Summary of the positive views (options 4-5) of the participants towards the training program

Perceptions of the program		N	Agree (4)		Strongly Agree (5)		Positive Response (Options 4-5)		*M*	*SD*
			n	%	*n*	%	*n*	%		
Perceived benefits [a]		146					127	87.0	4.44	0.44
1.	It has strengthened my understanding of the nature of adolescent development.	147	71	48.3	71	48.3	142	96.6	4.45	0.56
2.	It has helped me to cultivate positive attitude to adolescent development.	147	55	37.4	90	61.2	145	98.6	4.6	0.52
3.	It has strengthened my understanding of positive youth development, including its concept, design and research.	147	60	40.8	80	54.4	140	95.2	4.5	0.59
4.	It has helped me to understand the Project P.A.T.H.S., including its basic philosophy, design, implementation, and evaluation.	147	62	42.2	74	50.3	136	92.5	4.43	0.63
5.	It has strengthened me to understand the content of the Project P.A.T.H.S..	147	68	46.2	72	49.0	140	95.2	4.44	0.59
6.	It has helped me to acquire the attitude, knowledge and skills that are conducive to the successful implementation of the Project P.A.T.H.S..	147	76	51.7	57	38.8	133	90.5	4.29	0.65
7.	It has helped me to establish self-help support network and share teaching experiences among the program participants.	147	58	39.5	71	48.3	129	87.8	4.36	0.69
8.	It has promoted self-reflection.	147	65	44.2	78	53.1	143	97.3	4.5	0.55
9.	It has helped me to recognize factors affecting teaching.	146	71	48.6	67	45.9	138	94.5	4.4	0.59
Program quality [a]		145					121	83.4	4.39	0.48
1.	The training methods and activities are appropriate (e.g., lecture, games, group discussion).	147	64	43.8	80	54.8	144	98.6	4.53	0.53
2.	Training time is appropriate.	147	74	50.3	45	30.6	119	80.9	4.08	0.77
3.	It has met my expectation.	147	73	49.7	54	36.7	127	86.4	4.23	0.67
4.	There was much peer interaction amongst participants.	146	59	40.4	81	55.5	140	95.9	4.51	0.60
5.	Instructor(s) encouraged participants to do the best.	147	53	36.1	88	59.9	141	96.0	4.55	0.60

Table 2. (Continued)

Perceptions of the program		N	Agree (4)		Strongly Agree (5)		Positive Response (Options 4-5)		*M*	*SD*
			n	%	*n*	%	*n*	%		
Overall satisfaction [a]		145					130	89.7	4.33	0.54
1.	Overall speaking, I am satisfied with the training program.	147	73	49.7	67	45.5	140	95.2	4.41	0.58
2.	I think participants are satisfied with the training program.	145	72	49.7	55	37.9	127	87.6	4.25	0.68
Perceptions of the program (whole scale)[a]		143					116	81.1	4.42	0.43

Note: [a] Scores equal to or higher than 4 were treated as positive views.

Table 3. Summary of the positive views (options 4-5) of the participants towards the program instructor(s)

Perceptions of the program instructor(s)		N	**Agree (4)**		**Strongly Agree (5)**		**Positive Response (Options 4-5)**		*M*	*SD*
			n	%	*n*	%	*n*	%		
1.	The instructor(s) had good mastery of the curriculum.	147	73	49.7	71	48.3	144	98.0	4.46	0.54
2.	The instructor(s) understood the needs of participants.	147	69	46.9	60	40.8	129	87.7	4.29	0.67
3.	The instructor(s) showed good professional attitude.	147	35	23.8	110	74.8	145	98.6	4.73	0.47
4.	The instructor(s)' teaching was clear and easy to understand.	147	67	45.6	63	42.9	130	88.5	4.31	0.67
5.	Overall speaking, I have positive evaluation of the instructor(s)' teaching performance.	147	46	31.3	98	66.7	144	98.0	4.65	0.52
Total scale [a]		147					134	91.2	4.49	0.46

Note: [a] Scores equal to or higher than 4 were treated as positive views.

Table 4. Summary of the positive views (options 4-5) of participants towards their own performance in training

Perceptions of self-performance		N	**Agree (4)**		**Strongly Agree (5)**		**Positive Response (Options 4-5)**		*M*	*SD*
			n	%	*n*	%	*n*	%		
1.	I participated actively during discussion.	151	80	53.0	37	24.5	117	77.5	4.01	0.72
2.	I am willing to apply the specific skills and theories learnt from this training program.	151	76	50.3	69	45.7	145	96.0	4.42	0.57
3.	After attending the training program, I have confidence in program implementation.	151	85	56.3	49	32.5	134	88.8	4.21	0.63
4.	Overall speaking, I am satisfied with my performance.	150	85	56.7	33	22.0	118	78.7	3.97	0.74
Total scale [a]		150					112	74.7	4.15	0.53

Note: [a] Scores equal to or higher than 4 were treated as positive views.

Table 5. Summary of the positive views (options 4-5) of participants towards administrative arrangements

Perceptions of the administrative arrangements		N	Satisfied (4)		Very Satisfied (5)		Positive Response (Options 4-5)		*M*	*SD*
			n	%	*n*	%	*n*	%		
1.	Information obtained before attending the workshop.	151	76	50.3	55	36.4	131	86.7	4.23	0.69
2.	Workshop assigned.	150	74	49.3	64	42.7	138	92.0	4.35	0.62
3.	Location of the workshop.	151	75	49.7	71	47.0	146	97.7	4.44	0.56
4.	Reception provided by training team (e.g., transportation arrangement, refreshments).	151	59	39.1	88	58.3	147	97.4	4.56	0.55
5.	Facilities of the venue.	151	64	42.4	82	54.3	146	96.7	4.51	0.56
6.	Overall speaking, I am satisfied with the administrative arrangement.	151	61	40.4	89	58.9	150	99.3	4.58	0.51
Total scale [a]		150					130	86.7	4.44	0.49

Note: [a] Scores equal to or higher than 4 were treated as positive views.

Regarding perceived benefits, more than 90% of the respondents agreed or strongly agreed that they benefitted from the training, including a better understanding of adolescent development (96.6%) and positive youth development (95.2%), cultivation of positive attitude to adolescent development (98.6%), self-reflection (97.3%), and recognition of factors affecting teaching (94.5%). In addition, through the workshop, the teachers were more familiar with the project (92.5%), understood the content of the Tier 1 Program (95.2%), and acquired knowledge and skills implementing the program (90.5%). Nearly 90% of the respondents agreed that they established a self-help support network in the training.

The teachers in the training were also satisfied with the program quality. Almost all of them (98.6%) agreed that the training methods and activities were appropriate. They also held a positive view about peer interaction amongst teachers during the training (95.9%). Most participants had positive evaluation of program instructors. They agreed that the instructors were a professional team with good mastery of the curriculum (98%), clear understanding of the needs of the participants (87.7%), profession attitude (98.6%) and good teaching skills (88.5%). The participants also showed positive response toward the administrative arrangements of the program. After the training, 96% of the teachers expressed their willingness to use the theories and skills learnt through this training workshop.

To investigate whether there were differences between junior and senior secondary school teachers regarding their perceptions of the training workshop, a MANOVA analysis was performed. As demonstrated in Table 6, based on the omnibus F test, no statistically significant difference was found between the junior form and senior form programs in terms of the overall perception of the training ($F = 1.54$, $p > .05$).

Table 6. The comparison between junior and senior secondary school participants on the perceptions of the training program

Subjective Outcome Evaluation Scales	Senior			Junior			*F*
	N	*M*	*SD*	*N*	*M*	*SD*	1.54
Program content (16 items)	66	4.48	.40	77	4.36	.45	2.78
Perceived benefits (9 items)	66	4.51	.42	80	4.37	.45	3.81
Program quality (5 items)	67	4.45	.42	78	4.33	.52	2.29
Overall satisfaction (2 items)	67	4.42	.54	78	4.26	.54	2.98
Program instructor (5 items)	67	4.51	.44	80	4.47	.48	.36
Perceived self-performance (4 items)	69	4.30	.49	81	4.02	.54	11.16**
Administrative arrangements (6 items)	70	4.52	.45	80	4.37	.51	3.5
Total scale (31 items)	65	4.47	.36	76	4.34	.40	3.6

Note: $^{**}p < .01$.

Table 7. Pearson correlations among the key evaluation components

Variable	1	2	3	4	5	6
Perceived benefits (9 items)	-					
Perceived program quality (5 items)	.82***	-				
Instructor quality (5 items)	.64***	.60***	-			
Self-performance (4 items)	.54***	.50***	.38***	-		
Administrative arrangements (6 items)	.65***	.61***	.51***	.51***	-	
Overall satisfaction (2 items)	.69***	.76***	.50***	.44***	.58***	-

Note:$^{***}p < .001$.

Table 8. Multiple regression analyses predicting perceived benefits and overall satisfaction

Predictors	Perceived Benefits				Overall Satisfaction			
	B	*SE*	*β*	R^2	*B*	*SE*	*β*	R^2
Perceived program quality	0.53	.06	.57***	.74	0.64	.11	.55***	.60
Instructor quality	0.15	.06	.15**		0.03	.09	.023	
Self-performance	0.10	.04	.12*		0.04	.07	.03	
Administrative arrangements	0.15	.06	.16**		.16	.09	.14	
Perceived benefits					.13	.13	.11	

Note: $^*p < .05$; $^{**}p < .01$; $^{***}p < .001$.

The correlations among participants' perceptions of perceived benefits, program quality, instructor quality, self-performance, administrative arrangements, and overall satisfaction were examined using Pearson correlation analyses. The findings shown in Table 7 demonstrate that all related variables were significantly and positively associated to different extent (*r*s ranged from .38 to .82, *p*s < .001). In addition, a strong relationship was observed between perceived benefits and program quality ($r = .82$, $p < .001$).

To investigate the predictors of perceived benefits of the participants and factors associated with their overall satisfaction, two multiple regression analyses were performed. The findings in Table 8 show that program quality ($\beta = .57$, $p < .001$), instructor quality ($\beta = .15$, $p < .01$), self-performance ($\beta = .12$, $p < .05$) and administrative arrangements ($\beta = .16$, $p < .01$) could significantly predict the perceived effect of the program, with program quality as the strongest predictor of perceived benefits. Program quality also predicted overall satisfaction of the participants ($\beta = .55$, $p < .001$). However, other factors, including instructor quality, self-performance, administrative arrangements and perceived benefits did not significantly contribute to the overall satisfaction.

DISCUSSION

To promote the holistic and positive development in Chinese adolescents, the Project P.A.T.H.S. was transplanted to mainland China and has been implemented in over 30 secondary schools across the country (12, 29). Obviously, in-service training offered to school teachers is regarded as an indispensable part of this large scale implementation, because teachers usually play a crucial role in implementing the program in the front line (28, 30). In the training conducted in Changchun, participants showed enthusiasm towards the training by positive registering, learning, discussing, reflecting and sharing. In the present study, subjective outcome evaluation was used to examine the efficacy of this training program.

The present research findings demonstrate an overall success of the training program. Consistent with the previous training programs conducted in Hong Kong and other mainland cities, the training program received very positive feedbacks from the participants (25, 26, 28). Overall speaking, the quantitative evaluation results showed that a very high percentage of the participants were satisfied with the program content, instructors and administrative arrangement. Besides, majority of the participants agreed that they gained a higher level of competence in teaching PYD curriculums through this training and optimistic about the implementation of the project in the future. The present study also replicated previous evaluation findings that both junior and senior high school teachers held positive views towards the training program (15). Thus, we concluded that the training program was well-received in the mainland China. As some studies suggest a positive correlation between subjective outcome and objective outcome evaluation findings (31-33), it is conjectured that the teachers might possibly perform well in their actual teaching. Of course, future studies should examine whether teachers' positive perceptions of the training predict successful objective outcomes of the project in mainland China.

The present study also identified factors that contributed to a successful training program. Participants' perceived program quality as the strongest predictor of their perceived program benefits and their overall satisfaction, which was in line with the findings of previous trainings in mainland China

(34-36). The participants in Changchun training demonstrated an overall satisfaction with the program quality. This finding suggests that in future training programs, training implementers may use Changchun training design as a reference, such as using more interactive training methods and activities, being sensitive to teachers' needs and expectation, and encouraging peer interaction and self-reflection. In addition to the perceived quality of program and instructor, participants' self-performance and administrative arrangements of the training were also found to be important predictors of perceived program benefits. Hence, it is important for the trainers to have a holistic view when designing the training, and to take all these program components, including program quality, instructor quality, self-performance and administrative arrangements, into account (37).

Although the present study provides strong evidence that the training in Changchun is beneficial to the program participants, some limitations should be noted. First, subjective outcome evaluation in the present study was limited to quantitative data only. Although the quantitative approach is cost-effective and it favors objectivity, representativeness and generalization, qualitative approach is an important alternative or complementary evaluation method which can help to develop an in-depth understanding of the program benefits (38). Thus, qualitative evaluation of subjective outcomes (e.g., in-depth individual interview and focus group interview) should be included in future research to generate an integrated picture of effectiveness. Second, in addition to subjective evaluation, objective outcome evaluation is also recommended which can give a better understanding of training effectiveness in implementing the project in mainland China. Third, other factors that could affect participants' subjective evaluation of training, such as teachers' previous training attendance record and program implementation experiences, should be included in future studies. Despite the limitations above, the favorable evaluation findings suggest that the Changchun training program for the Project P.A.T.H.S. is well received in mainland China.

ACKNOWLEDGMENTS

The preparation for this paper and the Tin Ka Ping P.A.T.H.S. Project are financially supported by Tin Ka Ping Foundation. This chapter is a reprint with minor revisions of an earlier published paper in the *International Public Health Journal* 2018;10(1) issue with permission.

APPENDIX. CONTENT OF THE THIRD TRAINING PROGRAM IN THE 2015-2016 ACADEMIC YEAR IN CHANGCHUN, CHINA

Junior Group	
Day 1 (6.5 hours)	
Themes and objectives	Activities conducted
Introduce the latest progress of the Tin Ka Ping P.A.T.H.S. Project in the full implementation phase (2015-2016); Offer opportunities for junior and senior school delegates, principals, and teachers to share their experiences; and Familiarize the participants with the teaching units related to the constructs of "Cognitive Competence" (CC).	Introduce the Tin Ka Ping P.A.T.H.S. Project and the professional team; Introduce the training schedules of the Project; Guide the participants how to use the updated teaching materials and other online resources on the website; Introduce the Co-Walker Scheme; Report the results of evaluation of the second training program in Shaoguan; School sharing from Changchun on the implementation progress of senior programs; Warm-up activities; Lecture on the constructs of "Cognitive Competence" (CC) and the contents of units; Sharing session from participatory schools.
Day 2 (6.5 hours)	
Themes and objectives	Activities conducted
Offer opportunities for schools from Changchun and other participatory schools to share their teaching experiences and demonstrate teaching techniques; and Familiarize the participants with teaching method of the Tin Ka Ping P.A.T.H.S. Project.	Warm-up activities; Lesson demonstrations by experienced school teachers from participating schools; Group discussion and Q&A session.

Appendix (Continued)

Day 3 (6.5 hours)	
Themes and objectives	Activities conducted
Familiarize the teachers with the constructs and teaching units; Clarify participants' questions on project implementation; and Familiarize the participants with the teaching units related to the constructs of "Moral Competence" (MC) and "Self-Determination" (SD) Familiarize the participants with teaching method of the Tin Ka Ping P.A.T.H.S. Project.	Warm-up activities; Group discussions on "How to be a good P.A.T.H.S. teacher?", "How to teach a good lesson of P.A.T.H.S.?", and "How to implement P.A.T.H.S. much better?" Lecture on the constructs of "Moral Competence" (MC) and the contents of units; Sharing session from participatory schools.
Day 4 (6.5 hours)	
Themes and objectives	Activities conducted
Familiarize the teachers with the constructs and teaching units; Clarify participants' questions on project implementation; Familiarize the participants with teaching method of the Tin Ka Ping P.A.T.H.S. Project; and Familiarize the participants with the teaching units related to the constructs of "Self-Determination" (SD), "Spirituality" (SP), and "Clear and Positive Identity" (ID).	Warm-up activities; Lecture on the constructs of "Self-Determination" (SD) and the contents of the unit; Lecture on the constructs of "Spirituality" (SP) and the contents of the unit; Lecture on the constructs of "Clear and Positive Identity" (ID) and the contents of the unit; Sharing session from participatory schools; Interactive lecture on the teaching technique (Stress and fatigue for teachers); Introduce the evaluation results of 2015/16 academic year; Wrapping up and self-reflection; and Conclusion.
Senior Group	
Day 1 (6.5 hours)	
Themes and objectives	Activities conducted
Introduce the latest progress of the Tin Ka Ping P.A.T.H.S. Project during the full implementation phase (2015-2016); Familiarize the teachers with the constructs and teaching units.	Introduce the Tin Ka Ping P.A.T.H.S. Project and the professional team; Warm-up activities; Introduce the training schedules of the Project; Guide the participants how to use the updated teaching materials and other resources of Tin Ka Ping P.A.T.H.S. Project; Introduce the Co-Walker Scheme; Report the results of the second training program evaluation; Lecture on the constructs of "Social Competence (SC)" and the contents of the unit;

Day 1 (6.5 hours)	
Themes and objectives	Activities conducted
	Lecture on the constructs of "Emotional Competence (EC)" and the contents of the unit; Lecture on the constructs of "Behavioral Competence (BC)" and the contents of the unit; Sharing session from participatory schools; Group discussion and Q&A session
Day 2 (6.5 hours)	
Themes and objectives	Activities conducted
Offer opportunities for school delegates to share their implementation experiences and teaching plans; and Familiarize the participants with teaching method of the Tin Ka Ping P.A.T.H.S. Project.	Lesson demonstration by school teachers from participating schools; Group discussion and Q&A session.
Day 3 (6.5 hours)	
Themes and objectives	Activities conducted
Familiarize the teachers with the constructs and teaching units. Clarify participants' questions on project implementation; and Familiarize the participants with teaching method of the Tin Ka Ping P.A.T.H.S. Project.	Warm-up activities; Lecture on the constructs of "Cognitive Competence" (CC) and the contents of the unit; Lecture on the constructs of "Self-Efficacy" (SE) and the contents of the unit; Lecture on the constructs of "Moral Competence" (MC) and the contents of the unit; Lecture on the constructs of "Behavioral Competence" (BC) and the contents of the unit; Group discussion on "How to be a good P.A.T.H.S. teacher?", "How to teach a good lesson of P.A.T.H.S.?", and "How to implement P.A.T.H.S. much better?"
Day 4 (6.5 hours)	
Themes and objectives	Activities conducted
Familiarize the teachers with the constructs and teaching units; Clarify participants' questions on project implementation; and Familiarize the participants with teaching method of the Tin Ka Ping P.A.T.H.S. Project.	Warm-up activities; Lecture on the constructs of "Behavioral Competence" (BC) and the contents of the unit; Lecture on the constructs of "Social Competence" (SC) and the content of the unit; Lecture on the constructs of "Resilience" (RE) and the contents of the unit; Sharing session from participatory schools; Interactive lecture on the teaching technique (Stress and fatigue for teachers); Introduce the evaluation results of 2015/16 academic year; Wrapping up and self-reflection; and Conclusion.

REFERENCES

[1] Hesketh T, Ding QJ, Jenkins R. Suicide ideation in Chinese adolescents. Soc Psychiatry Psychiatr Epidemiol 2002;37(5):230-5.

[2] Xing XY, Tao FB, Wan YH, Xing C, Qi XY, Hao JH, et al. Family factors associated with suicide attempts among Chinese adolescent students: A national cross-sectional survey. J Adolesc Health 2010;46(6):592-9.

[3] China Youth Association for Network Development. Report on youth internet addiction. China: China Youth Association for Network Development, 2010. [Chinese].

[4] Daemon W. What is positive youth development?. Ann Am Acad Pol Soc Sci 2004;591:13-24.

[5] Shek DTL, Ma HK, Sun RCF. A brief overview of adolescent developmental problems in Hong Kong. ScientificWorldJournal 2011;11:2243-56.

[6] Catalano RF, Berglund ML, Ryan JA, Lonczak HS, Hawkins JD. Positive youth development in the United States: Research findings on evaluations of positive youth development programs. Ann Am Acad Pol Soc Sci 2004;591:98-124.

[7] Shek DTL, Sun RCF. Using student weekly diary to evaluation positive youth development programs: The case of Project P.A.T.H.S. in Hong Kong. Int J Child Adolesc Health 2008;1(2):93-102.

[8] Shek DTL, Sun RCF. Development, implementation and evaluation of a holistic positive youth development program: Project P.A.T.H.S. in Hong Kong. Int J Disabil Hum Dev 2009;8:107-18.

[9] Shek DTL, Ma CMS. Objective outcome evaluation of the Project P.A.T.H.S.: Longitudinal study based on indicators of positive youth development. In: Shek DTL, Sun RCF. eds. Development and evaluation of positive adolescent training through holistic social programs (P.A.T.H.S.), 2013:69-84.

[10] Shek DTL, Sun RCF. Positive youth development programs for adolescents with greater psychosocial needs: Subjective outcome evaluation over 3 years. J Pediatr Adolesc Gynecol 2014;27(S):S17-25.

[11] Shek DTL, Han XY, Lee TY, Yu L. Subjective outcome evaluation of a positive youth development program in China. Int J Disabil Hum Dev 2014;13:275-83.

[12] Shek DTL, Yu L, Sun RCF, Lee TY, Han XY, Li XX, et al. Objective outcome evaluation of a positive youth development program in China. Int J Disabil Hum Dev 2014;13:255-65.

[13] Shek DTL, Chak YLY. Design of training programs for a positive youth development program: Project P.A.T.H.S. in Hong Kong. Int J Adolesc Med Health 2010;22:345-67.

[14] Shek DTL, Leung H. Subjective outcome evaluation of the training program of the Project P.A.T.H.S.: Findings based on the revised training program. Int J Disabil Hum Dev 2014;13:267-74.

[15] Shek DTL, Lee TY, Wu J. Subjective outcome evaluation of a training program of Tin Ka Ping P.A.T.H.S. Project in China. Int Public Health J 2017;9(3), in press.

[16] Shek DTL, Leung JTY, Wu J. Subjective evaluation of a training program of the Tin Ka Ping P.A.T.H.S. Project in mainland China. Int Public Health J 2017;9(3), in press.

[17] Clarke N. The impact of in-service training within social services. Br J Soc Work 2001;31:757-74.

[18] Fullan M. This new meaning of education change, 3rd ed. New York: Teachers College Press, 2001.

[19] Shek DTL, Sun RCF. The Project P.A.T.H.S. in Hong Kong—Lessons learned and implications for positive youth development programs. ScientificWorldJournal 2012;2012:Article ID 687536. DOI: 10.1100/2012/687536.

[20] Scriven M. Evaluation thesaurus, 4th ed. Newbury Park, CA: Sage, 1991.

[21] Kirkpatrick DL, eds. Evaluating training programs: The four levels, 1st ed. San Francisco, CA: Berrett-Koehler, 2006.

[22] Salas E, Cannon-Bowers JA. The science of training: A decade of progress. Ann Rev Psychol 2001;52:471-99.

[23] Shek DTL, Wong KK. Qualitative evaluation of the training program of the Project P.A.T.H.S. in Hong Kong. Int J Adolesc Med Health 2010;22:413-23.

[24] Shek DTL, Wong KK. Subjective outcome evaluation of the training program of the Project P.A.T.H.S. based on qualitative findings. Int J Adolesc Med Health 2010;22:437-47.

[25] Shek DTL, Chak YLY. Training evaluation of the secondary 3 training program of the Project P.A.T.H.S. in Hong Kong. Int J Adolesc Med Health 2011;23:333-9.

[26] Shek DTL, Chak YLY. Evaluation of the training program of the Project P.A.T.H.S.: Findings based on the perspective of the participants from different cohorts. ScientificWorldJournal 2012;2012:Article ID: 687198. DOI: 10.1100/2012/687198

[27] Yang YJ, Guo ZQ. Evaluation on teacher training. Teach Dev Forum 2012;8:9-13.

[28] Shek DTL, Chak YLY. Subjective outcome evaluation of the secondary 2 training program of the Project P.A.T.H.S. in Hong Kong. Int J Adolesc Med Health 2011;23(4):325-32.

[29] Shek DTL, Han XY, Lee TY, Yu L. Impact of the Project P.A.T.H.S. in China. In: Shek DTL, Sun RCF, eds. Development and evaluation of Positive Adolescent Training through Holistic Social Programs (P.A.T.H.S.). Singapore: Springer Singapore, 2013:291-304.

[30] Shek DTL, Sun RCF. Implementation of a positive youth development program in a Chinese context: The role of policy, program, people, process, and place. ScientificWorldJournal 2008;8:980-96.

[31] Shek DTL. Subjective outcome and objective outcome evaluation findings: Insights from a Chinese context. Res Soc Work Pract 2009;20(3):293-301.

[32] Shek DTL. Is subjective outcome evaluation related to objective outcome evaluation? Insights from a longitudinal study in Hong Kong. J Pediatr Adolesc Gynecol 2014;27:S50-6.

[33] Shek DTL, Han XY. The relationship between subjective outcome evaluation and objective outcome evaluation findings: Evidence from China. Int J Disabil Hum Dev 2014;13(4):497-503.

[34] Shek DTL, Chung CK, Sun RCF. Evaluation of a training program of the Tin Ka Ping P.A.T.H.S. Project in mainland China. Int J Child Adolesc Health 2017, in press.

[35] Shek DTL, Pu EXP, Wu FKY. Evaluation of the training program of the Tin Ka Ping P.A.T.H.S. Project in mainland China. Int J Child Adolesc Health 2017, in press.

[36] Shek DTL, Zhu XQ, Leung JTY. Subjective outcome evaluation of the Tin Ka Ping P.A.T.H.S. project training program in mainland China. Int J Child Adolesc Health 2017, in press.

[37] Tan SC, Hu C, Wong SK, Wettasinghe CM. Teacher training on technology-enhanced instruction – a holistic approach. J Educ Techno Soc 2003;6(1):96-104.

[38] Shek DTL, Sun RCF. Qualitative evaluation of Project P.A.T.H.S.: An integration of findings based on program participants. ScientificWorldJournal 2012;2012:Article ID 528483: DOI:10.1100/2012/528483.

In: Advances in Chinese Children … ISBN: 978-1-53617-870-8
Editors: Ariel Tenenbaum et al. © 2020 Nova Science Publishers, Inc.

Chapter 11

TIN KA PING P.A.T.H.S. PROJECT IN MAINLAND CHINA: PRELIMINARY EVALUATION FINDINGS

Daniel TL Shek[1,*], PhD, FHKPS, BBS, SBS, JP, Tak-Yan Lee[2], PhD, Rachel CF Sun[3], PhD, Florence KY Wu[3], EdD and Janet TY Leung[1], PhD

[1]Department of Applied Social Sciences,
The Hong Kong Polytechnic University, Hong Kong, PR China
[2]Department of Social and Behavioral Sciences, Hong Kong, PR China
[3]Faculty of Education, The University of Hong Kong,
Hong Kong, PR China

* Corresponding Author: Professor Daniel TL Shek, PhD, FHKPS, BBS, SBS, JP, Associate Vice President (Undergraduate Programme) and Chair Professor of Applied Social Sciences, Department of Applied Social Sciences, The Hong Kong Polytechnic University, Hunghom, Hong Kong, PR China. Email: daniel.shek@polyu.edu.hk.

ABSTRACT

The Tin Ka Ping (TKP) P.A.T.H.S. Project is a pioneer positive youth development program implemented in China. In this study, subjective outcome evaluation data from two junior secondary schools in mainland China were used to reach a tentative understanding of students' opinions about program design, program instructors, and benefits of the program. Consistent with pervious findings in Hong Kong, the great majority of the students showed positive feelings of the program content, instructors, and program effectiveness. As predicted, program content, instructors, and effectiveness were significantly inter-correlated. Perceived program content and quality of instruction were also identified to be significant predictors of program effectiveness perceived by student participants. The present findings suggest that TKP P.A.T.H.S. program was well received by the students in mainland China.

INTRODUCTION

In the past few decades, positive youth development (PYD) approach has been widely used to promote holistic development for youths and young adults in Western countries (1, 2). Additionally, the approach is well adopted in the Chinese contexts (3, 4). In Hong Kong, the P.A.T.H.S. Project was designed utilizing 15 constructs of positive adolescent development recognized in the scientific literature (5). Systematic evaluation studies of the programs in the P.A.T.H.S. Project have shown that they have helped promote adolescent well-being and delayed the onset of risk behavior (6-8).

In terms of youth issues, it is noteworthy that adolescents in mainland China show many forms of risk behavior (9, 10). With a highly competitive education system, young people on the mainland also face very high academic stress. It is important to ask how we can promote holistic development for Chinese students in mainland China. Obviously, with the successful implementation experience of the P.A.T.H.S. Project in Hong Kong, it is expected that the project could be further transplanted to mainland China, where has similar cultural context with Hong Kong. Financially the P.A.T.H. Project was fully supported by Tin Ka Ping (TKP) Foundation. The P.A.T.H.S. Project was preliminary transplanted as a pilot scheme to four schools in Shanghai, Suzhou, Changzhou and Yangzhou in eastern China since 2011. During 2011-2014, teaching materials in simplified Chinese were developed by the Hong Kong Research Team, and teacher training and program evaluation were also implemented in mainland China. Because of the extensive support from TKP schools located throughout the country, the second phase (preparatory phase) of the project was launched in fall 2014, with the objective of providing systematic training and "trial" experience for the school teachers who are the potential instructors of the project (11). In 2014-15 school year, four training programs had been offered in three different cities in eastern or western China, including Shanghai, Suzhou and Chongqing (12-15). Besides attending the training programs, some schools also tried out the program.

To facilitate systematic evaluation of the TKP P.A.T.H.S. Project, the Research Team briefed the teachers in the training programs regarding the three major project evaluation strategies: (a) objective outcome evaluation using validated scales; (b) subjective outcome evaluation on the base of the replies in Form A (for the program participants) and Form B (for the program implementers), and (c) qualitative evaluation such as collection of students' diaries. With particular reference to the views of the program participants, the instrument used in evaluation (i.e., Form A) has three primary dimensions (program content, program instructors, and program effectiveness), which had excellent psychometric properties (16). The adoption of Form A as an evaluation tool has three advantages. First, we can aggregate data from multiple years that can show a general profile of the responses of participants. Second, the tool has been validated with excellent psychometric properties. Finally, subjective outcome evaluation is a relatively economical way to conduct program evaluation (17, 18).

The objective of the present study was to investigate the views of the student participants' on the TKP P.A.T.H.S. program implemented in mainland China. Three sets of research questions were addressed in the study:

- Question 1: What are student participants' perceptions of the program content, program instructors (teachers), and program effectiveness? Based on previous studies conducted in Hong Kong, it was predicted that the participants would be satisfied with the program content, program instructors and program effectiveness (Hypothesis 1).

- Question 2: What are the inter-relationships amongst program content, quality of instruction, and program effectiveness perceived by the participants? Based on the literature, it was expected that there would be a correlation between perceived program content and program instructors (Hypothesis 2a), perceived program content and program effectiveness (Hypothesis 2b), and perceived program instructors and program effectiveness (Hypothesis 2c).
- Question 3: What are the predictors of perceived program effectiveness? Based on previous findings, we predicted that perceived program content and program instructors would predict program effectiveness (Hypothesis 3a and 3b).

OUR STUDY

In the 2014–15 school year, data was collected using the questionnaire Form A from two schools (N = 521). Both schools followed the standardized instructions regarding student data collection and data entry that were given in Form A and provided by the Research Team. Passive informed consent was obtained from the student participating in the program at the beginning of the survey. The students could withdraw from the study if they did not want to participate. All students filled out the survey in a self-administered manner.

Instruments

Form A assesses the subjective views of the program participants. It was widely used in different schools in the Hong Kong P.A.T.H.S. Project. Program participants were invited to use Form A to share their perceptions of program content, program instructors (teachers, social workers, other workers), and program effectiveness after participating in TKP P.A.T.H.S. Project. From the findings in previous evaluation research, it has been found that Form A possesses excellent psychometric properties (16). Form A includes five parts:

- *Part 1 (participants' evaluations of the program content).* There are 10 items, which include students' perceptions of the curriculum objectives, course design, interaction with the instructors, and student participation in learning. Details of the items are shown in Table 1.
- *Part 2 (participants' evaluation of the program instructors).* There are 10 items including students' perception of the teaching, class preparation, the teachers' professional attitude, and the teachers' caring and supportive attitude. Details of the items are shown in Table 2.
- *Part 3 (participants' evaluation of program effectiveness).* There are 16 items assessing students' perception of the program benefits to their PYD, such as promotion of bonding, emotional competence, social skills and competence, or moral competence. Details of the items are shown in Table 3.
- *Part 4 (participants' overall satisfaction with the program).* There are three items measuring satisfaction. They inquire whether the students will recommend their friends to join the program, whether the students would like to participate in similar programs again, and the students' global satisfaction with the TKP P.A.T.H.S. program.
- *Part 5 (four open-ended questions).* Students are invited to share their views and feelings on things they learned and appreciated, to give suggestions to the teachers, and recommendations for the program.

Data analyses

SPSS 23 (IBM SPSS Statistics, IBM Corp, Somers, NY) was used for all the data analyses. Four subscale variables were created: (a) "program content (VC)" was the mean score of the 10 items in Part 1; (b) "program instructors (VI)" was the mean score of the 10 items in Part 2; (c) "program effectiveness (EF)" was the mean score of the 16 items in Part 3; (d) "total effectiveness" was calculated as the overall mean score of all the 36 items in Part 1, 2, and 3. Data analyses in this study only covered the quantitative data in Part 1 to Part 4.

Descriptive analyses were conducted to calculate the mean and standard deviations of each subscale. Reliability analyses were performed to measure the internal consistency of the above subscales and the overall scale. Pearson correlation coefficients were also calculated to examine interrelationships amongst the variables. Lastly, multiple regression analyses were performed to examine whether perceived program content and instructors predict program effectiveness. All the above analyses were conducted for the two schools (School 1 and School 2) separately and aggregately.

FINDINGS

Form A showed good psychometric properties. As the findings shown in Table 4, the scale had good internal consistency in School 1, School 2, and the overall sample. In the overall sample ($N = 521$), the reliability estimates were good: the Cronbach's alpha value for the total effectiveness scale was .96, and the Cronbach's alpha values for the subscales of program content, program instructors, and program effectiveness were .88, .93 and .94 respectively; the mean of inter-item correlation for the scale and subscales above, respectively was .38, .42, .56, and .51.

Table 1. Descriptive statistics of the participants' evaluations of the program content

	Respondents with positive responses (Options 4-6)					
	School 1		School 2		Overall	
	n	%	*n*	%	*N*	%
1) The objectives of the curriculum are very clear.	117	95.9	362	90.7	479	91.9
2) The design of the curriculum is very good.	119	97.5	349	87.5	468	89.8
3) The activities were carefully planned.	116	95.1	337	84.5	453	86.9
4) The classroom atmosphere was very pleasant.	110	90.2	325	81.5	435	83.5
5) There was much peer interaction amongst the students.	118	96.7	332	83.2	450	86.4
6) I participated actively during lessons (including discussions, sharing, games, etc.).	117	95.9	334	83.4	451	86.6
7) I was encouraged to do my best.	116	95.9	333	83.5	449	86.3
8) The learning experience I encountered enhanced my interest towards the lessons.	114	94.2	336	84.2	450	86.5
9) Overall speaking, I have a very positive experience of the program.	115	95.0	331	83.0	446	85.8
10)On the whole, I like this curriculum very much.	119	98.3	354	88.7	473	91.0

Note: All items are measured using a 6-point Likert scale where 1 = strongly disagree, 2 = disagree, 3 = slightly disagree, 4 = slightly agree, 5 = agree, 6 = strongly agree. Only respondents with positive responses (Options 4-6) are shown in the table. School 1: Shijiazhuang TKP school, School 2: Shanwei TKP school.

Descriptive analyses showed that the majority of the student participants evaluated the program positively regarding its content, instructors (teachers, social workers, other workers), as well as its effectiveness. As shown in Table 1, 89.8% of the participants had a positive view on the good design of the curriculum (item 2), 91.9% of the participants agreed that the curriculum objectives were very clear (item 1), and 91.0% of the participants had overall satisfaction of the curriculum (item 10). As shown in Table 2, amongst the top items rating program instructors, 96.0% of the participants agreed that the teachers had encouraged them to participate in different course activities (item 6), 95.0% of the participants agreed that they received timely help from the teachers (item 8) and 95.4% of the participants had a positive perception of the active involvement of the teachers (item 5).

Table 2. Descriptive statistics of the participants' evaluations of the program instructors

	Respondents with positive responses (Options 4-6)					
	School 1		School 2		Overall	
	n	%	*n*	%	*N*	%
1) The instructor(s) had a good mastery of the curriculum.	120	98.4	354	88.7	474	91.0
2) The instructor(s) was well prepared for the lessons.	121	99.2	362	90.7	483	92.7
3) The instructor(s)' teaching skills were good.	120	98.4	360	90.2	480	92.1
4) The instructor(s) showed good professional attitudes.	118	96.7	368	92.2	486	93.3
5) The instructor(s) was very involved.	119	98.3	377	94.5	496	95.4
6) The instructor(s) encouraged students to participate in the activities.	121	99.2	379	95.0	500	96.0
7) The instructor(s) cared for the students.	121	99.2	365	91.5	486	93.3
8) The instructor(s) was ready to offer help to students when needed.	121	99.2	374	93.4	495	95.0
9) The instructor(s) had much interaction with the students.	117	95.9	353	88.5	470	90.2
10)Overall speaking, I have a very positive experience of the instructors.	121	99.2	372	93.2	493	94.6

Note: All items are measured using a 6-point Likert scale where 1 = strongly disagree, 2 = disagree, 3 = slightly disagree, 4 = slightly agree, 5 = agree, 6 = strongly agree. Only respondents with positive responses (Options 4-6) are shown in the table. School 1: Shijiazhuang TKP school, School 2: Shanwei TKP school.

Table 3. Descriptive statistics of the participants' evaluations of the program effectiveness

	Respondents with positive responses (Options 3-5)					
	School 1		School 2		Overall	
	n	%	*n*	%	*N*	%
1) It has strengthened my bonding with teachers, classmates, and my family.	112	91.8	284	71.2	396	76.0
2) It has strengthened my resilience in adverse conditions.	111	91.0	316	79.2	427	82.0
3) It has enhanced my social competence.	114	93.4	328	82.2	442	84.8
4) It has improved my ability in handling and expressing my emotions.	115	94.3	324	81.2	439	84.3
5) It has enhanced my cognitive competence.	115	94.3	325	81.5	440	84.5
6) My ability to resist harmful influences has been improved.	116	95.1	344	86.2	460	88.3
7) It has strengthened my ability to distinguish between the good and the bad.	118	96.7	346	86.7	464	89.1
8) It has increased my competence in making sensible and wise choices.	115	94.3	333	83.5	448	86.0
9) It has helped me to reflect my life.	113	93.4	310	77.7	423	81.3
10)It has reinforced my self-confidence.	113	92.6	319	79.9	432	82.9
11)It has increased my self-awareness.	117	96.7	344	86.2	461	88.7
12)It has helped me to face the future with a positive attitude.	119	97.5	334	83.7	453	86.9
13)It has helped me to cultivate compassion and care for others.	114	93.4	321	80.5	435	83.5
14)It has encouraged me to care about the community.	101	82.8	256	64.2	357	68.5
15)It has promoted my sense of responsibility in serving the society.	110	90.9	320	80.2	430	82.7
16)It has enriched my overall development.	119	97.5	355	89.2	474	91.2

Note: All items are measured using a 5-point Likert scale where 1 = unhelpful, 2 = not really helpful, 3 = slightly helpful, 4 = helpful, 5 = very helpful. Only respondents with positive responses (Options 3-5) are shown in the table. School 1: Shijiazhuang TKP school, School 2: Shanwei TKP school.

Table 4. Mean, standard deviations, Cronbach's alphas, and the mean of inter-item correlations

	School 1		School 2		Overall	
	M (SD)	α (Mean#)	M (SD)	α (Mean#)	M (SD)	α (Mean#)
Program content (10 items)	5.46 (.66)	.90 (.48)	4.60 (.71)	.83 (.33)	4.80 (.79)	.88 (.42)
Program instructors (10 items)	5.68 (.53)	.93 (.59)	4.90 (.77)	.91 (.50)	5.08 (.79)	.93 (.56)
Program effectiveness (16 items)	4.34 (.76)	.96 (.63)	3.51 (.77)	.92 (.42)	3.70 (.84)	.94 (.51)
Total effectiveness (36 items)	5.02 (.59)	.97 (.45)	4.20 (.62)	.94 (.30)	4.39 (.70)	.96 (.38)

Note: School 1: Shijiazhuang TKP school, School 2: Shanwei TKP school.
Mean inter-item correlations.

Table 5. Other aspects of subjective outcome evaluation based on the participants' perception

If your friends have needs and conditions similar to yours, will you suggest him/her to join this course?

Respondents with positive responses (Options 3-4)					
School 1		School 2		Overall	
n	%	*n*	%	*N*	%
121	100.0	365	91.5	486	93.5

Note: The item is measured using a 4-point Likert scale where 1 = definitely will not suggest, 2 = will not suggest, 3 = will suggest, 4 = definitely will suggest. Only respondents with positive responses (Options 3-4) are shown in the table. School 1: Shijiazhuang TKP school, School 2: Shanwei TKP school.

Would you participate in similar courses again in the future?

Respondents with positive responses (Options 3-4)					
School 1		School 2		Overall	
n	%	*n*	%	*N*	%
119	98.3	371	93.0	490	94.2

Note: The item is measured using a 4-point Likert scale where 1 = definitely would not participate, 2 = would not participate, 3 = would participate, 4 = definitely would participate. Only respondents with positive responses (Options 3-4) are shown in the table. School 1: Shijiazhuang TKP school, School 2: Shanwei TKP school.

On the whole, are you satisfied with this course?

Respondents with positive responses (Options 4-6)					
School 1		School 2		Overall	
n	%	*n*	%	*N*	%
121	100.0	370	92.7	491	94.4

Note: All items are measured using a 6-point Likert scale where 1 = very dissatisfied, 2 = moderately dissatisfied, 3 = slightly dissatisfied, 4 = satisfied, 5 = moderately satisfied, 6 = very satisfied. Only respondents with positive responses (Options 4-6) are shown in the table. School 1: Shijiazhuang TKP school, School 2: Shanwei TKP school.

Regarding students' perception on their personal growth after the program, some items received high ratings. As Table 3 shows, 89.1% of the participants agreed that the program had improved their ability to distinguish between the good and the bad (item 7), 88.7% of the participants had a positive perception of their increased self-awareness (item 11), and 91.2% of the participants agreed that the program had enriched their overall development (item 16). In Table 5 we can see that 93.5% of the students would suggest their friends to join the program, 94.2% would participate in a similar program in the future, and 94.4% were satisfied with the program they participated. These findings provided support to hypothesis 1.

Table 6. Pearson correlations among program content, instructors, and effectiveness

School 1: Variable	**1**	**2**	**3**
1) Program content (10 items)	-		
2) Program instructors (10 items)	.71**	-	
3) Program effectiveness (16 items)	.59**	.58**	-

** $p < .01$.

School 2: Variable	**1**	**2**	**3**
1) Program content (10 items)	-		
2) Program instructors (10 items)	.60**	-	
3) Program effectiveness (16 items)	.51**	.45**	-

** $p < .01$.

Table 6. (Continued)

Overall : Variable	**1**	**2**	**3**
1) Program content (10 items)	-		
2) Program instructors (10 items)	.69**	-	
3) Program effectiveness (16 items)	.61**	.56**	-

** $p < .01$.

Table 7. Multiple regression analyses predicting program effectiveness by program content and instructors

	Predictors			
	Program content	Program instructors	Model	
	ß[a]	ß[a]	R	R^2
School 1	.36**	.33**	.64	.40
School 2	.37***	.23***	.54	.28
Overall	.44***	.26***	.64	.41

a Standardized coefficients.
** p < .01, *** p < .001.

Pearson correlation analyses (see Table 6) showed that program content (VC), instructors (VI) and effectiveness (EF) were all positively and significantly correlated: VC and VI ($r = .69, p < .01$); VC and EF ($r = .61, p < .01$); VI and EF ($r = .56, p < .01$). This means that hypotheses 2a, 2b, 2c were all supported. Multiple regression analyses (see Table 7) demonstrated that how the students' perceived the program content (VC) and program instructors (VI) significantly predicted their perceived program effectiveness (EF). In the total sample, both VC ($\beta = .44, p < .001$) and VI ($\beta = .26, p < .001$) significantly predicted EF, and accounted for 41% of the total variance of EF. These findings provided support for hypothesis 3a and hypothesis 3b.

Discussion

Similar to previous evaluations in Hong Kong (16, 19-21), Form A was shown to be a reliable evaluation tool of subjective outcome to assess the views of the student participants on the P.A.T.H.S. program implemented in the two middle schools in mainland China. Most important of all, the students had a very positive view on the program content, instructors, and benefits brought to their personal development. The evaluation findings clearly give preliminary support that TKP P.A.T.H.S. Project is an effective and promising program in the two schools which participated in the preparatory phase in 2014-15 school year.

With regard to the inter-relationships amongst the three aspects of subjective outcome evaluation, results of Pearson correlation analyses showed that program content, program instructors (teachers, social workers, other workers), and program effectiveness are the "holy trinity" of the subjective outcome evaluation (22). Besides, results showed that student participants' perceived program content and instructor quality significantly predicted their perceived program effectiveness, which covered different aspects of PYD. From the student participants' perspective, the P.A.T.H.S. curriculum was perceived as very beneficial to the development of adolescent.

The present study is a pioneer evaluation study of the project in mainland China. However, it has several limitations. First, common method variance may account for the significant inter-relationships amongst the different components of subjective outcome evaluation. Second, as only two schools were involved in the evaluation, the findings should be treated as tentative in nature. Third, in addition to subjective outcome evaluation, other forms of evaluation (such as qualitative methods) should be included in the evaluation model. Finally, besides students, other major stakeholders should be included to achieve a more comprehensive view of the impact of the program.

ACKNOWLEDGMENTS

The preparation for this chapter and Tin Ka Ping P.A.T.H.S. Project were financially supported by Tin Ka Ping Foundation. This chapter is a reprint with minor revisions of an earlier published paper in the *International Journal of Child and Adolescent Health* 2018;11(1) issue with permission.

REFERENCES

[1] Catalano RF, Berglund ML, Ryan JA, Lonczak HS, Hawkins JD. Positive youth development in the United States: Research findings on evaluations of positive youth development programs. Prev Treat 2002;5(1):15a.

[2] Catalano RF, Berglund ML, Ryan JA, Lonczak HS, Hawkins JD. Positive youth development in the United States: Research findings on evaluations of positive youth development programs. Ann Am Acad Pol Soc Sci 2004;591(1):98-124.

[3] Shek DTL, Sun RCF. The Project PATHS in Hong Kong – Lessons learned and implications for positive youth development programs. ScientificWorldJournal 2012;2012:Article ID 687536.

[4] Shek DTL, Sun RCF. The Project P.A.T.H.S. in Hong Kong: Development, training, implementation, and evaluation. J Pediatr Adolesc Gynecol 2013;26(3):S2-9.

[5] Shek DTL. Editorial: Construction of a positive youth development project in Hong Kong. Int J Adolesc Med Health 2006;18(3):299-302.

[6] Sun RCF, Shek DTL. Life satisfaction, positive youth development and problem behaviour among Chinese adolescents in Hong Kong. Soc Indic Res 2010;95(3):455-74.

[7] Sun RCF, Shek DTL. Positive youth development, life satisfaction and problem behaviour among Chinese adolescents in Hong Kong: A replication. Soc Indic Res 2012;105:541-59.

[8] Sun RCF, Shek DTL. Longitudinal influences of positive youth development and life satisfaction on problem behavior among adolescents in Hong Kong. Soc Indic Res 2013;114(3):1171-97.

[9] Mak KK, Lai CM, Watanabe H, Kim DI, Bahr N, Ramos M, et al. Epidemiology of Internet behaviors and addiction among adolescents in six Asian countries. Cyberpsychol Behav Soc Netw 2014;17(11):720-8.

[10] Xing XY, Tao FB, Wan YH, Xing C, Qi XY, Hao JH, et al. Family factors associated with suicide attempts among Chinese adolescent students: A national cross-sectional survey. J Adolesc Health 2010;46:592-9.

[11] Ross JG, Luepker RV, Nelson GD, Saavedra P, Hubbard BM. Teenage health teaching modules: Impact of teacher training on implementation and student outcomes. J Sch Health 1991;61(1):31-4.

[12] Shek DTL, Liang L, Lee TY. Evaluation of a training program of Tin Ka Ping P.A.T.H.S. Project in China (Shanghai). Int J Child Adolesc Health 2017;10(2):165-76.

[13] Shek DTL, Chung CK, Sun RCF. Evaluation of a training program of the Tin Ka Ping P.A.T.H.S. Project in mainland China (Shanghai). Int J Child Adolesc Health 2017;10(2):177-87.

[14] Shek DTL, Pu X, Wu FKY. Evaluation of the training program of the Tin Ka Ping P.A.T.H.S. Project in mainland China (Suzhou). Int J Child Adolesc Health 2017;10(2):189-99.

[15] Shek DTL, Zhu X, Leung JTY. Subjective outcome evaluation of the Tin Ka Ping P.A.T.H.S. Project in mainland China (Chongqing). Int J Child Adolesc Health 2017;10(2):210-11.

[16] Shek DTL, Ma CMS. Validation of a subjective outcome evaluation tool for participants in a positive youth development program in Hong Kong. J Pediatr Adolesc Gynecol 2014;27:S43-9.

[17] Trotter C. What does client satisfaction tell us about effectiveness? Child Abuse Rev 2008;17(4):262-74.

[18] Dominici G, Palumbo F. How to build an e-learning product: Factors for student/customer satisfaction. Bus Horiz 2013;56(1):87-96.

[19] Shek DTL. Secondary data analyses of subjective outcome evaluation data based on nine databases. ScientificWorldJournal 2012;2012:Article ID 346369.

[20] Shek DTL, Law MYM. Evaluation of the Project P.A.T.H.S. based on the client satisfaction approach: View of the students. J Pediatr Adolesc Gynecol 2014;27:S2-9.

[21] Shek DTL, Sun RCF. Participants' evaluation of the Project P.A.T.H.S.: Are findings based on different datasets consistent? ScientificWorldJournal 2012;2012:Article ID 187450.

[22] Shek DTL, Liang, J. (2015). Subjective outcome evaluation of a university subject on service leadership. Int J Disabil Hum Dev 2015;14(4):385-92.

In: Advances in Chinese Children … ISBN: 978-1-53617-870-8
Editors: Ariel Tenenbaum et al.

Chapter 12

Evaluation findings of Tin Ka Ping P.A.T.H.S. Project implemented in junior secondary schools: Implementers' views

Daniel TL Shek**, PhD, FHKPS, BBS, SBS, JP, Xiaoqin Zhu, PhD and Janet TY Leung, PhD
Department of Applied Social Sciences, The Hong Kong Polytechnic University, Hong Kong, PR China

Abstract

After the Project P.A.T.H.S. was successfully implemented in the pilot stage in four cities in East China, the project was implemented on a full-scale basis since 2015-2016 academic year. The present paper outlines the evaluation findings of the first year during the full implementation based on the views of the implementers using the subjective outcome evaluation approach. A total of 144 implementers from 13 secondary schools joined the current research. On the whole, results showed that the implementers

* Corresponding Author's E-mail: daniel.shek@polyu.edu.hk.

were highly satisfied with the implementation regarding program content, their own performance, and program benefits. As expected, perceptions of program content and implementers' own performance were positively associated with perceived program benefits. Together with previous evaluation findings in Hong Kong and China mainland, the current study suggests that the Project P.A.T.H.S. has been well received by participants and implementers, and it promotes positive development in adolescents in different Chinese communities.

INTRODUCTION

Positive youth development (PYD) programs are intended to promote all-round development among teenagers by providing them opportunities to recognize, utilize and enhance their strengths, which would establish a solid foundation for healthy adjustment which would eventually prevent youth problems, such as substance abuse, juvenile delinquency, and violent crimes (1). The beneficial influence of PYD programs has been widely recognized globally. For instance, sport camps in the United Kingdom (UK) have been shown to promote competence, confidence, and care amongst students (2). In South Africa, a narrative-based program was found to promote youth development and it successfully reduced alcohol use and HIV infection among the youngster (3). In a comprehensive review of efficacious youth programs around the world, researchers concluded that implementing preventive and PYD programs effectively is a promising way to reduce adolescent problem behaviors (4).

Although PYD programs are popular among Western countries, systematic and large-scale PYD programs are rarely developed and implemented in Chinese contexts (5). To fill this information gap, a curriculum-based PYD program entitled "Positive Adolescent Training through Holistic Social Programmes" (Project P.A.T.H.S.) was developed and carried out in Hong Kong since 2005-2006 academic year with the financial support of The Hong Kong Jockey Club Charities Trust. This is the first large-scale and holistic PYD program in different Chinese communities. During the past decade, this project has achieved a great success in competence building and problem prevention among Hong Kong adolescents. Specifically, empirical findings showed that the project successfully enhanced multiple developmental assets and well-being (e.g., self-confidence, spirituality, prosocial involvement, and social competence) in students while simultaneously reduced adolescents' engagement in maladaptive behaviors, such as drug abuse, delinquency, and self-harm activities (6-8). Consistently, the program was positively evaluated and regarded as effective by both adolescent participants and program implementers (9-11)

There is also an urgent need to design and launch evidence-based PYD programs in mainland China because there are growing trends of youth problems in China. For example, with rapid economic growth in the past decades in mainland China, materialism became prevalent among Chinese adolescents. According to a research conducted by Ipsos (12), China is now the most materialistic country among 20 countries including the United States, UK, Japan, Korea, and so on. Under this atmosphere, the younger generation in China is becoming more materialistic when compared to the older generation and their counterparts in other countries (13). It is noteworthy that materialism was adversely associated with healthy adolescent development, such as self-esteem, mental health, and life satisfaction (14). Similarly, an orientation of materialism also exerts negative impacts on students' intrinsic learning motivation, school performance, and developmental outcomes (15). All these findings take place alongside with the growing trends of external and internal problems among the Chinese youths (16).

To promote health development in Chinese adolescents in mainland China, the Project P.A.T.H.S. was adapted and implemented in mainland China in 2011, with financial support from Tin Ka Ping Foundation. Although the Project P.A.T.H.S. has benefited thousands of secondary students in Hong Kong, its effectiveness in mainland China remains uncertain due to several reasons. First, although the junior secondary school programs adopted in mainland China were based on those implemented in Hong Kong, their applicability is unclear because there are cultural or sub-cultural differences involved.

Second, the pedagogy of Project P.A.T.H.S. was based on experiential learning, which requires teachers to let students learn from their firsthand experience rather than only passively receiving knowledge from teachers (17). In particular, it emphasizes reflection since it allows students to introspect challenges and integrate new information to their existing schema (17). Obviously, such a student-centered pedagogy is quite different from the traditional teacher-centered one adopted in China. This stimulating pedagogy requires both teachers and students to make adaptations to their changing roles in the classroom. In this sense, both teachers and students may have difficulties in adjusting to the new teaching and learning styles, which might also potentially affect the effectiveness of the project.

Third, implementing and participating in such a PYD program might require extra working and schooling hours from teachers and students. Given that academic achievement is morbidly emphasized by schools, parents, and the society in China (18), school teachers and students may still have a mindset that the Project P.A.T.H.S. is competing for resource with other academic courses, which might possibly hinder students' academic achievement. Despite the strong evidence that effective PYD programs can actually enhance adolescents' school performance and academic achievement (19), schools might still have hesitation to devote sufficient effort in implementing the project.

In view of the above issues, a 3-year pilot implementation (i.e., from 2011-2012 to 2013-2014 academic year) was carried out in four secondary schools located in East China and different evaluation strategies were utilized to investigate the implementation effectiveness. Results revealed highly positive findings regarding the program effectiveness in promoting adolescent holistic development (20, 21). These encouraging findings motivated the Foundation to support the project for three more years (2015-2016 to 2017-2018 school years) after one-year of preparation (i.e., 2014-2015 school year).

Although the pilot implementation showed the benefits of the Tin Ka Ping Project P.A.T.H.S. in China mainland, continuous program evaluation should be carried out, not only for the purpose of providing evidence-based support but also informing directions to improve future implementation. To this end, the present study attempted to evaluate program effectiveness in the first year of full implementation (i.e., 2015-2016 academic year). A subjective outcome evaluation method was used, in which data on the views from the program implementers toward three main aspects (program content, implementer's own performance, and program effectiveness) were collected. Program implementers' views should be considered and understood because they directly deliver the program. Moreover, their direct interactions with students allow them to understand the real need and actual change of students. Based on the previous positive evaluation findings (11, 22, 23), we proposed the following hypotheses:

- A majority of the program implementers would show positive perceptions on program content (Hypothesis 1a), their own performance (Hypothesis 1b), and program effectiveness (Hypothesis 1c). In subjective outcome studies, a program is commonly regarded as positive if more than 80% of the respondents respond in the positive direction. We used the same cutoff point in this study.
- Program implementers' satisfaction of program content (Hypothesis 2a) and self-perceived performance (Hypothesis 2b) would have positive relationships with the perceived program effectiveness.
- Program implementers' evaluation of program effectiveness would be positively predicted by perceived program content (Hypothesis 3a) and own performance (Hypothesis 3b).

OUR STUDY

Program implementers (e.g., teachers) from 13 participating schools were invited to complete a subjective outcome evaluation form for implementers (i.e., Form B) after the program was implemented in 2015-2016 academic year. A total of 144 implementers completed and returned the Form B. Among all the implementers, 80 implemented the program for Secondary 1, 45 for Secondary 1 and Secondary 2, and 19 for Secondary 1, Secondary 2, and Secondary 3. The number of implementers in each school ranged from 5 to 30, with an average of 11 (*SD* = 6.79). An evaluation manual with detail instructions was given to implementers to guide them to complete the Form B prior to program evaluation. The procedures for collecting data and the related instructions were also covered in the training workshops.

Instruments

The Form B used in the present study has been widely used in prior evaluation studies and proved to be valid and reliable (11, 24). In Form B, six parts were developed to measure implementers' subjective perceptions of several aspects of the program.

First, two subscales were included in Part 1. Each subscale adopted 10 items to measure perceptions of the implementers toward the program content (e.g., impression of the program, classroom atmosphere, and students' participation) and self-performance (e.g., implementers' understanding of the program, involvement, and teaching skills). For each statement, the implementers gave their response on a 6-point Likert scale (1= strongly disagree, 6 = strongly agree). The higher they rated, the more they agreed with the statement. The two subscales in the first part showed good reliability in the present study (see Table 1).

Table 1. Mean, standard deviation, Cronbach's alphas, and mean of inter-item correlations among variables

	M	SD	Cronbach's α	Mean#
Program content (10 items)	5.28	.49	.89	.44
Program implementers (10 items)	5.12	.56	.92	.52
Program effectiveness (16 items)	4.23	.59	.96	.59

Note. # Mean inter-item correlations

Second, 16 items were employed in Part 2 to evaluate the implementers' perceived program effectiveness (e.g., improvement in students' resilience, emotional competence, and social competence). This subscale utilized a 5-

point Likert scale (1 = not helpful at all, 5 = very helpful). Similarly, a higher rating in this subscale indicates a higher level of perceived program effectiveness. This subscale also had good reliability as shown in Table 1.

For Part 3 to Part 5, each part only contained one question. The third part asked the implementers to indicate their willingness to recommend the program to students having similar needs on a 4-point Likert scale (1 = definitely will not, 4 = definitely will). Using the same 4-point scale (1 = definitely will not, 4 = definitely will), the fourth part invited the implementers to express their willingness in teaching similar courses in the future. Lastly, the question in the fifth part was designed to assess the implementers' perception of the extent to which the program helped their professional development. Implementers gave their responses on a 5-point Likert scale (1 = not helpful at all, 5 = very helpful).

The sixth part contained three open questions about the most appreciated elements of the program, the areas need improvement, and suggestions for future development. In the present paper, the focus is put on the quantitative data derived from the first five parts.

Data analyses

A reliability test was done to measure the internal consistency of each subscale. Descriptive analyses were then performed to calculate the percentage of favorable responses of each part. We also examined correlations among respondents' views toward program quality, their own performance, and program effectiveness. Besides, a multiple regression analysis was performed to examine the predictive effect of perceived program qualities and self-perceived performance on the level of perceived program effectiveness.

FINDINGS

Using 80% as a cutoff, positive responses toward the program content were found among all items as shown in Table 2. For example, all implementers agreed that the objectives of the program were very clear and the program activities were carefully designed. Moreover, almost all implementers (99.3%) had a very positive overall evaluation on the program and agreed that their students like this program very much.

Table 2. Summary of the program implementers' perceptions toward the program content

	Positive responses (Options 4-6)	
	N	%
1. The objectives of the curriculum are very clear.	144	100.0
2. The design of the curriculum is very good	143	99.3
3. The activities were carefully planned	144	100.0
4. The classroom atmosphere was very pleasant.	142	98.6
5. There was much peer interaction amongst the students	137	95.1
6. Students participated actively during lessons (including discussions, sharing, games, etc.)	141	97.9
7. The program has a strong and sound theoretical support.	141	97.9
8. The teaching experience I encountered enhanced my interest towards the lessons	142	98.6
9. Overall speaking, I have very positive evaluation of the program	143	99.3
10. On the whole, students like this curriculum very much	143	99.3

Note. All items are on a 6-point Likert scale with 1 = strongly disagree, 2 = disagree, 3 = slightly disagree, 4 = slightly agree, 5 = agree, 6 = strongly agree. Only respondents with positive responses (Options 4-6) are shown in the table.

Similar positive results were found in self-perceived performance (see Table 3). All implementers stated that they were ready to offer help to student when needed. Most of them (99.3%) had a very positive overall evaluation on themselves. Highly positive responses were also found on other items (e.g., professional attitude, involved, and cared for students).

Table 3. Summary of the program implementers' perceptions toward their own performance

		Positive responses (Options 4-6)	
		N	%
1.	I have a good mastery of the curriculum.	136	94.4
2.	I prepared well for the lessons	138	95.8
3.	My teaching skills were good	137	95.1
4.	I have professional attitude	142	98.6
5.	I was very involved	141	97.9
6.	I gained a lot during the course of instruction	142	98.6
7.	I cared for the students	142	98.6
8.	I was ready to offer help to students when needed	144	100.0
9.	I had much interaction with the students	141	97.9
10.	Over speaking, I have very positive evaluation of myself as an instructor	143	99.3

Note. All items are on a 6-point Likert scale with 1 = strongly disagree, 2 = disagree, 3 = slightly disagree, 4 = slightly agree, 5 = agree, 6 = strongly agree. Only respondents with positive responses (Options 4-6) are shown in the table.

Table 4 presents the respondents' subjective views on perceived program effectiveness. Overall speaking, respondents gave highly positive responses on all items. More specifically, almost all participants (99.3%) agreed that the program helped their students build a stronger bonding with teachers, classmates and their families, and they perceived their students had a positive attitude to face the future after joining the program. Moreover, nearly 99% of the implementers indicated that the program strengthened students' ability in expressing emotions, helped students to distinguish between good and bad, and cultivated compassion and care about others.

Results of the program implementers' positive responses toward other aspects of the program are shown in Table 5. Most (99.3%) of the respondents indicated that they would recommend students with similar needs to participate this program.

Also, 96.5% of them expressed their willingness to teach similar program again in the future and agreed that the program promoted their professional growth. In sum, hypotheses 1a, 1b and 1c were supported by the results.

Table 4. Summary of the program implementers' perceptions toward the program effectiveness

	Positive responses (Options 3-5)	
	N	%
1. It has strengthened students' bonding with teachers, classmates and their families	143	99.3
2. It has strengthened students' resilience in adverse conditions	141	97.9
3. It has enhanced students' social competence	140	97.2
4. It has improved students' ability in handling and expressing emotions	142	98.6
5. It has enhanced students' cognitive competence	141	97.9
6. Students' ability to resist harmful influences has been improved	141	97.9
7. It has strengthened students' ability to distinguish between the good and the bad	142	98.6
8. It has increased students' competence in making sensible and wise choices	141	97.9
9. It has helped students to have life reflections	141	97.9
10. It has reinforced students' self-confidence	142	98.6
11. It has increased students' self- awareness	142	98.6
12. It has helped students to face the future with a positive attitude	143	99.3
13. It has helped students to cultivate compassion and care about others	142	98.6
14. It has encouraged students to care about the community	139	96.5
15. It has promoted students' sense of responsibility in serving the society	142	98.6
16. It has enriched the overall development of the students	138	95.8

Note. All items are on a 5-point Likert scale with 1 = unhelpful, 2 = not very helpful, 3 = slightly helpful, 4 = helpful, 5 = very helpful. Only respondents with positive responses (Options 3-5) are shown in the table.

Table 5. Summary of the program implementers' positive perceptions on other aspects

Items	Positive responses (Options 3-4)	
	N	%
Willingness to suggest other students to participate in the program[a]	143	99.3
Willingness to teach similar programs in future[a]	139	96.5
The extent to which the program helped implementers' professional growth[b]	139	96.5

Note. [a] A 4-point Likert scale was used, with 1 = definitely will not, 2 = will not, 3 = will, 4 = definitely will. Only respondents with positive responses (Options 3–4) are shown in the table.

[b] A 5-point Likert scale was used, with 1 = unhelpful, 2 = not very helpful, 3 = slightly helpful, 4 = helpful, 5 = very helpful. Only respondents with positive responses (Options 3–5) are shown in the table.

Table 6 shows the results of Pearson correlation analyses. Both perception of program quality ($r = .58$, $p < .001$) and view toward own performance ($r = .66$, $p < .001$) showed a significant and positive linkage with implementers' perception of program effectiveness. These results provided support for hypotheses 2a and 2b.

Table 6. Correlations among perceptions on program content, implementers, and program effectiveness

Variable	Program effectiveness		
	1	2	3
1. Program content (10 items)	--		
2. Program implementers (10 items)	.74***		
3. Program effectiveness (16 items)	.58***	.66***	--

***$p < .001$.

To further investigate the relationship between perceived program content, self-perceived performance and perceived program effectiveness, a multiple regression analysis was done and the results are depicted in table 7. Both implementers' self-perceived performance ($\beta = .50$, $p < .001$) and perceived program content ($\beta = .20$, $p < .05$) significantly predicted program effectiveness. The two predictors accounted for 45% of the variance of program effectiveness. In short, both hypotheses 3a and 3b were supported.

Table 7. Multiple regression analysis predicting program effectiveness

Predictors		Model	
Program content	Program implementers		
β^a	β^a	R	R^2
.20*	.50***	.67	.45

Note. [a] Standardized coefficients. ***p < .001. *p < .05.

Discussion

The present research investigated evaluation findings based on implementers' views toward the Tin Ka Ping P.A.T.H.S. Project implemented in mainland China in 2015-2016 academic year. The current study employed a valid and reliable subjective outcome evaluation measurement (i.e., Form B) to assess the implementers' views toward the program implementation. The Form B mainly included three multi-item subscales that assessed implementers' perceptions of program content, their own performance and program effectiveness, respectively. The information of implementers' willingness to recommend the program to other students, willingness to implement similar programs in future, and the extent the experience promoted teachers' professional growth was also gathered in the present study. The present findings not only demonstrated that the program was effective. It also informed us about the possible factors that contributed to the implementation effectiveness.

Overall speaking, the implementers held positive perceptions of the program implemented in 2015-2016 school year. Notably, over 95% of the respondents gave positive ratings on all aspects of the program content; all of them regarded the curriculum objectives as clear and activities as meticulously designed; over 99% of them perceived that the curriculum was well designed and agreed that students loved the program a lot. In addition, the implementers held favorable views toward their own performance. Nearly or over 95% of them rated themselves as having good performance in all aspects. For instance, over 98% of the respondents perceived that they had professional attitudes, cared for the students, and were willing to offer help to the students.

Regarding perceived program effectiveness, results showed that the implementation of program was effective in cultivating students' myriad positive attributes, such as positive bonding with significant adults and peers, resilience, self-awareness, beliefs in the future, emotional and moral competence, and so on. Implementers' responses to the three questions illustrated in Table 5 reinforced the positive evaluation. Almost all respondents were willing to suggest other students to join the program, and approximately 97% of the implementers wished to teach similar course in future and felt that teaching the program had benefited themselves a lot regarding professional development. All these results coincide with the positive evaluation findings for the P.A.T.H.S. Project implemented in Hong Kong (11, 24), suggesting that the transplanting and adaptation of the project from Hong Kong to mainland China is successful.

Theoretically speaking, the well-designed program content and quality delivery of the content by implementers as well as some supportive external conditions (e.g., policy support) collaboratively ensure the great benefits enjoyed by program participants (25). In line with this argument, perceptions of program content and program implementers' performance were both significantly correlated with and functioned as two significant predictors of perceived program effectiveness. The existing literature suggests that several factors may contribute to the quality of program content and implementers' good performance in delivering program content.

First of all, the curriculum of the project was developed based on PYD theory that maintains adolescents as "assets to be developed" instead of "problems to be solved" (26). Based on this positive view of adolescents, course content was carefully selected to fulfill adolescents' developmental needs through promoting a wide range of psychosocial competencies, including self-efficacy, emotional competence, spirituality, and resilience (27). In addition to the strong theoretical basis, the curriculum also included a reflective and experiential learning pedagogy, which contends that students can learn by "experiencing, reflecting, thinking, and acting" (17). In line with the active learning philosophy, the center of teaching shifted from teachers to students; the method of teaching ranged from merely lecturing to a combination of diverse ones, including group work, role play, debate, and reflection. It is noteworthy that an encouraging learning environment as well as a collaborative atmosphere created by such an inspirational and innovative pedagogy are very helpful in promoting students' positive learning attitude, student engagement, and learning achievement (28, 29). These two unique features of the program content lay a solid foundation for the success of the program implementation in mainland China.

Besides the solid groundwork linked to program content, the qualified implementer constitutes another indispensable prerequisite of effective program delivery. It was evident that the characteristics of teacher, such as teaching experience and support for students, could significantly affect student learning (30, 31). Theories and empirical findings in the field of program evaluation also revealed that the quality of program implementers was a significant predictor of program effectiveness (5, 32). In view of the critical role of program implementers in program implementation, a series of training program was rigorously designed based on a theoretical framework proposed by Shek and Wai (33) and offered to implementers in the preparation year and during the full implementation phase. As expected, these training programs helped implementers better understand the PYD theory and the curriculum design, cultivate the positive and enthusiastic attitude toward program implementation, and master the required teaching skills (34, 35). Certainly, the comprehensive training enables the implementers to deliver the program effectively, which subsequently guarantees the benefits of the program.

While implementers gained confidence and experience in using experiential teaching method through training programs, positive findings of the present study also demonstrated that adolescents in mainland China can well adapt to the active learning style. In fact, instead of resisting the active pedagogy, students actually favored the student-centered approach and were able to actively participate in in-class activities involving interactions, critical thinking, self-reflections, sharing, and expression of personal views. This encouraging conclusion suggests that implementing

PYD programs with active and experiential teaching and learning methods is a very promising way to promote holistic development in Chinese adolescents.

Despite the very positive findings, the present study has several limitations. First, our study only considered the implementers' views. Besides, the sample size (N = 144) was not very large. To provide a full picture of program effectiveness and validate the present findings, future studies should involve other informants such as students and increase the sample size. Second, while acknowledging the advantages of subjective outcome evaluation approach, we also admit its inherent disadvantages. For example, reliability of subjective measures is affected by several factors that are hard, if not impossible, to control, such as item order and social desirability. Therefore, future studies could also include objective measures to offset these shortcomings. Third, although the present quantitative findings are very positive, it will certainly be illuminating to include qualitative methods such as focus group interview in future studies, as qualitative evaluation gives insight into the comprehensive picture of program effectiveness as well as mechanisms that underline the positive quantitative findings.

ACKNOWLEDGMENTS

The preparation for this paper and the Tin Ka Ping P.A.T.H.S. Project are financially supported by Tin Ka Ping Foundation. This chapter is a reprint with minor revisions of an earlier published paper in the *International Journal of Child and Adolescent Health* 2018;11(1) issue with permission.

REFERENCES

[1] Roth JL, Brooks-Gunn J. What exactly is a youth development program? Answers from research and practice. Appl Dev Sci 2003;7(2):94-111. doi: 10.1207/s1532480xads0702_6.

[2] Jones MI, Dunn JG, Holt NL, Sullivan PJ, Bloom GA. Exploring the '5Cs' of positive youth development in sport. J Sport Behav 2011;34(3):250-67.
[3] Hamby A, Pierce M, Daniloski K, Brinberg D. The use of participatory action research to create a positive youth development program. Soc Mar Q 2011;17(3):2-17.
[4] Catalano RF, Fagan AA, Gavin LE, Greenberg MT, Irwin CE, Ross DA, et al. Worldwide application of prevention science in adolescent health. Lancet 2012;379(9826):1653-64. doi: 10.1016/S0140-6736(12)60238-4.
[5] Shek DTL, Yu L. A review of validated youth prevention and positive youth development programs in Asia. Int J Adolesc Med Health 2011;23(4):317-24. doi: 10.1515/IJAMH.2011.028.
[6] Shek DTL, Yu L. Impact of the Project P.A.T.H.S. on adolescent risk behavior: A five-year longitudinal study. In: Shek DTL, Sun RCF, eds. Development and evaluation of Positive Adolescent Training through Holistic Social Programs (P.A.T.H.S.). Singapore: Springer, 2013:85-106.
[7] Shek DTL, Ma CMS. Impact of the Project P.A.T.H.S. in the junior secondary school years: Objective outcome evaluation based on eight waves of longitudinal data. ScientificWorldJournal 2012;2012:Article ID 170345. doi: 10.1100/2012/170345.
[8] Shek DTL, Ma CMS. Impact of the Project P.A.T.H.S. in the junior secondary school years: Individual growth curve analyses. ScientificWorldJournal 2011;11:253-66. doi: 10.1100/tsw.2011.6.
[9] Shek DTL, Yu L. Longitudinal impact of the project P.A.T.H.S. on adolescent risk behavior: What happened after five years? ScientificWorldJournal 2012;2012:Article ID 316029. doi: 10.1100/2012/316029.
[10] Shek DTL, Sun RCF. Participants' evaluation of the Project P.A.T.H.S.: Are findings based on different datasets consistent? ScientificWorldJournal 2012;2012:Article ID 187450. doi: 10.1100/2012/187450.
[11] Shek DTL, Ma CMS. Program implementers' evaluation of the Project P.A.T.H.S.: Findings based on different datasets over time. ScientificWorldJournal 2012;2012:Article ID 918437. doi: 10.1100/2012/918437.
[12] Ipsos. Global attitudes on materialism, finances and family. 2013. Accessed 2017 Feb 6. URL: http://www.ipsos-na.com/news-polls/pressrelease.aspx?id=6359
[13] Gu FF, Hung K. Materialism among adolescents in china: A historical generation perspective. J Asia Bus Stud 2009;3(2):56-64. doi: 10.1108/15587890980000411.
[14] Kasser T, Rosenblum KL, Sameroff AJ, Deci EL, Niemiec CP, Ryan RM, et al. Changes in materialism, changes in psychological well-being: Evidence from three longitudinal studies and an intervention experiment. Motiv Emotion 2014;38(1):1-22. doi: 10.1007/s11031-013-9371-4.
[15] Ku L, Dittmar H, Banerjee R. Are materialistic teenagers less motivated to learn? Cross-sectional and longitudinal evidence from the United Kingdom and Hong Kong. J Educ Psychol 2012;104(1):74-86. doi: 10.1037/a0025489.

[16] Auerbach RP, McWhinnie CM, Goldfinger M, Abela JRZ, Zhu X, Yao S. The cost of materialism in a collectivistic culture: Predicting risky behavior engagement in Chinese adolescents. J Clin Child Adolesc Psychol 2010;39(1):117-27. doi: 10.1080/15374410903401179.

[17] Kolb DA. Experiential learning: Experience as the source of learning and development. 2nd ed. Upper Saddle River, NJ: FT Press, 2014.

[18] Chen C, Uttal DH. Cultural values, parents' beliefs, and children's achievement in the United States and China. Hum Dev 1988;31(6):351-8. doi: 10.1159/000276334.

[19] Durlak JA, Weissberg RP, Dymnicki AB, Taylor RD, Schellinger KB. The impact of enhancing students' social and emotional learning: A meta-analysis of school-based universal interventions. Child Dev 2011;82(1):405-32. doi: 10.1111/j.1467-8624.2010.01564.x.

[20] Shek DTL, Han XY, Lee TY, Yu L. Impact of the Project P.A.T.H.S. in China. In: Shek DT, Sun RC, eds. Development and evaluation of Positive Adolescent Training through Holistic Social Programs (P.A.T.H.S.). Singapore: Springer, 2013:291-304.

[21] Shek DTL, Yu L, Sun RCF, Lee TY, Han XY, Li XX, et al. Objective outcome evaluation of a positive youth development program in China. Int J Disabil Hum Dev 2014;13(2):255-65. doi: 10.1515/ijdhd-2014-0311.

[22] Shek DTL, Chak YLY. Subjective outcome evaluation of the secondary 2 training program of the Project P.A.T.H.S. in Hong Kong. Int J Adolesc Med Health 2011;23(4):325-32. doi: 10.1515/IJAMH.2011.029.

[23] Shek DTL, Yu L, Ho VYT. Subjective outcome evaluation and factors related to perceived effectiveness of the Project P.A.T.H.S. in Hong Kong. ScientificWorldJournal 2012;2012:Article ID 490290. doi: 10.1100/2012/490290.

[24] Shek DTL, Ma CMS, Zhu X. Evaluation of a community-based positive youth development program in Hong Kong: Views of program implementers. Int J Disabil Hum Dev 2017;16(4):377-86. doi: 10.1515/ijdhd-2017-7006.

[25] Shek DTL, Sun RCF. Implementation of a positive youth development program in a Chinese context: The role of policy, program, people, process, and place. ScientificWorldJournal 2008;8:980-96. doi: 10.1100/tsw.2008.120.

[26] Lerner RM, Dowling EM, Anderson PM. Positive youth development: Thriving as the basis of personhood and civil society. Appl Dev Sci 2003;7(3):172-80. doi: 10.1207/S1532480XADS0703_8.

[27] Shek DTL, Sun RCF, eds. Development and evaluation of Positive Adolescent Training through Holistic Social Programs (P.A.T.H.S.). Singapore: Springer; 2013.

[28] Burch GF, Batchelor JH, Heller NA, Shaw J, Kendall W, Turner B. Experiential learning-What do we know? A meta-analysis of 40 years of research. Dev Bus Simul Exp Learn 2014;41(1):279-83.

[29] Jiusto S, DiBiaso D. Experiential learning environments: Do they prepare our students to be self-directed, life-long-learners? J Eng Educ 2006;95(3):195-204. doi: 10.1002/j.2168-9830.2006.tb00892.x.

[30] Bundick MJ, Tirri K. Student perceptions of teacher support and competencies for fostering youth purpose and positive youth development: Perspectives from two countries. Appl Dev Sci 2014;18(3):148-62. doi: 10.1080/10888691.2014.924357.

[31] Harris DN, Sass TR. Teacher training, teacher quality and student achievement. J Public Econ 2011;95(7):798-812. doi: 10.1016/j.jpubeco.2010.11.009.

[32] Forman SG, Olin SS, Hoagwood KE, Crowe M, Saka N. Evidence-based interventions in schools: Developers' views of implementation barriers and facilitators. School Ment Health 2009;1(1):26-36. doi: 10.1007/s12310-008-9002-5.

[33] Shek DTL, Wai CLY. Training workers implementing adolescent prevention and positive youth development programs: What have we learned from the literature. Adolescence 2008;43(172):823-45.

[34] Shek DTL, Zhu X, Leung JTY. Subjective outcome evaluation of the Tin Ka Ping P.A.T.H.S. project training program in mainland China. Int J Child Adolesc Health 2017;10(2):201-11.

[35] Shek DTL, Leung JTY, Wu J. Subjective evaluation of a training program of the Tin Ka Ping P.A.T.H.S. Project in mainland China. Int Public Health 2017;9(3):311-23.

In: Advances in Chinese Children … ISBN: 978-1-53617-870-8
Editors: Ariel Tenenbaum et al.

Chapter 13

SUBJECTIVE OUTCOME EVALUATION OF THE TIN KA PING P.A.T.H.S. PROJECT: VIEWS OF SENIOR SECONDARY SCHOOL STUDENTS

Daniel TL Shek[1,*], PhD, FHKPS, BBS, SBS, JP, Rachel CF Sun[2], Irene Wu[1], PhD and Moon YM Law[3], DSW, RSW

[1]Department of Applied Social Sciences,
The Hong Kong Polytechnic University, Hong Kong, PR China
[2]School of Social Sciences, Faculty of Education,
The University of Hong Kong, Hong Kong, PR China
[3]Caritas Institute of Higher Education, Hong Kong, PR China

* Corresponding Author: Daniel TL Shek, PhD, FHKPS, BBS, SBS, JP, Associate Vice President (Undergraduate Programme) and Chair Professor of Applied Social Sciences, Department of Applied Social Sciences, The Hong Kong Polytechnic University, Hunghom, Hong Kong, P.R. China. Email: daniel.shek@polyu.edu.hk.

ABSTRACT

The Tin Ka Ping P.A.T.H.S. Project is an innovative positive youth development (PYD) program in mainland China with an aim to promote holistic development of Chinese secondary school students. Based on the subjective outcome evaluation approach, this study explored the effectiveness of the Tin Ka Ping P.A.T.H.S. Project in senior secondary schools in the 2015-2016 academic year from the perspective of students. A total of 1,762 senior secondary students from six participating schools completed the evaluation form. Findings suggested that a high proportion of the participants expressed positive attitudes towards the program, instructors' performance, and benefits of the program. Compared with Grade 11, Grade 10 students reported higher levels of satisfaction in all three aspects. In line with previous studies, the three dimensions had significant inter-relationships, and both program quality and instructor performance were found to be significant predictors of perceived program benefits. As a pioneering attempt, this study provides evidence supporting the success of the Tin Ka Ping P.A.T.H.S. Project.

INTRODUCTION

Adolescence is a unique time of life before teenagers step into adulthood (1). In this transition period, internalizing and externalizing problems are common (2). Traditionally, adolescent behavioral problems such as delinquency, substance abuse, and violence have attracted much attention from researchers (1, 3). With rapid changes in the contemporary world, there is an emergence of new types of adolescent developmental issues such as obesity, eating disorders, unhealthy sexual behaviors, materialization, and low academic motivation (4, 5). Besides externalizing behaviors, internalizing symptoms also exist (6, 7). For instance, adolescents' problematic eating behaviors and associated problems (e.g., overweight and obesity) were largely triggered by their weight and body dissatisfaction (8), which in turn probably cause emotional processing difficulties (4). In the same vein, depressive symptoms, anxiety symptoms, and life stress could also result in unhealthy dietary patterns (9, 10).

Given these rising concerns, prevention and treatment concentrating on one single problem is the common approach in the past to deal with adolescent problematic behaviors and symptoms (11). However, realizing the co-existence of internalizing and externalizing problems and the overlapping causes, ecological models have been commonly adopted in understanding adolescent developmental issues (12). Among which, positive youth development (PYD) is an approach that aims to prevent problematic behaviors and symptoms through promoting adolescents' positive development adopting a "whole-person" perspective (13). PYD contends that adolescents are "resources to be developed" with their strengths in the developmental process (14). In Western societies, evidence from previous research supported that PYD programs are effective in reducing the probability of adolescent problem behaviors (15, 16).

With particular reference to China, adolescent externalizing behavior continues to rise in the face of complex and ever-changing environment. For example, the latest findings of adolescent sexual behavior study in Hong Kong showed that adolescent sexual behavior and their intention to engage in sexual behavior both gradually increased over time (17). Similarly, statistics from the National Health and Family Planning Commission in mainland China suggested that the average age for first-time sex behaviors was 15.9, with more than 45 percent of the participants not using contraceptives (18). Regarding health risk behaviors, findings from China Nationwide Nutrition and Health Survey in 2016 pointed out that adolescent obesity rates are rising dramatically in the last 30 years with prevalence rates of overweight and obese boys increased to 11.1% in 2014 from 0.2% in 1985 (19). Besides, in the area of unhealthy sleep behavior among adolescents, findings from an eight-year longitudinal study showed that nearly all students experienced at least one type of sleep problems (20). Another study conducted in southeast China found that the prevalence rate of less-than-5-hours sleep among adolescents (aged 13 to 20) was 5.6% (21). Meanwhile, short sleep among Chinese adolescents was associated with lower health-related quality of life (22), which are related to defiant attitudes, poor academic performance, and even suicidal ideation and attempts (20, 21). Although the highly comorbid externalizing and internalizing problems in

Chinese adolescents are severe, there are few PYD programs in different Chinese communities, particularly in mainland China.

Utilizing PYD constructs (14) to promote holistic development among Chinese adolescent, Shek and his research team (23) developed a PYD program entitled Project P.A.T.H.S. (Positive Adolescent Training through Holistic Social Programs) for junior secondary students in Hong Kong. Funded by The Hong Kong Jockey Club Charities Trust since 2005, this project has gone through over a decade's implementation (24). Later on, to benefit adolescents in mainland China, Tin Ka Ping Foundation introduced the Project P.A.T.H.S. in mainland China since 2011 (25), transplanting it into "Tin Ka Ping P.A.T.H.S. Project." With reference to the 15 positive youth development constructs identified by Catalano et al. (7), the research team developed school-based programs attempting to promote adolescent personal qualities (e.g., clear and positive identity, self-efficacy) and various competences (e.g., moral competence, social competence).

With the encouraging outcomes achieved in junior secondary students (26), the Tin Ka Ping P.A.T.H.S. Project was further extended into senior secondary schools since 2014. In response to specific developmental issues in Chinese adolescents, the TKP P.A.T.H.S. Project designed senior curriculum to strengthen the personal abilities and developmental assets among mainland senior secondary students. For example, in Unit EC 5.1 (emotional competence) named "Youth in Full Bloom," through taking part in both individual and group activities, students would learn to recognize different ways of expressing anger and its corresponding consequences, as well as to master effective anger management skills. As the senior curricula-based programs are new to both implementers and participants, the research team is quite concerned about its impact on the students. Thus, it is necessary to test out its effectiveness for further nationwide implementation.

Multiple evaluation methods have been employed to examine the effectiveness of the Project P.A.T.H.S. in Hong Kong since its inception, including objective and subjective outcome evaluation, process evaluation, qualitative assessment, as well as student products that include student reflection diaries and drawings (27). Longitudinal evaluation findings further confirmed the long-term positive effect of the project in promoting adolescent holistic development. Meanwhile, different stakeholders (e.g., participants, implementers) recognized the effectiveness of the program (24). Extensive studies have indicated that previous P.A.T.H.S. programs explicitly achieved the whole-person development goals. For example, Shek and Yu (28) found that through participating in Project P.A.T.H.S., adolescents reported a slower rate of increase in sexual behavior. Nevertheless, as the Tin Ka Ping Project is a new project implemented in China, the question of how useful the Tin Ka Ping P.A.T.H.S. Project in nurturing mainland Chinese adolescents needs to be answered. Hence, there is a need to conduct systematic evaluation studies.

Shek et al. (29) pointed out that participants' subjective satisfaction could yield useful information since it is highly associated with the objective PYD attribute scores after program implementation. Therefore, in the present study, subjective outcome evaluation was employed to assess the effectiveness of the Tin Ka Ping P.A.T.H.S. Project. Three dimensions of the program were covered, including perceived program content quality, perceived instructor quality, and perceived benefits of the program. Previous studies have identified factors affecting the effectiveness of school-based programs. Payne and Eckert (30) demonstrated that program structure was the most important factor than program providers and school climate in predicting program implementation quality. However, there is a consensus that teaching quality strongly predicts valued intended learning outcomes (31). Hence, the importance of factors that predict program effectiveness still needs further investigation.

Against the background mentioned above, several objectives were intrinsic to the current study. First, descriptive profiles on the responses of the participants to the program were presented. Based on past findings, it was predicted that a high proportion (at least 80%) of the respondents would show positive responses (Hypothesis 1). Second, the association among these three dimensions of subjective outcome evaluation was investigated. Based on previous findings, we predicted that there would be significant correlations amongst the three dimensions of subjective outcome evaluation (Hypotheses 2a to 2c). Third, the predictive effects of students' satisfaction with program content and instructor quality on perceived program benefits were examined. It was predicted that both perceived program quality and implementer would predict perceived program effectiveness (Hypotheses 3a and 3b). Finally, grade differences in participants' subjective evaluation on different indicators were also analyzed. Based on previous findings (32), it was expected that Grade 10 students would have more satisfaction than did Grade 11 students (Hypothesis 4).

OUR STUDY

In the 2015-2016 academic year, a total of 20,358 students from 30 schools participated in the Tin Ka Ping P.A.T.H.S. Project. Among which, 5,784 participants were senior secondary students from 17 schools, locating in both developed areas like Shanghai, Jiangsu and underdeveloped area like Gansu, and Guizhou. With encouraging findings in the initial implementation (26), the research team collected feedback from six participating schools. Correspondingly, the current study examined participants' perceptions of the effectiveness of the Tin Ka Ping P.A.T.H.S. senior secondary program in the 2015-2016 academic year.

After one year, all students were invited to respond to a subjective outcome evaluation form. Research findings in previous studies strongly supported the validity and reliability of this assessment tool (25, 29). Before the data collection process, participants were informed of the evaluation purpose and confidentiality of the data. With clear guidelines and adequate time to complete the assessment form, participants responded in a self-administration format. A total of 1,762 completed questionnaires were collected from senior students, including 1,433 from Grade 10 and 329 from Grade 11.

Instruments

Adopted from the Subjective Outcome Evaluation Form for participants (Form A) of Project P.A.T.H.S. in Hong Kong, the evaluation form employed in this study used the same wording but translated all items into simplified Chinese characters.

This subjective outcome evaluation form is comprised of three parts. The first part contained three rating scales measuring different aspects: participants' perceptions of the program content using 6-point Likert scale (1 = "strongly disagree"; 6 = "strongly agree") with 10 items, the performance of program instructors with same scale structures covering 10 items, and the perceived program benefits using 5-point Likert scale (1 = "unhelpful"; 5 = "very helpful") with 16 items. The second part employed three extra items to understand participants' overall attitudes (e.g., the willingness to participate in similar courses again in the future). The last part used four open-ended questions to examine participants' gains and opinions (e.g., the most important things that the participants learned from the program).

The present study only analyzed and investigated the quantitative parts (overall 39 items) of this evaluation form, while participants' responses to the open-ended questions will be discussed elsewhere.

Data analysis

Findings on the percentages of responses to the program content, instructors' performance, and program benefits as well as their overall satisfaction with the program were analyzed by descriptive statistical analyses in this study. By examining the percentages of responses to each response category, we can generate a picture on the satisfaction of the respondents on the different dimensions of the program.

Reliability analysis was conducted to investigate the internal consistency of the total scale and the subscales. Pearson correlation analysis was performed to examine the inter-relationships amongst the three domains of the program. A multivariate Analysis of Variance (MANOVA) was conducted to find out the differences of the three factors between Grade 10 and Grade 11. Lastly, to determine the predictors of the perceived program benefits, multiple regression analyses were employed. All the analyses were performed using SPSS 23.0.

FINDINGS

A total of 1,762 completed subjective evaluation forms were collected. As presented in Table 1, reliability analysis showed that the total scale and subscales had high internal consistency: 10 items on perceived program content (α = .94), 10 items on perceived instructor quality (α = .96), 16 items on perceived benefits (α = .97), and the overall 36 items measuring program effectiveness (α = .96).

Table 1. Reliability analyses and correlations among participants' perceptions on program content, instructors and program benefits

Subjective outcome evaluation Scales	M	SD	Cronbach's alphas	Mean of inter-item correlations	Inter-scale correlation		
					Program content	Program instructors	Program benefits
Program Content	5.25	.78	.94	.60	-	-	
Program Instructors	5.45	.72	.96	.71	.58***	-	
Program Benefits	4.23	.79	.97	.66	.36***	.25***	-
Total Effectiveness	4.86	.59	.96	.39	.77***	.70***	.81***

Note: *** $p < .001$.

Several observations based on descriptive statistical analyses can be highlighted from Tables 2 to 5. First, the findings in Table 2 revealed that over 93% of the participants expressed positive attitudes with all items scored 4 or above; 94.7% of the participants liked this program very much (item 10). Specifically, 96.4% participants recognized the "clear objectives of the curriculum" and 96.1% endorsed that the design of the curriculum was good. Second, Table 3 indicated that almost all students (97.6% of the participants) held positive views of the implementers (item 10) and they agreed that the instructors were well-prepared for class (97.9%). Almost all students also felt that the instructors were ready to help students. Regarding perceived program effectiveness (Table 4), 95.2% of the participants agreed that the program was able to promote their overall development, including improvement in "self-awareness" (95.7%), "ability to distinguish between good and bad" (95.2%), and "ability to face the future with a positive attitude" (95.1%). Table 5 further shows that 95.2% of the participants would potentially "recommend this program to their peers," 94.4% would consider "to join the similar program again," and 98.0% were satisfied with this program as a whole. In short, Hypothesis 1 was supported.

Consistent with our prediction, Pearson correlation analyses (Table 1) suggested that there was a strong relationship between perceived program content and perceived instructor quality ($r = .58$, $p < .001$). Such strong association could also be found in the relationships of these two domains with perceived program benefits (program content: $r = .36$, $p < .001$; instructor quality: $r = .25$, $p < .001$). In short, Hypotheses 2a to 2c were supported.

Multiple regression analysis was further performed to examine the predictors of perceived effectiveness. Results in Table 7 revealed that both perceptions of program content ($\beta = .32$, $p < .001$) and perceived quality of instructors ($\beta = .07$, $p < .05$) could positively predict perceived program benefits, explaining 8% and 38% of the variance in Grade 10 and Grade 11, respectively. The findings supported Hypotheses 3a and 3b.

Results based on MANOVA (Table 6) showed that significant differences in participants' satisfaction across grades were found for program content, instructor performance, and program benefits ($F = 60.69$, 18.86, and 56.47, $p < .001$, $\eta^2 = .035$, .011, and .032, respectively). In all three dimensions, Grade 10 students reported higher levels of satisfaction ($M = 5.32$, 5.49, and 4.30, respectively) compared with Grade 11 students ($M = 4.91$, 5.25, and 3.90, respectively). The findings provided support for Hypothesis 4.

Table 2. Descriptive statistics of the participants' evaluations on the program content

Items	Respondents with positive responses (Options 4-6)					
	Grade 10		Grade 11		Overall	
	N	%	*n*	%	*N*	%
The objectives of the curriculum are very clear.	1393	97.3	301	92.3	1694	96.4
The design of the curriculum is very good.	1384	96.6	305	93.8	1689	96.1
The activities were carefully planned.	1374	96.0	304	94.1	1678	95.7
The classroom atmosphere was very pleasant.	1367	95.5	300	93.5	1667	95.1
There was much peer interaction amongst the students.	1368	95.5	295	91.0	1663	94.7
I participated actively during lessons (including discussions, sharing, games, etc.).	1372	95.8	289	89.2	1661	94.6
I was encouraged to do my best.	1368	95.5	288	90.0	1656	94.5
The learning experience I encountered enhanced my interest towards the lessons.	1359	94.9	281	86.7	1640	93.4
Overall speaking, I have very positive evaluation of the program.	1363	95.2	291	90.4	1654	94.3
On the whole, I like this curriculum very much.	1372	95.8	292	89.6	1664	94.7

Note: All items are on a 6-point Likert scale with 1 = strongly disagree, 2 = disagree, 3 = slightly disagree, 4 = slightly agree, 5 = agree, 6 = strongly agree. Only respondents with positive responses (Options 4-6) are shown in the table.

Table 3. Descriptive statistics of the participants' evaluations on the program instructors

Items	Respondents with positive responses (Options 4-6)					
	Grade 10		Grade 11		Overall	
	n	%	*n*	%	*N*	%
The instructor(s) had a good mastery of the curriculum.	1402	98.0	305	93.6	1707	97.2
The instructor(s) was well prepared for the lessons.	1406	98.2	313	96.6	1719	97.9
The instructor(s)' teaching skills were good.	1393	97.4	308	94.8	1701	96.9
The instructor(s) showed good professional attitudes.	1392	97.3	309	94.8	1701	96.8
The instructor(s) was very involved.	1407	98.3	304	94.4	1711	97.5
The instructor(s) encouraged students to participate in the activities.	1393	97.3	310	95.7	1703	97.0

Items	Respondents with positive responses (Options 4-6)					
	Grade 10		Grade 11		Overall	
	n	%	*n*	%	*N*	%
The instructor(s) cared for the students.	1402	97.9	314	96.6	1716	97.7
The instructor(s) was ready to offer help to students when needed.	1401	97.8	313	96.6	1714	97.6
The instructor(s) had much interaction with the students.	1392	97.2	311	95.4	1703	96.9
Overall speaking, I have very positive evaluation of the instructors.	1400	97.8	315	96.6	1715	97.6

Note: All items are on a 6-point Likert scale with 1 = strongly disagree, 2 = disagree, 3 = slightly disagree, 4 = slightly agree, 5 = agree, 6 = strongly agree. Only respondents with positive responses (Options 4-6) are shown in the table.

Table 4. Descriptive statistics of the participants' evaluations on the program benefits

The extent to which the course (i.e., the program that all students have joined) has helped you:	Respondents with positive responses (Options 3-5)					
	Grade 10		Grade 11		Overall	
	n	%	*n*	%	*N*	%
It has strengthened my bonding with teachers, classmates and my family.	1345	94.5	292	90.4	1637	93.8
It has strengthened my resilience in adverse conditions.	1336	93.9	291	90.7	1627	93.3
It has enhanced my social competence.	1345	94.5	294	91.6	1639	94.0
It has improved my ability in handling and expressing my emotions.	1358	95.4	295	92.5	1653	94.9
It has enhanced my cognitive competence.	1353	95.1	286	89.4	1639	94.0
My ability to resist harmful influences has been improved.	1362	95.8	293	91.6	1655	95.0
It has strengthened my ability to distinguish between the good and the bad.	1367	96.1	291	91.5	1658	95.2
It has increased my competence in making sensible and wise choices.	1347	94.7	286	89.4	1633	93.7
It has helped me to have life reflections.	1337	94.0	280	87.2	1617	92.8
It has reinforced my self-confidence.	1354	95.2	288	89.4	1642	94.1
It has increased my self- awareness.	1369	96.3	300	93.2	1669	95.7
It has helped me to face the future with a positive attitude.	1360	95.6	299	92.9	1659	95.1
It has helped me to cultivate compassion and care about others.	1345	94.5	290	90.6	1635	93.8

Table 4. (Continued)

The extent to which the course (i.e., the program that all students have joined) has helped you:	Respondents with positive responses (Options 3-5)					
	Grade 10		Grade 11		Overall	
	n	%	*n*	%	*N*	%
It has encouraged me to care about the community.	1299	91.3	267	83.2	1566	89.8
It has promoted my sense of responsibility in serving the society.	1341	94.6	293	91.3	1634	94.0
It has enriched my overall development.	1364	95.9	296	92.2	1660	95.2

Note: All items are on a 5-point Likert scale with 1 = unhelpful, 2 = not very helpful, 3 = slightly helpful, 4 = helpful, 5 = very helpful. Only respondents with positive responses (Options 3-5) are shown in the table.

Table 5. Summary of participants' subjective evaluations on other aspects

Items	Respondents with positive responses (Options 3-5)					
	Grade 10		Grade 11		Overall	
	n	%	*n*	%	*N*	%
Willingness to suggest friends with similar needs or conditions to participate in the program [a]	1381	96.4	294	90.2	1675	95.2
Willingness to participate in similar courses again in the future [a]	1370	95.6	290	89.0	1660	94.4
Satisfaction with this course on the whole [b]	1412	98.5	312	95.4	1724	98.0

Note: [a]: the item is on a 4-point Likert scale with 1 = definitely will not suggest, 2 = will not suggest, 3 = will suggest, 4 = definitely will suggest. Only respondents with positive responses (Options 3-4) are shown in the table.

[b]: the item is on a 6-point Likert scale with 1 = very dissatisfied, 2 = moderately dissatisfied, 3 = slightly dissatisfied, 4 = satisfied, 5 = moderately satisfied, 6 = very satisfied. Only respondents with positive responses (Options 4-6) are shown in the table.

DISCUSSION

The purpose of the current study was to explore senior students' evaluation of the Tin Ka Ping P.A.T.H.S. Project in its pilot extension phase. As there is a lack of PYD programs designed for Chinese adolescents and related evaluation attempts are scarce, this study could be regarded as a pioneering attempt.

The current study adds to the Chinese literature in several important aspects. First, the measuring instrument used in this study is a constructive response to the lack of validated evaluation tools in mainland China. Second, the sample size is sufficiently large to permit generalization to other populations. Third, concerning the externalizing and internalizing problems among adolescents (6), positive perceptions of the perceived benefits of the program indicated that the Tin Ka Ping P.A.T.H.S. Project could serve as a protective factor by promoting the psychosocial competence in adolescents (33). Furthermore, this study further investigated the predictors of perceived benefits, which could make a contribution to the advancement of the theories and applications of PYD programs in mainland China.

Several positive observations support the above-mentioned contributions. First, high values of Cronbach's coefficient and inter-scale correlation among three subscales gave support to the excellent psychometric properties of this subjective outcome evaluation instrument. Second, consistent with the previous findings from an evaluation of Project P.A.T.H.S. in Hong Kong (24), profiles of responses to all items echoed that the majority of senior secondary students participating in the program were fond of this PYD program. A considerable proportion of participants believed that this program has helped them promote different competencies (e.g., cognitive competence, sense of responsibility in serving the society). In particular, quality of the program instructor was more recognized as revealed by the high endorsement rate (97%). Generally speaking, the findings supported Hypothesis 1. In line with other studies, different dimensions of subjective outcome evaluation were significantly correlated (Hypotheses 2a to 2c) and both perceived program quality and implementers were significant predictors of perceived program effectiveness (Hypotheses 3a and 3b). Similar findings also occurred in the evaluation studies on the Project P.A.T.H.S. in Hong Kong (34).

Similar to previous findings, grade differences existed in all three aspects (i.e., program content, instructor quality, and perceived benefits), with Grade 10 students showing more favorable satisfaction ratings. This finding is consistent with a previous study conducted by Shek and Law (34) that Grade 7 students maintained more positive attitudes compared with Grade 8 students.

Table 6. Comparisons of participants' subjective outcome evaluations on different aspects across grades

Subjective outcome evaluation	Grade 10		Grade 11		MANOVA	
Scales	*M*	*SD*	*M*	*SD*	*F*	η^2
Program Content	5.32	.75	4.91	.83	60.69 [a]	.035
Program Instructors	5.49	.70	5.25	.74	18.86 [a]	.011
Program Benefits	4.30	.78	3.90	.77	56.47 [a]	.032

Note: [a]: $p < .001$.

Table 7. Multiple regression analyses predicting perceived program benefits by perceived program content and perceived instructors quality

	β [a]		Model	
	Program Content	Program Instructors	*F*	R^2
Grade 10	$.23^{***}$	$.09^{**}$	63.80^{***}	.083
Grade 11	$.77^{***}$	$.22^{***}$	82.94^{***}	.381
Overall	$.32^{***}$	$.07^{*}$	125.13^{***}	.130

Note: [a] Standardized coefficients. * $p < .05$. ** $p < .01$. *** $p < .001$.

Although this paper presents the first study of subjective outcome evaluation of the Tin Ka Ping Project in China, several limitations of this study are worth mentioning. First, the disparity in sample size between different grades deserves serious consideration before making solid conclusions. Second, senior secondary students in Grade 12 were not involved since they were busy with preparation for examination. However, they are also important targets who may encounter intense challenges physically and mentally in the face of the college entrance examination. Third, as subjective outcome evaluation only provides evidence from one perspective, objective outcome evaluation regarding participants' development in real life situations is also required. Despite these limitations, the positive findings in the present study could be interpreted as evidence supporting the effectiveness of the Tin Ka Ping P.A.T.H.S. Project in mainland China.

ACKNOWLEDGMENTS

The present paper and the Tin Ka Ping P.A.T.H.S. Project are financially supported by Tin Ka Ping Foundation. This chapter is a reprint with minor revisions of an earlier published paper in the *International Journal of Child and Adolescent Health* 2018;11(1) issue with permission.

REFERENCES

[1] Arbeit MR, Johnson SK, Champine RB, Greenman KN, Lerner JV, Lerner RM. Profiles of problematic behaviors across adolescence: Covariations with indicators of positive youth development. J Youth Adolesc 2014;43(6):971-90. doi:10.1007/s10964-014-0092-0.

[2] Shek DTL, Sun RCF, Merrick J. Development of Chinese adolescents: Assessment, issues, and intervention. ScientificWorldJournal 2012;2012:Article ID 935096. doi:10.1100/2012/935096.

[3] Shek DTL, Lin L. What predicts adolescent delinquent behavior in Hong Kong? A longitudinal study of personal and family factors. Soc Indic Res 2016;129(3):1291-318. doi:10.1007/s11205-015-1170-8.

[4] Walther M, Hilbert A. Emotional ppenness, problematic eating behaviours, and overweight in adolescents. Eat Behav 2015;17:111-4. DOI:10.1016/j.eatbeh.2015.01.004.

[5] Shek DTL, Ma HK, Sun RCF. Development of a new curriculum in a positive youth development program: The Project P.A.T.H.S. in Hong Kong. ScientificWorldJournal 2011;11:2207-18. doi:10.1100/2011/289589.

[6] Boylan K, Vaillancourt T, Boyle M, Szatmari P. Comorbidity of internalizing disorders in children with oppositional defiant disorder. Eur Child Adoles Psy 2007;16(8):484-94. doi:10.1007/s00787-007-0624-1.

[7] Catalano RF, Fagan AA, Gavin LE, Greenberg MT, Irwin CE, Ross DA, et al. Worldwide application of prevention science in adolescent health. Lancet 2012;379(9826):1653-64. doi:10.1016/S0140-6736(12)60238-4.

[8] Chen H, Jackson T. Predictors of changes in weight esteem among mainland Chinese adolescents: A longitudinal analysis. Dev Psychol 2009;45(6):1618-29. doi:10.1037/a0016820.

[9] Hou FL, Xu SJ, Zhao YQ, Lu QY, Zhang SC, Zu P, et al. Effects of emotional symptoms and life stress on eating behaviors among adolescents. Appetite 2013;68:63-8. doi:10.1016/j.appet.2013.04.010.

[10] O'Neil A, Quirk SE, Housden S, Brennan SL, Williams LJ, Pasco JA, et al. Relationship between diet and mental health in children and adolescents: a systematic review. Am J Public Health 2014;104(10):e31-42. doi:10.2105/AJPH.2014.302110.

[11] O'Connell ME, Boat T, Warner KE, eds. Preventing mental, emotional, and behavioral disorders among young people: Progress and possibilities. Washington, DC: National Academies Press, 2009.

[12] Ling Y, Huebner ES, He YS, Zhong MT. Three subtypes of internalizing and externalizing behaviors in Chinese adolescents: Results of a latent class analysis. Appl Res Qual Life 2016;11(4):1309-20. doi:10.1007/s11482-015-9438-3.

[13] Benson PL, Scales PC, Syvertsen AK. The contribution of the developmental assets framework to positive youth development theory and practice. Adv Child Dev Behav 2010;41:197-230. doi:10.1016/B978-0-12-386492-5.00008-7.

[14] Lerner RM, Almerigi JB, Theokas C, Lerner JV. Positive youth development a view of the issues. J Early Adolescence 2005;25(1):10-6. doi:10.1177/0272431604273211.

[15] Masten AS. Invited commentary: Resilience and positive youth development frameworks in developmental science. J Youth Adolesc 2014;43(6):1018-24. DOI:10.1007/s10964-014-0118-7.

[16] Weiss MR, Stuntz CP, Bhalla JA, Bolter ND, Price MS. 'More than a game': Impact of The First Tee life skills programme on positive youth development: Project introduction and Year 1 findings. Qual Res Sport Exercise Health 2013;5(2):214-44. doi:10.1080/2159676X.2012.712997.

[17] Shek DTL, Leung H. Do adolescent sexual behavior and intention to engage in sexual behavior change in high school years in Hong Kong? J Pediatr Adolesc Gynecol 2016;29(1):S49-60. doi:10.1016/j.jpag.2015.10.008.

[18] National Health and Family Planning Commission. Chinese family panel studies: Report on Chinese family development 2015. Beijing: China Population Press, 2015 [Chinese].

[19] Liu Y. Report on nutrition and health of Chinese Adolescent was published, which reminds adolescent to remember "52110" for healthy life [Chinese]. Xinhua news 2016. URL: http://news.xinhuanet.com/health/2016-05/15/c_128983274.htm.

[20] Lin WH, Yi CC. Unhealthy sleep practices, conduct problems, and daytime functioning during adolescence. J Youth Adolesc 2015;44(2):431-46. doi:10.1007/s10964-014-0169-9.

[21] Guo L, Xu Y, Deng JX, Huang JH, Huang GL, Gao X, et al. Association between sleep duration, suicidal ideation, and suicidal attempts among Chinese adolescents: The moderating role of depressive symptoms. J Affect Disorders 2017;208:355-62. doi:10.1016/j.jad.2016.10.004.

[22] Xu F, Chen G, Stevens K, Zhou HR, Qi SX, Wang ZY, et al. Measuring and valuing health-related quality of life among children and adolescents in mainland China–a pilot study. PLoS One 2014;9(2):e89222. doi:10.1371/journal.pone.0089222.

[23] Shek DTL. Effectiveness of the Tier 1 Program of the Project P.A.T.H.S.: Preliminary objective and subjective outcome evaluation findings. ScientificWorldJournal 2006;6:1466-74. doi:10.1100/tsw.2006.238.

[24] Shek DTL, Wu FKY. The Project P.A.T.H.S. in Hong Kong: Work done and lessons learned in a decade. J Pediatr Adolesc Gynecol 2016;29(1):S3-S11. doi:10.1016/j.jpag.2015.10.003.

[25] Shek DTL, Han XY, Lee TY, Yu L. Subjective outcome evaluation of a positive youth development program in China. Int J Disabil Hum Dev 2014;13(2):275-83. doi:10.1515/ijdhd-2014-0313.

[26] Shek DTL, Han XY, Lee TY, Yu L. Impact of the Project P.A.T.H.S. in China. In: Shek DTL, Sun RCF, eds. Development and evaluation of Positive Adolescent Training through Holistic Social Programs (P.A.T.H.S.). Singapore: Springer,2013:291-304. doi:10.1007/978-981-4451-54-3_19.

[27] Shek DTL, Ma HK, Merrick J. Effectiveness of the Project P.A.T.H.S. in Hong Kong: Evaluation based on different strategies and different studies over time. ScientificWorldJournal 2012;2012:Article ID 427801. doi:10.1100/2012/427801

[28] Shek DTL, Yu L. Longitudinal impact of the Project P.A.T.H.S. on adolescent risk behavior: What happened after five years? ScientificWorldJournal 2012;2012:Article ID 316029. doi:10.1100/2012/316029.

[29] Shek DTL, Yu L, Sun RCF, Lee TY, Han XY, Li XX, Zhao X. Objective outcome evaluation of a positive youth development program in China. Int J Disabil Hum Dev 2014;13(2):255-65. doi:10.1515/ijdhd-2014-0311.

[30] Payne AA, Eckert R. The relative importance of provider, program, school, and community predictors of the implementation quality of school-based prevention programs. Prev Sci 2010;11(2):126-41. doi:10.1007/s11121-009-0157-6.

[31] Spooren P, Brockx B, Mortelmans D. On the validity of student evaluation of teaching: The state of the art. Rev Educ Res 2013;83(4):598-642. doi:10.3102/0034654313496870.

[32] Shek DTL, Ng CSM, Law MYM. Positive youth development programs for adolescents with greater psychosocial needs: Evaluation based on program implementers. Int J Adolesc Med Health 2015;29(1):33-9. DOI:10.1515/ijamh-2017-3005.

[33] Shek DTL. The role of positive youth development and family functioning in Chinese adolescent well-being: Theoretical considerations and empirical evidence. In:

Maggino F, ed. A life devoted to quality of life. Cham: Switzerland: Springer International Publishing, 2016:43-58. doi:10.1007/978-3-319-20568-7_3.

[34] Shek DTL, Law MYM. Evaluation of the Project P.A.T.H.S. based on the client satisfaction approach: View of the students. J Pediatr Adolesc Gynecol 2014;27:S2-9. doi:10.1016/j.jpag.2014.02.006.

In: Advances in Chinese Children … ISBN: 978-1-53617-870-8
Editors: Ariel Tenenbaum et al.

Chapter 14

IMPLEMENTATION OF THE TIN KA PIN PROJECT IN TWO CHINESE CITIES: STUDENTS' SUBJECTIVE OUTCOME EVALUATION

***Lu Yu*[1,*], *PhD and Esther YW Shek*[1,2]**

[1]Department of Applied Social Sciences, The Hong Kong Polytechnic University, Hong Kong, PR China

[2]Department of Psychology, University of Exeter, Devon, United Kingdom

ABSTRACT

In this chapter we investigated the subjective outcome of a positive youth development program, the Tin Ka Ping project, among secondary school students in two relatively underdeveloped cities in China mainland. A total of 1,573 students who participated in the project responded to an evaluative form upon completion of the project. The findings showed that the majority of the participants were highly satisfied with the project. Regardless of

* Corresponding Author's E-mail: lu.yu@polyu.edu.hk.

their grade, students consistently rated the program content and the instructors positively, and they perceived the project as beneficial to their personal development in multiple areas. Participants' perceptions about the program content and the instructors both significantly predicted their perceived effectiveness of the project. Similar to previous findings based on adolescents living in economically developed Chinese cities, the present study suggests that the Tin Ka Ping project was equally welcomed by youth in underdeveloped areas in China, and provides evidence for the usefulness of the project in promoting Chinese adolescents' holistic development.

INTRODUCTION

The Project P.A.T.H.S. is a curriculum-based positive youth development program designed for Chinese adolescents in Hong Kong (1). Adopting a strengths-based approach, the program focuses on promoting the development of 15 well-established positive youth development attributes among youth, including bonding (BO), social competence (SC), emotional competence (EC), cognitive competence (CC), behavioral competence (BC), moral competence (MC), self-efficacy (SE), Prosocial Norms (PN), Resilience (RE), Self-Determination (SD), Spirituality (SP), clear and positive identity (ID), belief in the future (BF), prosocial involvement (PI) and recognition of positive behaviour (RB) (2). It is believed that by nurturing these attributes, youth behavioral problems, such as delinquency, alcohol use, and Internet addiction, can be effectively prevented (3, 4). With the fund by The Hong Kong Jockey Club, the project P.A.T.H.S. has been widely implemented in secondary schools in Hong Kong since 2006, to promote adolescents' holistic development. So far, a total of 280 secondary schools with more than 200,000 students in Hong Kong have participated in the project. To examine the effectiveness of the program, multiple evaluative strategies have been adopted and the findings converged to suggest that the project P.A.T.H.S. was well received by different stakeholders, and had significant impact on Hong Kong adolescents' development (1, 5-7).

The success of the project P.A.T.H.S. in Hong Kong has provided evidence for the applicability and effectiveness of using positive youth development approach to promote Chinese adolescents' development.

However, such program is almost non-existent in China mainland, although it has the largest youth population in the world. In particular, the rapid economic and social development that has recently taken place in the country has significant influence on adolescent psychological well-being. A recent review of the current status of youth mental health in China mainland showed that adolescent behavioral problems, mood disorders, substance use, and youth suicide are all on the rise (8). Besides, similar to Hong Kong youth, adolescents in China mainland are facing a wide range of developmental issues (9, 10), which could lead to various risk behaviors and problems, if not handled well (11). For example, Chinese parents' high expectation on their children's academic performance and the increased competition have created high academic stress in adolescents. According to a survey by China Youth Social Service Centre, around 70% of secondary school students considered academic stress as their major source of pressure (12). In another study, perceived academic stress was found to significantly predict high school students' depressive symptoms, while this relationship could be moderated by positive school climate with low level of achievement orientation (9). This suggests that promoting a healthy school culture or nurturing positive values among students regarding achievement may effectively prevent their mental health problems even the academic stress remains. These findings point to the pressing need of developing and implementing effective prevention and intervention programs to help Chinese young people tackle with the challenges and have healthy holistic development. Positive youth development program, like the Project P.A.T.H.S., may serve this purpose.

Against this background, with the financial support of the Tin Ka Ping foundation, the research team of the project P.A.T.H.S. started to adapt the project for Chinese young people since 2010, collaborating with a university in China mainland. The new project, entitled the Tin Ka Ping (TKP) project, was developed based on the theoretical framework of P.A.T.H.S., whereas took into account the specific cultural context in China Mainland (4). The project was first piloted in four secondary schools in East China and then further promoted and formally implemented in 30 secondary schools across 27 cities in China (4). A series of training sessions were provided to school teachers and social workers by the research team before the program implementation to ensure the quality of implementation. To evaluate the effectiveness of the TKP project, similar evaluative studies were conducted. Both qualitative and quantitative findings supported that the TKP project was highly welcomed by teachers and students, and effectively promoted Chinese secondary school students' positive development (13-17).

While the TKP project has been offered in a number of Chinese cities with different economic backgrounds, evaluative studies were mainly conducted in schools located in relatively developed areas, such as Shanghai, and its nearby cities like Suzhou and Yangzhou (4). There is a lack of research investigating the implementation quality and outcomes of the project for students in underdeveloped regions where educational resources are relatively limited as compared to big cities. Therefore, the present study aimed to examine the effectiveness of the TKP project for adolescents in two underdeveloped Chinese cities: Baiyin and Shaoguan. Both cities are characterized as "countdown" cities with declined population and economy in recent years. Baiyin used to be a prosperous city with abundant mineral resources, but its development has been slowing down as the mines are exhausted, and the local economy gradually declines. Another city, Shaoguan, had been famous for its steel, non-ferrous metal, electric power, machine, tobacco, pharmaceutical and toy industries. However, since 1980s, the industry development in Shaoguan became tardy and the city has been deindustrialized. These socio-economic changes have inevitably affected local people's life satisfaction, feeling of happiness and mental health (18-20), which may further influence the development of local youth, as well as the implementation and effectiveness of the TKP project in these areas. However, although the TKP project has been implemented in two secondary schools in the two cities for three years, it remains unclear whether the curriculum content of the project is appropriate for local adolescents, whether the project implementers, i.e., school teachers, are able to implement the project with high quality, and to what extent students perceive the project as beneficial to their development.

The present study was designed to address these questions through investigating students' perceptions about the project in two participating schools in Baiyin and Shaoguan. Specifically, we intended to 1) examine participant's subjective outcome evaluation about the TKP project in terms of their views on the program content, instructors and benefits; 2) to compare subjective outcome evaluations among students of different grades and 3), to investigate the predictive effects of students' perceptions about the program quality, the implementers, and benefits of the program on their overall satisfaction of the program.

OUR STUDY

Participants of the present study were recruited from students of two secondary schools in Baiyin (one school) and Shaoguan (one school) who joined the TKP project in the academic years of 2015/16 and 2016/17. Secondary 3 and 6 students (equivalent to Grade 9 and 12) didn't participate because of their heavy workload for the preparation of the entrance exams to high school and university. At the participating school in Baiyin, the program was implemented for senior students at Secondary 4 and 5 only (equivalent to Grade 10 and 11), while at the school in Shaoguan, the program was offered to both junior and senior students in Secondary 1, 2, 4, and 5 (equivalent to Grade 7, 8, 10, and 11).

After obtaining written consents from the school management, students, and their parents, all participating students completed a subjective outcome evaluation form on a voluntary basis upon completion of the project. The survey was administered by trained program workers in classroom settings with standardized instructions. Students were reassured about the confidentiality and anonymity of their responses. A total of 1,573 participants completed the questionnaires, including 481 students at Secondary 1 (only Shaoguan), 468 students at Secondary 2 (only Shaoguan), 392 students at Secondary 4 (173 from Baiyin, and 219 from Shaoguan), and 232 students at Secondary 5 (142 from Baiyin and 90 from Shaoguan).

Instruments

A validated subjective outcome evaluation form was used to assess students' perceptions about the TKP project. The form is consisted of six parts. The first subscale contains 10 items measuring participants' subjective evaluation about the program content. The second part also has 10 items but focusing on participants' perceptions about the program instructors. Items of both subscales were rated on a 6-point Likert scale (1 = strongly disagree, 6 = strongly agree). The third part measures students' perceived benefits of the project, consisted of 16 items evaluated on a 5-point rating scale (1 = unhelpful, 5 = very helpful). The fourth part has two questions asking 1) whether the participant would recommend the project program to their friends, and 2) whether the student would like to attend a similar program in the future. The fifth part asks students' overall satisfaction about the program based on a 6-point rating scale (1 = strongly dissatisfied; 6 = strongly satisfied). The final part is consisted of four open-ended questions about students' other experiences in the project, and the related findings would be reported elsewhere. The evaluation form shows good internal consistency on the present sample of students. As displayed in Table 1, Cronbach's alpha coefficients for the three subscales were all above .92, and mean inter-item correlations ranged between .52 and .65.

Table 1. Reliability analyses and correlations among participants' perceptions on program content, instructors, and program benefits

Subscales	M	SD	Cronbach's α	Mean inter-item correlations	1	2
Views about program content	4.84	.79	.92	.52	-	-
Views about instructors	5.11	.79	.95	.65	.45***	-
Perceived program benefits	3.84	.79	.94	.57	.36***	.31***

Note: *** $p < .001$.

Data analyses

Descriptive statistics were used to depict students' subjective outcome evaluation about the TKP project. Particularly, percentages of students with positive ratings were summarized in terms of their views about program content, program implementers/instructors, and perceived benefits. To compare students' subjective outcomes across grades, Multivariate Analysis of Variance (MANOVA) was conducted with participants' perceptions about program, perceptions about instructors, and perceived benefits of the project as three dependent variables, and students' grade as the independent variable. Lastly, to determine the predictive effects of students' perceptions of program content and instructors on students' perceived benefits of the program, multiple regression analyses were conducted. In the model, perceived program benefits served as the dependent variable, students' grade, perceptions about the program content, and views about instructors served as three independent variables. All the analyses were performed using SPSS 23.0.

FINDINGS

Means and standard deviations of students' subscale scores were summarized in Table 1. Tables 2 to 5 further report the percentages of students with positive responses to different aspects of the project. First, the majority of students had positive ratings on the program content. As can be seen in Table 2, students of different grades consistently showed favorable evaluation about various aspects of the program content. For instance, 92.3% of students at Secondary 1, 88.5% of students at Secondary 2, 92.6% and 86.6% of the Secondary 4 and 5 students agreed that they liked the curriculum very much. Based on the whole sample, more than 92% of the participants expressed that "the design of the curriculum is very good", and that "the activities were carefully planned"; 89.3% of the participants reported that they participated actively during lessons and "have very positive evaluation of the program". Second, in terms of participants' evaluation about the program instructor, the percentage of students with positive ratings was overwhelmingly high (see Table 3). More than 93% of the students perceived the instructors as having a good mastery of the curriculum (93.8%), being well prepared for the lessons (93.4%), having good teaching skills (93.4%), and showing good professional attitudes (93.6%). Students also appreciate teachers' encouragement and care for the students. Over 95% of the participants agreed that the instructor was ready to offer help when needed, and had very positive evaluation of the instructors.

Table 2. Percentage of participants with positive ratings on program content

Items	Respondents with positive responses (Options 4-6)									
	Secondary 1		Secondary 2		Secondary 4		Secondary 5		Overall	
	n	%	*n*	%	*n*	%	*n*	%	*N*	%
The objectives of the curriculum are very clear.	450	93.6	444	94.9	367	93.6	211	90.9	1472	93.6
The design of the curriculum is very good.	442	91.9	438	93.6	365	93.1	213	91.8	1458	92.7
The activities were carefully planned.	443	92.1	424	90.6	369	94.1	212	91.4	1448	92.1
The classroom atmosphere was very pleasant.	404	84.0	426	91.0	363	92.6	215	92.7	1408	89.5
There was much peer interaction amongst the students.	424	88.1	426	91.0	350	89.3	210	90.5	1410	89.6
I participated actively during lessons (discussions, sharing, games, etc.).	430	89.4	425	90.8	346	88.3	203	87.5	1404	89.3
I was encouraged to do my best.	416	86.5	410	87.6	343	87.5	202	87.1	1371	87.2
The learning experience I encountered enhanced my interest towards the lessons.	435	90.4	412	88.0	358	91.3	196	84.5	1401	89.1
Overall speaking, I have very positive evaluation of the program.	426	88.6	416	88.9	349	89.0	208	89.7	1404	89.3
On the whole, I like this curriculum very much.	444	92.3	414	88.5	363	92.6	201	86.6	1422	90.4

Note: All items are on a 6-point Likert scale with 1 = strongly disagree, 2 = disagree, 3 = slightly disagree, 4 = slightly agree, 5 = agree, 6 = strongly agree. Only respondents with positive responses (options 4-6) are shown in the table.

Table 3. Percentage of participants with positive ratings on program instructors

Items	Respondents with positive responses (Options 4-6)									
	Secondary 1		Secondary 2		Secondary 4		Secondary 5		Overall	
	n	%	*n*	%	*n*	%	*n*	%	*N*	%
The instructor(s) had a good mastery of the curriculum.	446	92.7	446	95.3	370	94.4	213	91.8	1475	93.8
The instructor(s) was well prepared for the lessons.	447	92.9	435	92.9	371	94.6	216	93.1	1469	93.4
The instructor(s)' teaching skills were good.	443	92.1	442	94.4	366	93.4	218	94.0	1469	93.4
The instructor(s) showed good professional attitudes.	447	92.9	441	94.2	368	93.9	217	93.5	1473	93.6
The instructor(s) was very involved.	443	92.1	443	94.7	374	95.4	218	94.0	1478	94.0
The instructor(s) encouraged students to participate in the activities.	456	94.8	442	94.4	366	93.4	221	95.3	1485	94.4
The instructor(s) cared for the students.	453	94.2	448	95.7	369	94.1	223	96.1	1493	94.9
The instructor(s) was ready to offer help to students when needed.	457	95.0	450	96.2	372	94.9	219	94.4	1498	95.2
The instructor(s) had much interaction with the students.	445	92.5	440	94.0	359	91.6	218	94.0	1462	92.9
Overall speaking, I have very positive evaluation of the instructors.	459	95.4	451	96.4	373	95.2	220	94.8	1503	95.5

Note: All items are on a 6-point Likert scale with 1 = strongly disagree, 2 = disagree, 3 = slightly disagree, 4 = slightly agree, 5 = agree, 6 = strongly agree. Only respondents with positive responses (options 4-6) are shown in the table.

Third, Table 4 reports students' perceived benefits of the project. As shown in the table, 92.5% of the participants agreed that the program has enriched their overall development, 91.3% of the participants perceived that the program helped them to face the future with a positive attitude, and 92.1% of the pariticpants reported that the programme has strenghthened their ability to distinghish between the good and the bad. Moreover, Table 5 indicates that 94.8% of the participants were willing to recommond their friends to participate in this program and 92.9% of the participants would consider joining a similar program in the future. The overall satisfaction was also high, with 95.3% of the participants expressing that they were satisfied or very satisfied with the project as a whole. Overall speaking, these findings suggest that the TKP project has been welcomed by adolescents in Baiyin and Shaoguan, which provide positive evidence for the successful implementation of the project underdeveloped regions.

Table 4. Percentage of participants with positive ratings on program benefits

Items The extent to which the course (i.e., the program that all students have joined) has helped you:	Respondents with positive responses (Options 3-5)									
	Secondary 1		Secondary 2		Secondary 4		Secondary 5		Overall	
	n	%	*n*	%	*n*	%	*n*	%	*n*	%
It has strengthened my bonding with teachers, classmates and my family.	406	84.4	405	86.5	359	91.6	211	90.0	1381	87.8
It has strengthened my resilience in adverse conditions.	413	85.9	418	89.3	369	94.1	202	87.1	1402	89.1
It has enhanced my social competence.	424	88.1	418	89.3	366	93.4	214	92.2	1422	90.4
It has improved my ability in handling and expressing my emotions.	427	88.8	421	90.0	368	93.9	214	92.2	1430	90.9
It has enhanced my cognitive competence.	422	87.7	423	90.4	372	94.9	209	90.1	1426	90.7
My ability to resist harmful influences has been improved.	427	88.8	438	93.6	372	94.9	208	89.7	1445	91.9
It has strengthened my ability to distinguish between the good and the bad.	434	90.2	439	93.8	369	94.1	207	89.2	1449	92.1
It has increased my competence in making sensible and wise choices.	430	89.4	411	87.8	365	93.1	206	88.8	1412	89.8
It has helped me to have life reflections.	409	85.0	409	87.4	361	92.1	199	85.8	1378	87.6
It has reinforced my self-confidence.	422	87.7	403	86.1	362	92.3	204	87.9	1391	88.4
It has increased my self-awareness.	420	87.3	419	89.5	371	94.6	210	90.5	1420	90.3
It has helped me to face the future with a positive attitude.	423	87.9	437	93.4	367	93.6	209	90.1	1436	91.3
It has helped me to cultivate compassion and care about others.	422	87.7	416	88.9	365	93.1	210	90.5	1413	89.8
It has encouraged me to care about the community.	374	77.8	375	80.1	356	90.8	200	86.2	1305	83.0
It has promoted my sense of responsibility in serving the society.	413	85.9	418	89.3	368	93.9	212	91.4	1411	89.7
It has enriched my overall development.	436	90.6	442	94.4	371	94.6	206	88.8	1455	92.5

Note: All items are on a 5-point Likert scale with 1 = unhelpful, 2 = not very helpful, 3 = slightly helpful, 4 = helpful, 5 = very helpful. Only respondents with positive responses (options 3-5) are shown in the table.

Table 5. Percentage of participants with positive ratings on other aspects of the program and overall satisfaction

Items	Respondents with positive response (options 3-5)									
	Secondary 1		Secondary 2		Secondary 4		Secondary 5		Overall	
	n	%	n	%	n	%	n	%	N	%
1. Willingness to suggest friends with similar needs or conditions to participate in the program [a]	450	93.6	449	95.9	376	95.9	216	93.1	1491	94.8
2. Willingness to participate in similar courses again in the future [a]	449	93.3	436	93.2	364	92.9	213	91.8	1462	92.9
3. Satisfaction with this course on the whole [b]	449	93.3	451	96.4	381	97.2	218	94.0	1499	95.3

Note: [a]The two items are rated on a 4-point scale with 1 = definitely will not suggest, 2 = will not suggest, 3 = will suggest, 4 = definitely will suggest. Only respondents with positive responses (options 3-4) are shown in the table.

[b]The item is rated on a 6-point scale with 1 = very dissatisfied, 2 = moderately dissatisfied, 3 = slightly dissatisfied, 4 = satisfied, 5 = moderately satisfied, 6 = very satisfied. Only respondents with positive responses (options 4-6) are shown in the table.

Table 6. Comparisons of participants' subjective outcome evaluations across grades

Subscales	Secondary 1		Secondary 2		Secondary 4		Secondary 5		Tests of Between-Subjects Effects		
	M	*SD*	*M*	*SD*	M	SD	M	SD	*F*	*p*	Partial η^2
Views about program content	4.83	.83	4.82	.68	4.86	.84	4.84	.87	0.12	.95	.00
Views about instructors	5.14	.79	5.12	.70	5.05	.86	5.16	.82	1.14	.33	.00
Perceived program benefits	3.84	.84	3.76	.70	3.93	.77	3.84	.89	3.26	.01	.01

Ratings by students of different grades

To compare students' ratings across grades, MANOVA was employed and the results showed a significant multivariate effect for the three dependent variables as a group in relation to students' grade, $F(9, 3765.14) = 2.02$,

$p = .03$, Wilk's lambda = 0.99. As seen in Table 6, univariate analyses further suggest that the effect of grade was only significant for students' perceived benefits of the project, but not for their perceptions about program content and instructors. Post hoc tests revealed that students at Secondary 4 had significantly higher ratings on perceived program benefits than students of Secondary 2 ($p = .01$). No significant differences were detected among students of other grades. It seemed that participants at Secondary 4 level perceived the TKP project as more beneficial to their development than did students of Secondary 2. Overall speaking, the findings suggest that students of different grades had generally consistent ratings about the TKP project.

Prediction of students' perceived benefits

Person correlation coeffections among subscales were reported in Table 1. As expected, participants' views about program content, instructors, and perceived benefits were moderately and positively correlated with each other (rs ranged between .31 and .36, $p < .001$) in expected directions. High ratings of the program content and implementers were significantly associated with high level of perceived benefits of the program. Results of multiple regression analysis further showed that after controlling for the effects of grade ($\beta = .04$, $p = .12$), both students' views about program content ($\beta = .27$, $p < .001$) and their perceptions about the instructors ($\beta = .19$, $p < .001$) significantly predicted project benefits. The two predictors explained 15.9% of the variance in students' perceived benefits of the project, $F(2, 1549)_{change} = 146.60$, $p < .001$.

Discussion

The aim of this study is to examine whether the TKP project can be well implemented in relatively underdeveloped cities in mainland China to promote positive development of local adolescents, based on subjective outcome evaluation. Using data collected in two years, the findings suggest that the vast majority of the participants perceived the program content positively and had favorable views about the program implementers. Students viewed the project as being beneficial to their development in multiple areas, and expressed their willingness to attend similar programs in the future and to recommend the program to other young people. More than 95% of the participants were satisfied with the project on the whole. These findings support the applicability of positive youth development program in different Chinese contexts (13, 14), and provide preliminary evidence for the effectiveness of the TKP project in promoting adolescents' development in less developed Chinese cities.

Consistent with findings based on secondary school students in Hong Kong and in other Chinese metropolis (15), the current sample of participants showed very positive attitude towards both program content and instructors. Aside from the reason that the TKP project was adapted from a successful youth program with evident outcomes (the project P.A.T.H.S.), the desirable feedbacks from students may also be due to the systematic training conducted by the research team for program implementers (21). Before each school formally launches the TKP project, the school teaching team is required to attend a series of intensive training workshops in which the theoretical framework of the project, lesson plans for each topic, previous evaluative methods and findings, were introduced by experienced researchers and teachers, through experiential learning and various interactive teaching approaches. The research team also spent time to discuss with program implementers on the appropriateness of the curriculum content, the pedagogy, and possible difficulties in teaching specific topics. Necessary adaption of the teaching content would be made based on the discussion between researchers and the school teacher. In addition, similar to the project P.A.T.H.S. in Hong Kong, a co-walker scheme has been incorporated in the implementation of the TKP project. For each school, at least one scholar from the research team serves as the co-walker, who keeps constant communication with the school teaching team and provides advice throughout the program implementation in the particular school. All these strategies help the instructors to have extensive preparation and teach the curriculum with confidence, which may contribute to the successful implementation of the project (22). This also echoes our finding that students' views about the program content and about the instructors significantly predicted their perceived effectiveness of the program.

When we compare students' evaluation across different grades, no significant differences were identified, except that students of Secondary 4 appeared to be more positive when rating the perceived program benefits than did students of Secondary 2. One possible reason may be that Secondary 4 students just successfully passed the entrance exams to high school. These students may have less academic stress and are able to participate in the project more actively than Secondary 2 students who remain facing the problem of entering a high school. It should be noted that as the effect size was quite small (partial $\eta^2 = 0.01$), the finding needs to be further validated in the future based on a larger sample of participants. Generally, students at different grades consistently showed favorable perceptions about the program.

While the findings are encouraging, several limitations of the study must be acknowledged. First, although the sample size of the present study was not small, the participants were from only two schools of the two cities, which may affect the generalizability of the findings. In the future, when the project is implemented on a larger scale, a more representative sample of students from different grade and schools shall be recruited to participate in the evaluation study. Second, this study only gathered student's opinions and did not collect feedbacks from other stakeholders, such as program implementers, other school personnel, and parents. Data provided by other informants on the effectiveness of the project would triangulate the subjective evaluation findings based on students, and offer new insights for researchers to understand the program implementation and its outcomes (23). Third, apart from the subjective evaluation indicators, more objective outcomes should be measured in the future to evaluate the impact of the program on adolescents' real development (13). For example, whether students' perceived stress, anxiety, and depression reduced, and their life satisfaction and happiness increased after participating in the program, could be investigated in further studies. Last but not least, other evaluative methods, such as individual interview, focus groups, and reflective journals

(16) could be adopted to gain a deeper understanding about how the project plays a role in youth life and helps an adolescent to develop.

To conclude, the present study provides preliminary evidence on the successful implementation of the TKP project in two secondary schools located in less developed regions in China. As there is a lack of evaluation findings focusing on the effectiveness of positive youth development program for Chinese adolescents in these areas (24), the present study makes a useful contribution to the field. The findings suggest that although the positive youth development approach was originally developed in the West (3), it can be well applied in different Chinese contexts to promote the holistic development of adolescents. With the present evidence, we advocated that more youth programs based on positive youth development approach could be designed and implemented to benefit more Chinese young people.

ACKNOWLEDGMENTS

The preparation for this paper and the Tin Ka Ping P.A.T.H.S. Project were financially supported by the Tin Ka Ping Foundation. The authorship is equally carried between the first author and the second author. This chapter is a reprint with minor revisions of an earlier published paper in the *International Journal of Child and Adolescent Health* 2019;12(2) issue with permission.

REFERENCES

[1] Shek DTL, Sun RCF. Implementation quality of a positive youth development program: Cross-case analyses based on seven cases in Hong Kong. ScientificWorldJournal 2008;8:1075-87.

[2] Catalano RF, Berglund ML, Ryan JAM. Positive youth development in the United States: Research findings on evaluations of positive youth development programs. Ann Am Acad Polit Soc Sci 2004;591:98-124.

[3] Fergus S, Marc AZ. Adolescent resilience: A framework for understanding healthy development in the face of risk. Annu Rev Public Health 2005;26:399-419.

[4] Shek DTL, Han XY, Leung JTY. Review on child youth and family social work. Shanghai: East Chia University of Science and Technology Press, 2018.

[5] Shek DT, Ma CM. Program implementers' evaluation of the project P.A.T.H.S.: findings based on different datasets over time. ScientificWorldJournal 2012;2012:918437.

[6] Shek DTL. Objective Outcome Evaluation of the Project P.A.T.H.S. in Hong Kong: Findings Based on Individual Growth Curve Models. ScientificWorldJournal 2010;10:182-91.

[7] Shek DTL, Ma CMS. Impact of the Project P.A.T.H.S. in the junior secondary school years: Individual growth curve analyses. ScientificWorldJournal 2011;11:253-66.

[8] Zheng Y, Zheng X. Current state and recent developments of child psychiatry in China. Child Adolesc Psychiatry Ment Health 2015;9:10. doi:10.1186/s13034-015-0040-0

[9] Liu Y, Lu Z. Chinese high school students' academic stress and depressive symptoms: Gender and school climate as moderators. Stress Heal J Int Soc Investig Stress 2012;28:340-6.

[10] Ling Y, Huebner ES, He Y, Zhong M. Three Subtypes of Internalizing and Externalizing Behaviors in Chinese Adolescents: Results of a Latent Class Analysis. Appl Res Qual Life 2016;11:1309-20.

[11] Chen X, Glaude MW. Academic stress among Chinese adolescents: Can psychological stress theory explain this tragedy ? Int J Human Soc 2017;7:17-25.

[12] Sun J, Dunne MP, Hou X, Xu A. Educational stress among Chinese adolescents: Individual, family, school and peer influences. Educ Rev 2013;3:284-302.

[13] Shek, DTL, Yu L, Ma CMS. The students were happy but did they change positively? Yes, they did. Int J Disabil Hum Dev 2014;13(4):505-11.

[14] Shek, DTL, Leung, H. Subjective outcome evaluation of the training program of the Project P.A.T.H.S.: Findings based on the revised training program. Int J Disabil Hum Dev 2014;13(2):267-274.

[15] Shek, DTL, Han, XY, Lee, TY, Yu, L. Subjective outcome evaluation of a positive youth development program in China. Int J Disabil Hum Dev 2014;13(2):275-83.

[16] Shek, DTL, Wu, FKY. Quantitative evaluation of the revised training program Project P.A.T.H.S. in Hong Kong. Int J Adolesc Med Health 2012;24(3):267-72.

[17] Shek DTL, Yu L. Subjective Outcome Evaluation of the project P.A.T.H.S: Descriptive Profiles and Correlates. ScientificWorldJournal 2010;10:211-23.

[18] Fraser C, Jackson H, Judd F, Komiti A, Robins G, Murray G, et al. Changing places: The impact of rural restructuring on mental health in Australia. Health Place 2005;11:157-71.

[19] Maxwell P. The economic decline of large remote mining towns: Does the Broken Hill experience offer lessons for Kalgoorlie Boulder? Miner Econ 2015;28(3):83-101.

[20] Audureau E, Rican S, Coste J. From deindustrialization to individual health-related quality of life: Multilevel evidence of contextual predictors, mediators and modulators across French regions, 2003. Heal Place 2013;22:140-52.

[21] Shek, DTL, Ng, CSM. Secondary 1 program of project P.A.T.H.S.: process evaluation based on the co-walker scheme. ScientificWorldJournal 2009;9:704-14.

[22] Shek, DTL, Law, MYM. Implementation of the extension phase of the Project P.A.T.H.S. in Hong Kong: observations based on the Co-Walker Scheme. Int J Adolesc Med Health 2013;25(4):459-66.

[23] Shek, DTL, Yu, L. A stakeholder-collaborative evaluation of intervention for students with greater psychosocial needs. Int J Adolesc Med Health 2012;24(3):223-30.

[24] Shek, DTL, Wu, FKY, Merrick, J. Editorial: Evaluation of positive youth development and leadership programs in Hong Kong. Int J Child Adolesc Health 2016;9(2):139-41.

In: Advances in Chinese Children … ISBN: 978-1-53617-870-8
Editors: Ariel Tenenbaum et al.

Chapter 15

SUBJECTIVE OUTCOME EVALUATION OF A SERVICE LEADERSHIP SUBJECT: FINDINGS BASED ON UNIVERSITY STUDENTS IN HONG KONG

Janet TY Leung*, PhD
and Daniel TL Shek, PhD, FHKPS, BBS, SBS, JP
Department of Applied Social Sciences,
The Hong Kong Polytechnic University, Hong Kong, PR China

ABSTRACT

In this chapter we assessed the subjective outcome evaluation of a credit-bearing subject entitled "Service Leadership" in a university in Hong Kong. The samples included 64 and 74 students who took the subject offered in the regular semester (Semester 1) and intensive summer semester (Semester 3) in 2016-2017 academic year, respectively. Students'

---

* Corresponding Author: Janet Leung, PhD, Associate Professor, Department of Applied Social Sciences, The Hong Kong Polytechnic University, Hunghom, Hong Kong, PR China. Email: janet.leung@polyu.edu.hk.

perceptions of the course content, instructor quality, benefits and global satisfaction of the subject were assessed at the end of the subject. Results indicated that majority of students had positive views toward course content, instructor quality, and benefits from the subject in enhancing their competencies in different aspects, such as social and emotional competence, self-confidence, resilience, and self-leadership. The two delivery modes (i.e., regular semester and intensive summer semester) also showed significant differences in the subjective outcomes, with the course conducted in regular term having higher scores than the course offered in summer term. As predicted, course content, instructor quality, and course benefits were inter-correlated significantly. While course content and instructor quality significantly predicted perceived subject benefits, course content and perceived benefits of the subject were significant predictors of students' global satisfaction.

INTRODUCTION

One may ask the question: why does a university teach "service leadership"? There are strong reasons to address the question. First, service-oriented industries are the skeleton of the Hong Kong economy, contributing to 92.4% of Gross Domestic Product (GDP) in 2017 in Hong Kong (1). Among the service industry components, import/export wholesale and retail trades, finance and insurance, and pubic administration, social and personal services cover 21.5%, 18.9% and 18.2% of the GDP respectively (1). As university graduates have potential tendency to be engaged in frontline and supervisory positions in these industries, service leadership education is important for preparing the students to contribute to these service industries. Second, Hong Kong is a metropolitan city where people from all over the world come in and out for business, vacation, education and other matters. Other than acquiring the discipline-related knowledge and skills, university students should build up a global perspective and develop the 21st Century skills to adapt to the dynamic environment in the service industries (2). Dede (2) highlighted four areas of competence in economic and social ecology of the 21st Century, namely: 1) global awareness; 2) economic and entrepreneurial literacy; 3) awareness of civic rights and responsibilities; and 4) health and wellness sensitivity. Besides, the 21st Century skills cover three sets of competency skills, including: learning and thinking skills (e.g., skills on problem-solving, communication, innovation, critical analyses, collaborative learning), information and communications technology (ICT) literacy, and life skills (e.g., leadership, social responsibility, adaptability, self-direction etc.) (2).

Third, service leadership education serves as a platform for building interpersonal and intrapersonal competencies of university students (3, 4), who are at the developmental transition from adolescence to adulthood. During emerging adulthood, individuals need to develop financial independence, shoulder civic responsibilities, establish connections with peers and romantic partners, and build up engagement with work and education (5). Service leadership education, which focuses on psychosocial competencies, character strengths and caring disposition, may foster positive youth development of university students in their life transition to adulthood (4).

Fourth, young people nowadays face different developmental and ecological challenges in adapting to the competitive and complex environment (6). Particularly, millennials growing up in a relatively prosperous and protective era are portrayed as egocentric, narcissistic and unempathetic (7). Also, the rise of materialism has shifted one's values from concentrating on intrinsic motives (e.g., purpose in life, satisfaction from helping others) to extrinsic ones (e.g., money, prestige) (8). Hence, there is a need to reinforce the emphases in service leadership (including moral competence, character strengths, caring disposition) in university education, and give students more opportunities to reflect on their own life expectations and values.

Most importantly, university students are important stakeholders of Hong Kong future. They are expected to lead and contribute to the future social and economic development of Hong Kong. Thus, there is an urgent need to nurture the development of university students via service leadership education.

Table 1. Course content of "Service Leadership" subject

Lecture	Topic	Content
1	Introduction	• Overview of the subject • Definitions and conceptions of service leadership • Importance of service leadership in the global world • Relevance to university students
2	Core beliefs and components	• Core beliefs about service leadership
3	Intrapersonal competences	• IQ, EQ, AQ and SQ
4	Interpersonal competences	• Communication, relationship building, conflict resolution
5	Character strengths	• Moral character; basic character strengths
6	Caring disposition	• Social cognition (warmth and competence); primary elements of care (love, listening, and empathy)
7	Character strengths in Chinese philosophies	• Relevance of Confucian virtues to service leadership, e.g., integrity (lian), loyalty (zhong), filial piety (xiao), benevolence (ren) etc.
8	Contemporary leadership models and the dark side of leadership	• Review of contemporary models of leadership • Dark side of leadership
9	Factors leading to positive social relationship	• Trust, fairness, respect, care, behavioral consistency and loyalty
10	Self-leadership	• Self-monitoring, self-regulation, and self-improvement
11	Developmental assets	• Self-esteem; self-efficacy; purpose in life, and optimism about future
12	Review of Service Leadership qualities	• Comparisons between models of leadership • Potential application
13	Wrap-up; Group presentation	• Group presentation

In 2012, the Victor and William Fung Foundation and the Hong Kong Institute of Service Leadership and Management (HKI-SLAM) initiated the Fung Service Leadership Initiative in eight universities in Hong Kong that were funded by the University Grants Council. The Initiative aims at designing and implementing service leadership education courses and programs to university students. Employing a holistic positive development approach, it is expected that service leadership education can help to enhance leadership mentality, values and competencies among university students (9). As suggested by Shek and Chung (10), the ultimate goal of service leadership education is to promote students' service leadership attributes in order to "maintain Hong Kong's competitiveness in the global market and to develop leaders with a human face" (p. xix).

Adopting the SLAM framework on the main components of service leadership (i.e., relevant task management capabilities, character strengths and a caring personality) (10, 11), The Hong Kong Polytechnic University has designed and implemented a credit-bearing "Service Leadership" subject for undergraduate students. The program consists of 13 lectures highlighting the important attributes of service leadership (see Table 1). Prior studies showed that participants had positive views on course content, instructors, benefits and global satisfaction (12-14). To replicate previous findings, this study attempted to evaluate the effectiveness of "Service Leadership" subject offered to undergraduate students in a regular semester (Semester 1) and summer semester (with intensive teaching) of the 2016/17 academic year at The Hong Kong Polytechnic University. A subjective outcome evaluation approach was adopted to examine students' perception of (1) course content, (2) course implementers, (3) course benefits; (4) global satisfaction after completing the subject. There are five research questions:

1) What are the perceptions of the students on course content, implementers, benefits and global satisfaction after taking the subject?
2) Are there any differences in perceptions of course content, implementers, benefits, total effectiveness (combination of perceived course content, implementers and benefits) and global satisfaction between participants taking the subject in the regular semester (Semester 1) and intensive summer semester (Semester 3)? As the subject schedule offered in intensive summer semester is tight, it was hypothesized that participants taking the subject in the regular semester would have a more positive view on course content, implementers, benefits, total effectiveness and global satisfaction than those taking the subject in summer semester (Hypotheses 2a to 2e).

3) What are the interrelationships among perceptions of course content, course implementers, course benefits, total effectiveness and global satisfaction of participants of the subject? Based on the results of previous studies (12-14), it was hypothesized that perceived course content, course implementers, course benefits, total effectiveness and global satisfaction of participants would be interrelated with each other (Hypotheses 3a to 3j).
4) Do perceptions of course content and implementers predict perceived benefits of the participants? Based on the findings of previous studies (12-14), it was hypothesized that perceptions of course content and implementers of the participants would positively predict their perceived benefits respectively (Hypotheses 4a and 4b).
5) Do perceptions of course content, implementers and benefits predict global satisfaction of the participants? Based on the findings of previous studies (12), it was hypothesized that perceptions of course content, implementers, and benefits of the participants would positively predict their global satisfaction respectively (Hypotheses 5a to 5c).

OUR STUDY

The data was collected from the participants of two classes of "Service Leadership" subject offered in regular semester (Semester 1) and intensive summer semester (Semester 3) of 2016-2017 academic year. There were 64 and 74 university students enrolled into the subject during Semester One and intensive summer term, respectively. Written informed consent from students was obtained at the beginning of the course. The students were invited to fill out the Subjective Outcome Evaluation Scale that contained the measures during the last lecture of the course in an anonymous matter. The students were given adequate time to complete the evaluation form. A trained research assistant was responsible to conduct the evaluation, with the absence of the instructor.

Measures

A validated Subjective Outcome Evaluation Scale (SOES) was employed in the present study. The SOES consists of five parts: program content (PC), program implementer (PI), program benefits (PB), global satisfaction of the course and qualitative feedback of the course for further improvement. The present study focused on the first four parts of the SOES.

1) Program Content (PC) consists of 10 items, which assesses perceptions of students on course design, in-class activities, interactions among classmates, students' participation and global satisfaction on program content. The items are rated in a 5-point Likert scale on from 1 = "Strongly disagree" to 5 = "Strongly agree." A higher mean score of PC indicates a more positive view of program content from the students.
2) Program Implementer (PI) contains 10 items, which measures the students' perceptions of the attitudes, teaching strategies and skills of the instructors, engagement and interactions with the students, as well as global satisfaction on the instructors' teaching. The items are rated on a 5-point Likert scale on from 1 = "Strongly disagree" to 5 = "Strongly agree." A higher mean score of PI indicates a more positive view of program implementer from the students.
3) Program Benefits (PB) consists of 18 items, which assesses the students' perceptions of their changes on relevant task competencies (e.g., problem-solving, cognitive competence), care and compassion towards others, qualities of self-leadership and sense of civic responsibility. The items are rated in a 5-point Likert scale on from 1 = "Strongly disagree" to 5 = "Strongly agree." A higher mean score of PB indicates more benefits perceived by the students after participating in the course.
4) Global Satisfaction (GS) includes three questions on whether the participants will recommend their friends to select this course, whether they will enroll in similar course again in the future, and their rating of their global satisfaction of the course. For the first two

questions of GS, the respondents are requested to rate in a 5-point Likert scale on from 1 = "Definitely will not" to 5 = "Definitely will." Finally, the last question of GS is rated in a 5-point Likert scale on from 1 = "Very dissatisfied" to 5 = "Very satisfied."

Data analyses

Descriptive data analyses were performed to assess the perceptions of participants on their comments of program content (PC), program implementer (PI) and benefits from the course (PB). A composite variable of "Total Effectiveness" (TE) was created by averaging the scores of all items of PC, PI and PB. One-way ANOVAs were employed to compare between the participants' responses in two semesters. Correlation analyses were performed to examine the interrelationship of the 5 domains (PC, PI, PB, GS and TE). Finally, multiple regression analyses were conducted to assess the relative importance of different domains in affecting perceived benefits and global satisfaction of the participants respectively.

FINDINGS

Regarding program content, the mean score of perceived program content (PC) of total participants was 4.04 (SD = .46) (see Table 2). Most participants of the two classes showed positive responses (Options 4 and 5) on curriculum design, classroom atmosphere, class activities, peer interaction and their own involvement respectively (Table 3). Particularly, the clear course objectives, content design, classroom activities and interactions among peers were greatly appreciated by the students, with 91.3%, 87.7%, 88.4% and 87.7% of the participants rated positively on the relative items respectively. Overall, 89.9% of the participants showed very positive evaluation on the course, and 82.6% of the participants liked the course very much (see Table 3).

For students' perceptions of program implementer, the results showed very positive responses (Options 4 and 5) on the qualities of instructors, including their knowledge on service leadership, preparation, professional attitudes and involvement (see Table 4). Besides, the instructors showed positive engagement with the students by expressing their care, offering their help, giving encouragement to them, and facilitating interactions among students (see Table 3). Overall, 97.1% of total students from these two classes expressed a very positive evaluation on the instructors (see Table 4). The mean score of perceived program implementer (PI) of total participants was 4.33 (SD = .42), showing participants' positive responses on the program implementers (see Table 2).

Regarding students' perceptions of their benefits from the course, the participants showed positive views (Options 4 and 5) that the course enhanced their situational task competencies, care and compassion towards others, qualities of self-leadership and sense of responsibility to contribute to the society (see Table 5). 86.2% of the total respondents showed that the course promoted their overall development. Besides, the theories, research and concepts helped majority of students understand (88.4% of the students rated Options 4 or 5) and synthesize (89.1% of the students rated Options 4 or 5) the characteristics of successful service leaders (see Table 5). The mean score of perceived program benefits (PB) of total participants was 4.02 (SD = .47) (see Table 2), showing evidence of positive benefits perceived by the students after participating in the course.

On the whole, 86.3% of the students felt satisfied with the subject (Options 4 and 5; see Table 6). 78.3% of the students would invite their friends to enroll in the course, and 57.2% of the students would attend similar courses in the future (see Table 6). The mean score of global satisfaction (GS) of total participants was 3.90 (SD = .67) (see Table 2).

Table 2. Means, standard deviations, Cronbach's alphas, and mean of inter-item correlations among three samples

Subjective Outcome	**Semester 1 (n= 64)**				**Semester 3 (n= 74)**				**Overall (n= 138)**			
Evaluation Scales	Mean	*SD*	α	*Mean*[#]	Mean	*SD*	α	*Mean*[#]	Mean	*SD*	α	*Mean*[#]
Program Content (PC: 10 items)	4.20	.40	.88	.42	3.90	.47	.90	.50	4.04	.46	.90	.56
Program Implementer (PI: 10 items)	4.48	.42	.92	.54	4.21	.39	.90	.49	4.33	.42	.92	.67
Program Benefits (PB: 18 items)	4.19	.45	.95	.52	3.88	.45	.94	.48	4.02	.47	.95	.50
Total Effectiveness (TE: 38 items)	4.27	.36	.96	.38	3.97	.38	.96	.37	4.11	.40	.96	.45
Global Satisfaction (GS: 3 items)	4.07	.68	.85	.69	3.76	.63	.85	.67	3.90	.67	.86	.73

Note: *Mean*[#]: inter-item correlation.

Table 3. Summary of the participants' positive responses towards Program Content (PC)

Perceptions of program content [a]		Semester 1 ($n = 64$)				Semester 3 ($n = 74$)				Overall ($n = 138$)			
		M†	*SD*	Positive Responses [b]		M†	*SD*	Positive Responses [b]		M†	*SD*	Positive Responses [b]	
				n	%			n	%			n	%
1.	The objectives of the curriculum are very clear.	4.19	.59	60	93.8	3.95	.52	66	89.2	4.06	.56	126	91.3
2.	The content design of the curriculum is very good.	4.17	.58	60	93.8	3.89	.54	61	82.4	4.02	.57	121	87.7
3.	The activities were carefully arranged.	4.23	.53	61	95.3	3.92	.57	61	82.4	4.07	.57	122	88.4
4.	The classroom atmosphere was very pleasant.	4.14	.61	58	90.6	3.84	.74	55	74.3	3.98	.70	113	81.9
5.	There was much peer interaction amongst the students.	4.33	.59	60	93.8	3.99	.67	61	82.4	4.14	.66	121	87.7
6.	I participated in the class activities actively (including discussions, sharing, games, etc.).	3.98	.55	54	84.4	3.89	.77	55	74.3	3.93	.67	109	79.0
7.	I was encouraged to do my best.	4.20	.54	60	93.8	3.95	.62	60	81.1	4.07	.59	120	87.0
8.	The learning experience enhanced my interests towards the program.	4.16	.67	56	87.5	3.80	.66	53	71.6	3.96	.69	109	79.0
9.	Overall speaking, I have a very positive evaluation on the program.	4.28	.55	61	95.3	3.95	.64	63	85.1	4.10	.62	124	89.9
10.	On the whole, I like this program very much.	4.27	.57	60	93.8	3.82	.71	54	73.0	4.03	.68	114	82.6

Note. [a] Scores on the scale/subscale higher than or equal to 4 were treated as positive responses. [b] For every item, respondents with positive responses (options 4-5) are shown in the Table. † 1=Strongly Disagree; 2=Disagree; 3=Neutral; 4=Agree; 5=Strongly Agree.

Table 4. Summary of the participants' positive responses towards Program Instructors (PI)

Perceptions of program instructor [a]		Semester 1 ($n = 64$)				Semester 3 ($n = 74$)				Overall ($n = 138$)			
		$M^{\dagger}$	*SD*	Positive Responses [b]		$M^{\dagger}$	*SD*	Positive Responses [b]		$M^{\dagger}$	*SD*	Positive Responses [b]	
				n	%			n	%			n	%
1.	The instructor(s) had a good mastery of the program.	4.41	.56	62	96.9	4.15	.54	68	91.9	4.27	.56	130	94.2
2.	The instructor(s) was (were) well prepared for the lessons.	4.50	.53	63	98.4	4.19	.49	71	95.9	4.33	.53	134	97.1
3.	The teaching skills of the instructor(s) were good.	4.25	.56	60	93.8	3.96	.65	61	82.4	4.09	.63	121	87.7
4.	The instructor(s) showed good professional attitudes.	4.47	.53	63	98.4	4.20	.47	72	97.3	4.33	.51	135	97.8
5.	The instructor(s) was (were) very involved.	4.61	.52	63	98.4	4.20	.52	70	94.6	4.39	.56	133	96.4
6.	The instructor(s) encouraged students to participate in the activities.	4.56	.50	64	100.0	4.39	.54	72	97.3	4.47	.53	136	98.6
7.	The instructor(s) cared for the students.	4.41	.58	61	95.3	4.28	.51	72	97.3	4.34	.55	133	96.4
8.	The instructor(s) was (were) ready to offer help to students when needed.	4.52	.56	62	96.9	4.32	.50	73	98.6	4.41	.54	135	97.8
9.	The instructor(s) had much interaction with the students.	4.50	.62	60	93.8	4.19	.59	67	90.5	4.33	.62	127	92.0
10.	Overall speaking, I have a very positive evaluation on the instructor(s).	4.55	.50	64	100.0	4.20	.52	70	94.6	4.36	.54	134	97.1

Note. [a] Scores on the scale/subscale higher than or equal to 4 were treated as positive responses. [b] For every item, respondents with positive responses (options 4-5) are shown in the Table. † 1=Strongly Disagree; 2=Disagree; 3=Neutral; 4=Agree; 5=Strongly Agree.

Table 5. Summary of the participants' positive responses towards Program Benefits (PB)

Perceptions of program benefits [a]		Semester 1 (*n* = 64)				Semester 3 (*n* = 74)				Overall (*n* = 138)			
		M†	*SD*	Positive Responses [b]		M†	*SD*	Positive Responses [b]		M†	*SD*	Positive Responses [b]	
				n	%			n	%			n	%
1.	It has enhanced my social competence.	4.16	.57	60	93.8	3.99	.54	63	85.1	4.07	.56	123	89.1
2.	It has improved my ability in expressing and handling my emotions.	4.11	.59	56	87.5	3.88	.66	57	77.0	3.99	.64	113	81.9
3.	It has enhanced my critical thinking.	4.05	.63	55	85.9	3.82	.69	57	77.0	3.93	.67	112	81.2
4.	It has increased my competence in making sensible and wise choices.	4.19	.56	59	92.2	3.81	.66	56	75.7	3.99	.64	115	83.3
5.	It has helped me make ethical decisions.	4.27	.62	58	90.6	3.95	.72	59	79.7	4.09	.69	117	84.8
6.	It has strengthened my resilience in adverse conditions.	4.23	.61	58	90.6	3.78	.67	54	73.0	3.99	.68	112	81.2
7.	It has strengthened my self-confidence.	4.13	.65	54	84.4	3.82	.65	55	74.3	3.96	.67	109	79.0
8.	It has helped me face the future with a positive attitude.	4.23	.64	57	89.1	3.88	.64	58	78.4	4.04	.66	115	83.3
9.	It has enhanced my love for life.	4.03	.67	53	82.8	3.69	.64	46	62.2	3.85	.67	99	71.7
10.	It has helped me explore the meaning of life.	4.05	.65	54	84.4	3.69	.60	48	64.9	3.86	.65	102	73.9
11.	It has enhanced my ability of self-leadership.	4.33	.56	61	95.3	3.85	.66	54	73.0	4.07	.66	115	83.3
12.	It has helped me cultivate compassion and care for others.	4.19	.61	57	89.1	3.89	.61	60	81.1	4.03	.63	117	84.8
13.	It has helped me enhance my character strengths comprehensively.	4.30	.58	60	93.8	3.91	.58	62	83.8	4.09	.61	112	88.4
14.	It has enabled me to understand the importance of situational task competencies, character strength and caring disposition in successful leadership.	4.22	.55	60	93.8	4.03	.60	64	86.5	4.12	.58	124	89.9

Table 5. (Continued)

Perceptions of program benefits [a]		Semester 1 (n = 64)				Semester 3 (n = 74)				Overall (n = 138)			
		M[†]	*SD*	Positive Responses [b]		M[†]	*SD*	Positive Responses [b]		M[†]	*SD*	Positive Responses [b]	
				n	%			n	%			n	%
15.	It has promoted my sense of responsibility in serving the society.	4.19	.56	59	92.2	3.91	.58	60	81.1	4.04	.58	119	86.2
16.	It has promoted my overall development.	4.27	.65	57	89.1	3.97	.64	62	83.8	4.11	.66	119	86.2
17.	The theories, research and concepts covered in the program have enabled me to understand the characteristics of successful service leaders.	4.28	.58	60	93.8	3.97	.60	62	83.8	4.12	.60	122	88.4
18.	The theories, research and concepts covered in the program have helped me synthesize the characteristics of successful service leaders.	4.22	.60	58	90.6	4.00	.53	65	87.8	4.10	.57	123	89.1

Note. [a] Scores on the scale/subscale higher than or equal to 4 were treated as positive responses. [b] For every item, respondents with positive responses (options 4-5) are shown in the Table. [†] 1=Strongly Disagree; 2=Disagree; 3=Neutral; 4=Agree; 5=Strongly Agree.

Table 6. Summary of the participants' Global Satisfaction with the program

Satisfaction with the program [a]		Semester 1 ($n = 64$)				Semester 3 ($n = 74$)				Overall ($n = 138$)			
		M	*SD*	Positive Responses [b]		*M*	*SD*	Positive Responses [b]		*M*	*SD*	Positive Responses [b]	
				n	%			n	%			n	%
1.	Will you suggest your friends to take this program? [c]	4.11	.72	55	85.9	3.84	.78	53	71.6	3.96	.76	108	78.3
2.	Will you participate in similar programs again in the future? [c]	3.78	1.00	42	65.6	3.53	.80	37	50.0	3.64	.90	79	57.2
3.	On the whole, are you satisfied with this program? [d]	4.31	.53	62	96.9	3.90	.58	57	77.0	4.09	.59	119	86.2

Note. [a] Scores on the scale/subscale higher than or equal to 4 were treated as positive responses. [b] For every item, respondents with positive responses (options 4-5) are shown in the Table. [c] 1= Definitely will not, 2 = Will not, 3 = Not sure, 4 = Will, 5 = Definitely will. [d] 1= Very dissatisfied, 2 = Moderately dissatisfied, 3 = Neutral, 4 = Satisfied, 5 = Very satisfied.

The results of one-way ANOVAs showed that there were significant differences on perceptions of program content, program implementer, program benefits, total effectiveness and global satisfaction between students taking service leadership course in regular semester (Semester 1) and intensive summer term (Semester 3) respectively, with students participating in Semester 1 perceived better subjective outcomes than did those participating in intensive summer term (see Table 7). Hypotheses 2a to 2e were supported.

Table 7. One-way ANOVA comparing the evaluations on the program of participants in different semesters

Subjective Outcome Evaluation Scales	Semester 1 (n= 64)		Semester 3 (n= 74)		Comparison	
	Mean	*SD*	Mean	*SD*	*F*	*p*
Program Content	4.20	.40	3.90	.47	15.54	< .001
Program Implementer	4.48	.42	4.21	.39	15.10	< .001
Program Benefits	4.19	.45	3.88	.45	16.50	< .001
Total Effectiveness	4.27	.36	3.97	.38	21.62	< .001
Global Satisfaction	4.07	.68	3.76	.63	7.74	< .01

Table 8. Correlations coefficients among the variables

	1	2	3	4
1. Program Content	1			
2. Program Implementer	.60***	1		
3. Program Benefits	.71***	.54***	1	
4. Total Effectiveness	.87***	.76***	.93***	1
5. Global Satisfaction	.62***	.43***	.61***	.65***

Note: *** $p < .001$.

Furthermore, correlation analyses showed that all variables (PC, PI, PB, TE, GS) were all correlated with each other, with Pearson's r ranging from .43 to .93 (see table 8). Hypotheses 3a to 3j were supported. Multiple regression analyses further indicated that both program content and program implementer were significant predictors of perceived benefits of the students, with $\beta = .61$ ($p < .001$) and .17 ($p < .05$) respectively, explaining 53% of the total variance of perceived benefits (Table 9). Hypotheses 4a and

4b were supported. In addition, among the relationship of program content, program implementer and program benefits on global satisfaction of the students, both program content and program benefits were significant predictors of global satisfaction of the students, with $\beta = .36$ ($p < .001$) and .34 ($p < .001$). The predictor variables explained 44% of the total variance of global satisfaction of the participants (see table 9). Hypotheses 5a and 5c were supported.

Table 9. Multiple regression analyses predicting perceived benefits and global satisfaction

Predictors	Program Benefits				Global Satisfaction			
	B	*SE*	β	R^2	*B*	*SE*	β	R^2
Program Content	.68	.08	.61***	.53	.52	.14	.36***	.44
Program Implementer	.19	.08	.17*		.05	.13	.03	
Program Benefits					.48	.13	.34***	

Note: *$p < .05$; ***$p < .001$.

DISCUSSION

This study aimed at assessing the effectiveness of a service leadership subject in a university in Hong Kong. The findings echoed the results of previous studies (12-14), showing that the participants had positive views perceptions on course content, implementers, benefits and global satisfaction after participating in the subject. The findings reveal that the subject was able to introduce the theories and concepts of service leadership to the students and promoted their leadership competencies.

However, participants of subject offered in the regular semester (Semester 1) rated higher on the subjective outcomes in the four aspects (PC, PI, PB and GS) than did those participated in the intensive summer semester (Semester 3). As the summer semester lasted for seven weeks to cover 13 lectures, the students needed to attend two lectures each week. Thus, the students may have difficulties to fully comprehend the concepts and theories, and may exhibit pressure in preparing presentations and assignments. The tight program schedule and stresses may affect their perceptions of course arrangement, instructors, benefits and global satisfaction. As such, there is a need to refine the flow and content of the subject in order to meet the tight program schedule, and provide more support to the students on their preparation of presentations and assignments.

As predicted, course content and quality of implementers are important predictors of perceived benefits of the students. As such, it is important to develop a curriculum that can inspire students on the essential components of service leadership and enhance their competencies and character strengths in becoming a service leader. In particular, program activities and interactions among peers are essential elements for students to acquire the knowledge of service leadership. From the literature (15, 16), experiential learning involves direct experience, reflections and observation, abstract conceptualization, and active experimentation (15), which is a practical pedagogy to engage students in the leadership process, and encourage them to reflect and make meanings through their experiences and reflections (16). Hence, it is necessary to enrich the curriculum with more experiential activities for the students to experience and reflect on their leadership style. In addition, qualities of instructors are critical in transferring knowledge and practice to university students. In education literature, essential practices of student-teacher contacts, constructive feedback to students, high expectations, and respect for diverse potentials and learning paths of students are evident to facilitate student development and learning (17). Besides, instructors serve as role-models of a service leader for students. Their attitudes, behaviors and responses to students reflect the attributes of a service leader.

Furthermore, the findings indicated that program content and perceived benefits were predictors of students' global satisfaction, which echo the findings of previous research (12-14). Obviously, perceived benefits are important predictors in influencing students' global satisfaction, as the strengthening of students' competencies and character strengths fulfils participants' expectations of the course, which increases their satisfaction of the course. Moreover, the program content determines the "what" and "how" of service leadership theories and concepts are conveyed to the students, which affects their global satisfaction. Interestingly, program implementer, relative to program content and perceived benefits, was not a significant predictor of students' global satisfaction. Students felt satisfied with the course only when they acquired the knowledge of service leadership, and perceived changes of their intrapersonal and interpersonal competence. The performance of program instructors becomes secondary when compared with program content and perceived benefits. These findings are in line with previous findings (18).

There are several implications of the study. First, the findings indicated that students showed positive perceptions on course content, instructors, benefits and global satisfaction of the participants after participating in a service leadership subject. As commented by Eich (16) that "there has been little empirical research on student leadership program quality and program activities that contribute significantly to leadership development and learning" (p. 176), the present study shows empirical support on the effectiveness of a quality service leadership subject conducted in a university. Second, in the urging needs in equipping young people with 21st Century skills to face the present social and economic challenges (2), service leadership is proved to be essential in university education to enhance relevant task competencies, character strengths and a caring composition of the students (10). Third, while program content and quality of implementer contribute to the perceived benefits of the participants, program content and perceived benefits are predictors of participants' satisfaction of the course. The findings reaffirm Haworth and Conrad's (19) comments on the importance of interactive teaching and learning, well-structured curriculum and participatory atmosphere among students are essential attributes of a high-quality leadership education program. Last but not the least, program schedule may contribute to the difference on program effectiveness between subject offered in regular semester and intensive summer semester. Course implementer may need to refine the structure and content of the service leadership program, and provide more flexibility and support to the students to minimize the constraints caused by tight program schedule.

Despite the very positive evaluation findings, there are two main limitations of the study. First, the study employed a subjective outcome evaluation approach to examine the effectiveness of a service leadership subject in Hong Kong. There is a need to conduct objective outcome evaluation (20) to examine the changes of students' outcomes of task competencies, character strengths and caring attributes before and after participating in the subject. Along with this line, the findings are based on a cross-sectional data collected at the end of the semester, it is suggested to track the changes of students' outcomes. Actually, we have conducted such studies in the past (21). Second, qualitative studies can incorporate with subjective outcome evaluation to give a full picture of the experience and changes of the students after taking the subject. Focus group interviews, case study and reflective journals are useful qualitative methods to capture the processes of changes that the students experience (22).

Despite the limitations, this study provides empirical support on the importance of promoting service leadership education to college students in Hong Kong, and identifies key components necessary for designing and implementing a quality leadership subject. As suggested by Shek and Chung (23) that there are "unfinished tasks" of service leadership program evaluation and examination of factors leading to program success, the present study takes a humble step to the quest.

ACKNOWLEDGMENTS

The development of the Service Leadership subjects and preparation for this paper are financially supported by the Victor and William Fung Foundation and the Service Leadership Endowed Professorship in Service Leadership Education at The Hong Kong Polytechnic University. This chapter is a reprint with minor revisions of an earlier published paper in the *International Journal of Child Health and Human Development* 2019;12(3) issue with permission.

REFERENCES

[1] Census and Statistics Department. Hong Kong annual digest of statistics: 2019 edition. Hong Kong: Government of Hong Kong Special Administrative Region, 2019.

[2] Dede C. Comparing frameworks for 21st century skills. 21st century skills: Rethinking How Students Learn 2010;20:51-76.

[3] Kouzes JM, Posner BZ. Leadership is personal. In: Kouzes JM, Posner BZ, eds. A leader's legacy. San Francisco, CA: Wiley, 2006:50–5.

[4] Shek DTL, Leung H. Service leadership qualities in university students through the lens of student well-being. In: Shek DTL, Chung P, eds. Promoting leadership qualities in university students – The case of Hong Kong. Singapore: Springer, 2015: 1-17.

[5] Schulenberg, JE, Bryant AL, O'Malley PM. Taking hold of some kind of life: How developmental tasks relate to trajectories of well-being during the transition to adulthood. Dev Psychopathol 2004;16(4):1119-40.

[6] Shek DTL, Cheung BPM. Developmental issues of university students in Hong Kong. Int J Adolesc Med Health 2013;25(4):345-51.

[7] Twenge JM. Generation ME: why today's young Americans are more confident, assertive, entitled - and more miserable than ever before. New York: Free Press, 2006.

[8] King RB, Datu JAD. Materialism does not pay: Materialistic students have lower motivation, engagement, and achievement. Contemp Educ Psychol 2017;49:289-301.

[9] Chung, P. Distinguishing characteristics of service leadership and management education. Hong Kong Institute of Service Leadership and Management (HKI-SLAM) 2010. URL: http://hki-slam.org/index.php?r=article&catid=2&aid=29.

[10] Shek DTL, Chung P. Promoting leadership qualities in university students – The case of Hong Kong. Singapore: Springer, 2015.

[11] Shek, DTL, Chung, P, Leung, H. How unique is the service leadership model? Comparison with contemporary leadership approaches. Int J Disabil Hum Dev 2015;14(3):217-31.

[12] Shek DTL, Chi X, Lin L. Subjective outcome evaluation of a service leadership subject for university students in Hong Kong. Int J Child Adolesc Health 2017;10(2):213-21.

[13] Shek DTL, Liang J, Zhu, X. Subjective outcome evaluation of a service leadership subject for university students in Hong Kong. Int J Child Health Hum Dev 2016;9(2):225-32.

[14] Shek DTL, Lin L, Liu TT. Service leadership education for university students in Hong Kong: subjective outcome evaluation. Int J Disabil Hum Dev 2014;13(4):513-21.

[15] Kolb DA. Experiential learning: Experience as the source of learning and development. Englewood Cliffs, NJ: Prentice-Hall, 1984.

[16] Eich D. A grounded theory of high-quality leadership programs: Perspectives from student leadership development programs in higher education. J Leadersh Organ Stud 2008;15(2):176-87.

[17] Chickering AW, Gamson ZF. Applying the seven principles for good practice in undergraduate education: New directions for teaching and learning (No. 47). San Francisco, CA: Jossey-Bass, 1991.

[18] Shek DTL, Liang JQ. Subjective outcome evaluation of a university subject on service leadership. Int J Disabil Hum Dev 2015;14(4):385-92.

[19] Haworth JG, Conrad CF. Emblems of quality in higher education: Developing and sustaining high-quality programs. Needham Heights, MA: Allyn Bacon, 1997.

[20] Shek DTL. Subjective outcome and objective outcome evaluation findings: Insights from a Chinese context. Res Soc Work Pract 2010;20(3):293-301.

[21] Lin L, Shek DTL. Does service leadership education contribute to student well-being? A quasi-experimental study based on Hong Kong university students. Appl. Res. Qual. Life 2018. URL: https://doi.org/10.1007/s11482-018-9644-x.

[22] Morgan DL. Paradigms lost and pragmatism regained: Methodological implications of combining qualitative and quantitative methods. J Mix Methods Res 2007;1(1):48-76.

[23] Shek DTL, Leung H. (2015). Service Leadership Education for University Students: Seven Unfinished Tasks. In Shek DTL, Chung P, eds. Promoting leadership qualities in university students – The case of Hong Kong. Singapore: Springer, 2015:225-32.

In: Advances in Chinese Children … ISBN: 978-1-53617-870-8
Editors: Ariel Tenenbaum et al.

Chapter 16

STUDENT DEVELOPMENT UNDER A NEW GENERAL EDUCATION PROGRAM IN HONG KONG: A 3-YEAR LONGITUDINAL ASSESSMENT

Daniel TL Shek*, PhD, FHKPS, BBS, JP, Lu Yu, PhD and Xiaoqin Zhu, PhD

Department of Applied Social Sciences, The Hong Kong Polytechnic University, Hong Kong, PR China

ABSTRACT

Universities in Hong Kong have implemented general education programmes since September 2012 when the undergraduate education was formally extended from three years to four years. At The Hong Kong Polytechnic University (PolyU), a new general education curriculum entitled 'General University Requirements' (GUR) has been incorporated in its four-year undergraduate education, aiming to cultivate five desired graduate attributes (critical thinking, problem solving, effective

* Corresponding Author's E-mail: daniel.shek@polyu.edu.hk.

communication, ethical leadership, and lifelong learning). To investigate students' actual learning and development over time under the new general education programme, a yearly online survey was conducted for three consecutive years (N = 460). Results showed that students gained significant improvements in their development of the five desired generic competences after two-year university study, despite a slight decrease in some of these attributes in the second year of their university life. These findings suggest that the new general education programme at PolyU is effective in promoting students' personal development and its intended learning outcomes are largely achieved.

INTRODUCTION

Higher education system is undergoing changes in face of globalization and emergence of the knowledge economy. In Hong Kong, the University Grants Committee (UGC) mandated the extension of undergraduate education for one additional year (i.e., from 3-year to 4-year) in eight public universities starting from 2012/2013 academic year. The additional year allows the universities to implement their new general education (GE) programs, which aim to help students develop desirable generic attributes such as critical and higher-order thinking, effective communication, leadership, ethical reasoning, and lifelong learning (1), and thus promote students' all-round development. However, little is known about the actual impact of the GE reform on student learning and development. To address this question, the present study investigated how students change pertaining to five desirable generic attributes during their three-year study of one new GE program at The Hong Kong Polytechnic University (PolyU), one of the public universities in Hong Kong.

Educational changes and learning outcomes assessment

It is believed that higher education adds value to individual development (2). What university graduates have achieved from university learning has long-term effects of shaping their life and determining their career development

(3). Furthermore, as contemporary economy is primarily based on knowledge and service, competitiveness of citizens is crucial to competitiveness and success of a society (4). As such, the University Grants Committee of Hong Kong (UGC) (5) believed that Hong Kong's vision to be Asia's world city 'is only possible if it is based upon the platform of a very strong education and higher education sector'. It is this profound worth of higher education that calls for investigations on how university curriculum affects students and to use this information to increase effectiveness of higher education.

In recent years, employers and researchers criticize that what undergraduate students learned in college are falling well short of 21st Century's demands and higher education institutions may not effectively teach foundational skills that promote student success in contemporary knowledge society (6-7). These concerns prompted a great deal of research especially in North American, Europe, and Australia and the results suggest the importance of a systematic approach to embed a wide range of generic attributes beyond disciplinary expertise or knowledge across curricula in university education (8-10). In response, more and more higher education institutions have placed higher priority on cultivating students with more generic competences or 'soft skills', by revising teaching practice, implementing 'high-impact' educational programs or integrating General Education (GE) in university curricula. For instance, the Association of American Colleges and Universities (11) has launched a campaign to promote contemporary liberal education and proposed four learning outcomes essential for students to thrive in rapidly changing world, including 'knowledge of human cultures and the physical and natural world', 'intellectual and practical skills', 'personal and social responsibility', and 'integrative and applied learning'.

With these far-reaching educational changes comes research on assessment of actual student accomplishment as a result of university study (12-14). Particular across the United States, there has been a great deal of momentum behind student learning outcomes assessment. For example, according to two national surveys conducted by the National Institute for Learning Outcomes Assessment (NILOA) (15), most higher education institutions have applied various assessment approaches such as student surveys and classroom-based assessments to perform learning outcome assessment. Besides, researchers have explored the impacts of contemporary educational practice, especially liberal education on student achievement (13, 16-18). Basically, these studies suggest that numerous teaching and learning practices (e.g., first-year seminars, reflective learning, learning communities, group project, global learning, service learning, etc.) involved in liberal education are effective to foster essential learning outcomes in college, such as critical and higher-order thinking, moral reasoning, ethical leadership, civic and social responsibility, global looking and multicultural competences.

Education reform and emphasis on general education in Hong Kong

In recent decades, Hong Kong has experienced significant economic and social-cultural changes, including the historical change from a British colony to a Special Administrative Region of China, an increase in economic development and living standards, and the structural shift from a manufacturing-oriented economy to a knowledge- and service-based economy (19). All these factors make quality higher education particularly important for developing people with a broad knowledge base and multiple competences to sustain Hong Kong's development (20). However, the 3-year undergraduate education under the British framework in Hong Kong has long been criticized for its over-specialization and emphasis on passive learning (21). University curricula that concentrate on specialist knowledge upon student enrollment might successfully help students develop intellectual competence, yet they were inadequate to nurture other generic attributes such as critical thinking, leadership, and communication skills. Just as pointed out by Freake (1), Hong Kong university graduates were 'technically knowledgeable upon entry to the workforce, but with limited ability to develop over time and adapt to new situations'. Similar concern was indicated by a market survey which found that over 80% of Hong Kong employers were not confident that Hong Kong students developed sufficient generic attributes such as creativity, analytical thinking, leadership and interpersonal skills (22). The survey also revealed that approximately 90% of the employers thought that Hong Kong students performed worse than their North American counterparts.

As a result, education reform is in great need to address these concerns and respond to demands of today's society. To this end, Hong Kong Education Commission raised education reform proposals in 2000 and UGC mandated the formal structural change in higher education system in 2012/2013. Specifically, the eight public universities funded by UGC extended the length of their undergraduate education from three to four years and incorporated GE programs in the new curricula. It is expected that the new 4-year undergraduate curricula would contribute to the development of qualified graduates with holistic competences to form a solid foundation for Hong Kong's economy, development of society, and its place in the fast-changing world (23).

As UGC did not mandate a formal structure for GE in Hong Kong, each university independently developed their own GE programs (1, 21). Despite divergence in some specific common core requirements of GE curricula in different universities, three features were commonly shared (21). First, a set of intended learning outcomes were emphasized to cultivate desirable graduate attitudes, which focused on multidisciplinary knowledge, multi-perspective, critical thinking, communication, problem-solving, civic responsibility, ethic reasoning, leadership, lifelong learning, and global outlook (1). Second, to align with the intended learning outcomes, traditional teacher-centered pedagogy emphasizing book learning and rote memorization was altered to a more engaging and student-centered pedagogy, such as individual project and group presentation. Third, more authentic forms of assessment were adopted accordingly to motivate student leaning and support leaning outcomes (21).

Basically, the GE curricula in Hong Kong are based on a US-style general education framework (21). In fact, most teaching and learning practices involved in Hong Kong GE curricula were similar to that being regarded as 'good practices' or 'high-impact educational practices' in the

United States (13, 24). As mentioned earlier, these practices adopted in general education have been widely studied in USA and vetted as positively contributing to university students' holistic development and growth (e.g., 3, 13). However, whether they are also effective in Hong Kong remains unknown.

Compared with the long history of general education in the United States, Hong Kong GE program represents an entirely new curricular structure and educational philosophy. As a result, it may have 'less legitimacy as a valued education undertaking and thus will be more difficult to develop as an integral component of undergraduate education' (21). On the other hand, Hong Kong students are used to Chinese culture and learning styles, such as didactic training, thus they may have reluctance and difficulties in adapting to the more active mode of pedagogies associated with GE subjects. Just as asked by Jaffee (21): 'will the students suddenly be prepared to engage, interact, debate, participate, discuss, and criticize?'. Concerning these challenges, it cannot be taken for granted that GE programs in Hong Kong are effective as they were in USA. As a result, there is a need to investigate the actual changes of students and provide evidence for the effectiveness of general education in Hong Kong.

Assessment of student learning outcomes under general education in Hong Kong

As GE programs in Hong Kong vary in structure in eight universities, assessment of students' learning outcomes should accordingly pertain to the specific GE curriculum. Despite the importance of effective assessment of student achievement under the new GE curricula, only a few universities have carried out evaluation projects, among which most were preliminary and focused on pilot courses of new GE curricula. For example, one institution formally evaluated a general education foundation course during its pilot stage, while did not report any evaluation findings in formal implementation (25). Another university launched a 2-year study to assess the effectiveness of pilot courses of its GE program (26), but no evaluative findings were published.

At The Hong Kong Polytechnic University (PolyU), a five-year longitudinal evaluation project involving multiple evaluation strategies to systematically investigate the effectiveness of its new GE program has been implemented since 2012/13 academic year (27). At PolyU, the new GE curriculum entitled 'General University Requirements' (GUR) includes six core components: Freshman Seminar, Language and Communication Requirements, Leadership and Intrapersonal Development, Cluster Area Requirements, Service Learning and Healthy Lifestyle. These GUR components cover a wide range of subjects and intended learning outcomes, which are aligned with five desired graduate attributes defined by PolyU: problem solving, critical thinking, lifelong learning, ethical leadership, and effective communication (28). Despite the challenges in implementing GE in Hong Kong we mentioned before, the GUR subjects were overall well-received by both students and teaching staff (27, 29-31). Evaluation findings on one specific subject developed to satisfy the Leadership and Intrapersonal Development requirement also showed that students were not only satisfied with the course (32, 33), but also demonstrated positive changes after taking the course (34).

While the abovementioned findings could support effective implementation of the GUR at PolyU, it is still not clear whether students had significant personal development not just in a single course. To answer this question, the current study sought to assess students' learning and development during GUR study by comparing their ratings on five desired graduate attributes of PolyU across three years. This longitudinal objective outcome evaluation would provide more convincing evidence on students' changes and personal growth over time (35).

OUR STUDY

Participants of the longitudinal study are PolyU undergraduate students under the 4-year curriculum enrolled in 2012-2013 academic year when the

GUR was first implemented. Students are invited to complete an online survey every year and their informed consent are obtained before the first wave of data collection. Up to 2014-2015 academic year, three waves of data have been collected.

In the first wave of data collection, a pool including 1,000 students from eight faculties/schools at PolyU was initially selected based on a stratified random sampling method. These 1,000 students were invited through emails and/or phone calls to complete the online survey in November 2012 (i.e., 2012-2013 academic year), and 687 of them responded to the invitation while 543 completed the survey, resulting in a response rate of 54.30%. The second wave of data collection was conducted in November 2013 (i.e., 2013-2014 academic year). Those 687 students who responded to the invitation in first wave were invited again and 643 students completed the survey, resulting in a response rate of 93.59%. In the third wave of data collection conducted in November 2014 (i.e., 2014-2015 academic year), an invitation was sent to 643 students who participated in the second wave of online survey. A total of 566 students completed the online survey in the third wave, indicating a response rate of 88.02%.

In order to investigate longitudinal development of students across three years, data collected in the three waves were matched which resulted in 460 students (M_{age} = 20.12, SD_{age} = .54) who completed all three waves of online survey. Among these participants, 182 (39.57%) were male, and 278 (60.43%) were female. A total of 333 (72.39%) participants were born in Hong Kong, 113 (24.57%) were born in mainland China, and the remaining 14 (3.04%) were born in other places. Most participants reported that their parental marital status was first marriage (82.83%). Preliminary analyses showed that there were no significant differences in measures of demographic information including age, gender composition, place of birth and parental marriage status between the matched sample (N = 460) and those students who dropped out of the survey after the first wave of data collection (N = 83).

Instruments

Table 1. Alignments between subscales and desired graduate attributes at PolyU

Desired attributes	Instruments	Indicators
Problem Solving	CPYDS	Problem Solving
Critical Thinking	CPYDS	Critical Thinking
Lifelong Learning	CPYDS NSSE	Life-long Learning Higher Order Learning Reflective and Integrative Learning Learning Strategies Quantitative Reasoning
Ethical Leadership	C-IRI CPYDS	Empathy Ethical Leadership Self-leadership
Effective Communication	CPYDS NSSE	Social Competence Collaborative Learning Discussions with Diverse Others

Note. CPYDS: Chinese Positive Youth Development Scale. C-IRI: Chinese-Interpersonal Reactivity Index. NSSE: National Survey of Student Engagement.

Table 2. Reliabilities of each instrument used in three waves

Instru-ments	Subscales	# of items	Reliability					
			2012-2013		2013-2014		2014-2015	
			α	mean inter-item correlation	α	mean inter-item correlation	α	mean inter-item correlation
C-IRI	Empathy	11	.72	.19	.69	.17	.71	.19
CPYDS	Problem Solving	3	.67	.42	.65	.38	.76	.51
	Social Competence	3	.84	.65	.86	.68	.86	.68
	Critical Thinking	3	.68	.42	.77	.53	.83	.61
	Ethical Leadership	15	.83	.25	.89	.36	.87	.33
	Self-leadership	5	.68	.30	.71	.33	.72	.35
	Life-long Learning	2	.46	.30	.59	.42	.63	.47
NSSE	Higher Order Learning	4	.77	.45	.77	.46	.82	.54
	Reflective and Integrative Learning	7	.82	.40	.84	.43	.88	.51
	Learning Strategies	3	.70	.43	.75	.50	.78	.54
	Quantitative Reasoning	3	.71	.45	.70	.43	.79	.56
	Collaborative Learning	4	.70	.37	.75	.42	.76	.44
	Discussions with Diverse Others	4	.66	.33	.62	.29	.69	.36

Note. CPYDS: Chinese Positive Youth Development Scale. C-IRI: Chinese-Interpersonal Reactivity Index. NSSE: National Survey of Student Engagement.

To measure student development regarding the five desired graduate attributes defined by PolyU, three core instruments were used: a) Chinese Interpersonal Reactivity Index (C-IRI), b) Chinese Positive Youth Development Scale (CPYDS), and c) National Survey of Student Engagement (NESS) which has been updated in 2013. A total of 13 subscales of these instruments were adopted as indicators of the five desired attributes. The alignment of each subscale with corresponding attribute to be measured is shown in Table 1 and Cronbach's alpha for each subscale in each wave is shown in Table 2.

Chinese-Interpersonal Reactivity Index (C-IRI)

Since ethical reasoning and empathy are important competences of an ethical leader (36), the present study used the Empathy (EM, 11 items) subscale of the C-IRI that adapted by Siu and Shek (37) as one measure of ethical leadership. Using a 4-point Likert scale, average score across 11 items was computed as one indicator of ethical leadership. The C-IRI has been widely used and demonstrated good reliability in previous studies (e.g., 38, 39). In the present study, Cronbach's alpha coefficients of the EM subscale in three waves ranged from .68 to .72, indicating good reliability.

Chinese Positive Youth Development Scale (CPYDS)

The Chinese Positive Youth Development Scale (CPYDS) was developed by Shek, Siu, and Lee (40) to measure Chinese adolescents' positive youth development (PYD) attributes. The original scale contains 90 items related to 15 constructs of PYD, and has been found to be valid and reliable as a global measure of PYD in Chinese adolescents in previous studies (34, 41). In the present study, 6 subscales of the CPYDS including Problem Solving (PS), Social Competence (SC), Critical Thinking (CT), Ethical Leadership (EL), Self-leadership (SL), and Life-long Learning (LL) were adopted to measure student developmental qualities. Using 6-point Likert scale, average scores across items in each subscale were used to form indexes reflecting students' performance in the desired graduate attributes. In the present study, the internal consistencies of the subscales were from acceptable to good as reflected by the medium to large Cronbach's alpha coefficients across three waves.

National Survey of Student Engagement (NSSE)

Another instrument used in the present study was a locally adapted version of the (NSSE which assesses student engagement in high levels of learning and development. The NSSE has been widely used at universities in many countries, including USA, Canada, Australia, and China (42-44). The NSSE consists of 47 items pertaining to 10 Engagement Indicators (EIs) (45), including Higher-Order Learning (HO), Reflective & Integrative Learning (RI), Learning Strategies (LS), Quantitative Reasoning (QR), Collaborative Learning (CL), Discussions with Diverse Others (DD), Student- Faculty Interaction (SF), Effective Teaching Practices (ET), Quality of Interactions (QI), and Supportive Environment (SE). The present study used 6 EIs (i.e., HO, RI, LS, QR, CL, and DD) to indicate student competence in lifelong learning and effective communication (see Table 1). We adopted a 4-point Likert scale for all items in 6 subscales and calculated average scores in each subscale. In the present study, the Cronbach's alpha coefficients for these subscales ranged from .62 to .88 across three waves, suggesting good internal consistencies of adapted subscales.

FINDINGS

To explore student development over three years, 13 repeated measures analysis of variance (ANOVA) with Bonferroni post hoc tests were performed, each using one indicator of the five desired attributes at PolyU as the dependent variable. The independent variable was time, operationalized as the academic year when the data were collected and extracted (i.e., 2012-2013, 2013-2014 and 2014-2015). Results of ANOVA are summarized in Table 3.

Table 3. Comparisons of students' performance in three waves (N = 460)

Desired Attributes	Indicators	2012-2013		2013-2014		2014-2015		Repeated Measures ANOVA	
		M	*SD*	*M*	*SD*	*M*	*SD*	F	η^2_p
Problem Solving	Problem Solving[a]	4.28	.70	4.24	.66	4.47	.64	28.80^{***}	.06
Critical Thinking	Critical Thinking[b]	4.65	.62	4.59	.67	4.67	.69	3.95^{*}	.01
Lifelong Learning	Life-long Learning	4.66	.77	4.59	.73	4.63	.74	1.83	.004
	Higher Order Learning[ad]	2.42	.57	2.51	.55	2.77	.57	65.46^{***}	.13
	Reflective and Integrative Learning[a]	2.34	.48	2.28	.47	2.64	.51	120.63^{***}	.21
	Learning Strategies[a]	2.49	.61	2.46	.58	2.60	.61	11.27^{***}	.02
	Quantitative Reasoning[ad]	2.06	.57	2.16	.55	2.40	.61	56.54^{***}	.11
Ethical Leadership	Empathy[c]	2.94	.37	2.88	.36	2.92	.36	5.63^{**}	.01
	Ethical Leadership[c]	4.67	.45	4.57	.53	4.63	.49	10.72^{***}	.02
	Self-leadership[b]	3.83	.56	3.79	.56	3.86	.57	3.21^{*}	.01
Effective Communi-cation	Social Competence	4.59	.76	4.58	.73	4.61	.74	.31	.001
	Collaborative Learning[a]	2.43	.54	2.39	.53	2.59	.54	26.27^{***}	.05
	Discussions with Diverse Others[a]	2.27	.54	2.24	.51	2.46	.60	34.67^{***}	.07

Note.[a] Post hoc Bonferroni test indicated that rating in Wave 3 was significantly higher than rating in both Wave 1 and Wave 2. [b] Post hoc Bonferroni test indicated that rating in Wave 3 was significantly higher than rating in Wave 2. [c] Post hoc Bonferroni test indicated that rating in Wave 2 was significantly lower than rating in Wave 1. [d] Post hoc Bonferroni test indicated that rating in Wave 2 was significantly higher than rating in Wave 1.

* $p < .05$, ** $p < .01$, *** $p < .001$.

Problem solving

Students' ability in problem solving was assessed by the CPYDS Problem Solving (PS) subscale. Results of repeated measures ANOVA showed that there were significant differences in participants' scores of PS across three academic years (F (2, 918) = 28.80, $p < .001$, $\eta^2_p = .06$). Bonferroni post hoc tests further revealed that the rating in 2014-2015 (M = 4.47, SD = .64) was significantly higher than the ratings in 2012-2013 (M = 4.28, SD = .70, $p < .001$) and 2013-2014 (M = 4.24, SD = .66, $p < .001$). These results suggested that participants had significant growth in their problem solving competence after two years of GUR study.

Critical thinking

Students' critical thinking was measured by the CPYDS Critical Thinking (CT) subscale. Significant differences in participants' scores of CT across three years were also observed (F (2, 918) = 3.95, $p = .02$, $\eta^2_p = .02$). Participants had higher CT scores in 2014-2015 (M = 4.67, SD = .69) than in 2013-2014 (M = 4.59, SD = .67, $p = .02$). The results provided evidence for positive development in students' critical thinking from their second year to third year of university study.

Lifelong learning

Students' capacity of lifelong learning was measured by five indicators: Life-long Learning (LL) subscale of CPYDS, and four subscales of NSSE including Higher-Order Learning (HO), Reflective and Integrative Learning (RI), Learning Strategies (LS), and Quantitative Reasoning (QR). While no significant differences were observed in ratings of LL among three waves (F (2, 918) = 1.83, $p = .16$, $\eta^2_p = .004$), significant differences were found in ratings of HO (F (2, 918) = 65.46, $p < .001$, $\eta^2_p = .13$), RI (F (2, 918) = 120.63, $p < .001$, $\eta^2_p = .21$), LS (F (2, 918) = 11.27, $p < .001$, $\eta^2_p = .02$), and QR (F (1.97, 905.99) = 56.54, $p < .001$, $\eta^2_p = .11$). For these four indicators, post hoc tests further revealed that student scores in 2014-2015 were significantly higher than their scores in both 2012-2013 and 2013-2014. Besides, for HO and QR, scores in 2013-2014 were also significantly higher than that in 2012-2013. Means and standard deviations for the four indicators are listed in Table 3. These findings suggested that students' competence of lifelong learning has been significantly improved in the third year of their university study.

Ethical leadership

Three indicators were used to measure ethical leadership: Empathy (EM) subscale of C-IRI, the Ethical Leadership (EL) and Self-leadership (SL) subscales of CPYDS. Results of repeated measures ANOVA indicated that student scores in these three subscales had significant differences in three academic years (see Table 3). Post hoc analyses further indicated that EM score in 2013-2014 (M = 2.88, SD = .36) was significantly lower than that in 2012-2013 (M = 2.94, SD = .37, p = .002). For EL, the score in the second year (M = 4.57, SD = .53) was significantly lower than that in the first year (M = 4.67, SD = .45, $p < .001$) while marginally lower than that in the third year (M = 4.63, SD = .49, p = .05). Moreover, student SL score in 2014-2015 (M = 3.86, SD = .57) was significantly higher than that in 2013-2014 (M = 3.79, SD = .56, p = .03). These findings suggested that students tended to give lower ratings for their empathy and ethical leadership in their second year. Nevertheless, the ratings rebounded in third year of university study.

Effective communication

Three subscales were adopted to assess students' effective communication including Social Competence (SC) subscale of CPYDS, Collaborative Learning (CL) subscale and Discussions with Diverse Others (DD) subscale of NSSE. Repeated measures ANOVA showed that there was no significant difference in students' scores on SC among three waves (F (2, 918) = .31, p = .73). However, students scored higher on CL (F (1.97, 905.62) = 26.27, $p < .001$, $\eta^2_p = .05$) and DD (F (1.96, 900.05) = 34.67, $p < .001$, $\eta^2_p = .07$) in 2014-2015 as compared to 2012-2013 and 2013-2014. In other words, in the third year of university study, students had more collaborative learning and were more likely to discuss with diverse others in their study.

Discussion

In Hong Kong, GE curricula usually have two sets of intended learning outcomes (46). One is 'program intended learning outcomes' which incorporate goals of all general education subjects, such as five desired graduate attributes of PolyU, and the other is 'course intended learning outcomes' which are more specific and should support 'program intended learning outcomes'. The rationale behind two-level design is that it is impossible to achieve all program-level outcomes through one single GE course (47). Such a framework used in designing intended learning outcomes requires two-level assessment accordingly: course-level and program-level (47-48). While course-level assessment of student learning outcomes have been carried out in each GE course in all universities in Hong Kong (21), including PolyU (32-34, 49), program-level assessment showing how the students learn and develop as a result of the whole general education curriculum is scanty. In this case, the present study represents a pioneering work in conducting program-level assessment in Hong Kong to reveal how well the students achieve the intended learning outcomes on program-level. Such an attempt would benefit universities and program designers in terms of continuously improving the quality of general education curricula and the whole higher education system (47, 50).

Specifically, the present study investigated learning outcomes of students enrolled in a new general education (GE) curriculum, i.e., the General University Requirements (GUR) at Hong Kong Polytechnic University (PolyU). Based on comparisons of student self-reported ratings on indicators of five desirable generic competences across three academic years, results suggest that students showed significant improvement in most developmental indicators after two-year university study. These findings strongly support previous findings that the implementation of the GUR at PolyU was successful and effective (27, 29). Furthermore, on top of the positive findings based on subjective outcome evaluations reported in previous studies (e.g., 30, 31), students' actual development and personal growth as measured by the current objective outcome evaluation provide much stronger evidence for the accountability and value of the GUR incorporated in the 4-year undergraduate curriculum.

Regarding students' scores on indicators of the desirable graduate attributes across three years, it seems that most developmental indicators followed a U-shaped trajectory over the period. This distribution features a visible dip on the ratings during the second year of the 4-year curriculum. For example, students tended perceive themselves as having lower level of capacity in critical thinking, life-long learning, reflective and integrative leaning, empathy, and ethical leadership in the second year (i.e., 2013-2014 academic year) than in the first year, although the tendency was significant in only two indicators (i.e., empathy and ethical leadership). It is possible that such a trend was a result of setbacks encountered in students' first year university life, such as difficulties in adjusting to new educational demands, social environments, and life styles. This reasoning is in line with great challenges revealed in research on university transition in first year (e.g., 51). These challenges could continue to exist in sophomore year, resulting in identity confusion, low self-evaluation due to academic stress, and other social pressures, which may cause a decline in learning outcomes among sophomores (52).

Nevertheless, ratings on developmental indicators rebounded at the third year. It might be possible that students have already well adapted to university life after two years. For example, students may have developed sufficient skills and supporting networks to deal with academic and other types of stress in the third year of university life, as suggested by students' highest scores in collaborative leaning and higher order leaning strategies in the academic year of 2014-2015. It is noteworthy that students had obtained significant improvement in different aspects of generic competences after two years of university study. The improved areas included problem solving, critical thinking, higher order learning, reflective and integrative learning, learning strategies, quantitative reasoning, self-leadership, collaborative learning, and discussions with diverse other, which cover all five desired graduate attributes of PolyU. Previous research has demonstrated that good practices in general education help students develop desirable generic capacities in Western cultures (e.g., 13, 53). Findings of the present study indicate that a US-style general education curriculum is also effective in facilitating student development in a holistic manner in Chinese culture.

Taken together, while the present finding suggests that the unique characters of GE program at PolyU help promote student generic competences, for example, more engaging pedagogies are more effective in facilitating student learning than teacher-centered lecturing method (e.g., 54), it should be noted that such a positive effect might be hindered during the first year of students' university life. In other words, students may have difficulties in accepting such a totally new teaching and learning method at the very beginning of their university life. This is consistent with some scholars' concerns that interactive pedagogies might not be readily well received by Chinese students who are largely influenced by cultural traditions (21). As a result, universities and faculties need to develop more effective approaches to incorporate interactive teaching and learning strategies in GE curricula that take into account Chinese students' characteristics. For example, nurturing student critical thinking through writing assignment may be more easily accepted by Chinese students than asking them to make critical comments in front of all students in the class. Furthermore, more assessment studies should be conducted to reveal strengths and weakness of such approaches in Chinese contexts and use the results to improve the quality of teaching and learning. Besides, additional projects or programs aiming to help freshmen adapt to university life and requirements would help students benefit from general education curricula.

The present study also provides evidence for the effectiveness of using longitudinal self-reported data to assess student learning and personal development during university study. To carry out effective program-level assessment of learning outcomes, balancing efficiency, accuracy and cost in measuring student outcomes is a great challenge. Asking students to report how much they have achieved during a certain period is an inexpensive and efficient method while students may not always be able to accurately judge their own growth (55). In contrast, longitudinal assessments of objective outcomes would be more accurate in revealing student achievement during the period. In longitudinal design, objective outcomes can be measured either with actual tests (e.g., some tasks measuring critical thinking) or self-reported questionnaire. Given that the former method should require great financial and human resources (e.g., more standardized and controlled measuring environment), and students are reasonably accurate in estimating their current attributes or skills (55), combining longitudinal design and self-reported measures represents a cost-effective and relatively accurate method to examine student personal development.

Several limitations of the present study should be noted. First, the study only measured student outcomes in three time points and used analysis of variance (ANOVA) to examine changes, which despite of its merits cannot reveal systematic change rates across different waves over time (56). As a result, future research should follow up student development for a longer time period and using more powerful statistical techniques such as growth curve modeling to identify the developmental trajectory of students (56). Second, the present study examined student development in one university in Hong Kong. Therefore, the relative advantages and disadvantages of the GUR as compared to other GE curricula in other high education institutions were unknown. Future assessments could conduct comparisons on student learning outcomes across different universities in Hong Kong and abroad (e.g., universities in mainland China). Third, the present study is quantitative research in nature, which is not able to provide students' in-depth perceptions on their experience (i.e., qualitative data) during university study to help researchers interpret and reflect on the findings. To gain a more comprehensive understanding of student learning outcomes and to triangulate the current findings, multiple research methods including qualitative studies should be used in future assessment of student learning outcomes.

Fourth, as no control group was used in this study, it is possible that the change is simply a result of developmental maturation. While it is a logical possibility, it is noteworthy that there is no research suggesting that university students necessarily show a rise in developmental indicators in this study (e.g., 3, 57).

Finally, while we interpret the present findings in terms of the beneficial effect of the GUR at PolyU, the changes may also be due to the beneficial effect of the overall four-year programme (i.e., including the effects of Major Programme). Since both the GUR and the discipline-specific program are offered at the same time, it is difficult, if not impossible, to separate their specific effects. However, two points should be noted when we interpret the findings. Primarily, evaluation of specific GUR subjects, such as leadership subjects, shows their contribution to the development of desired graduate attributes of PolyU students. Besides, as GUR subjects concentrate more in the first two years of the 4-year undergraduate program, it is more likely that the beneficial effect is a result of students' GUR study.

ACKNOWLEDGMENTS

This work and 'The Longitudinal Evaluation of the General University Requirements under the New 4-year Curriculum Project' are supported by The Hong Kong Polytechnic University under Learning and Teaching Development Grant. The authors declare that there is no conflict of interest with any financial organisations regarding the material reported in this manuscript. This chapter is a reprint with minor revisions of an earlier published paper in the *International Public Health Journal 2018;10*(1) issue with permission.

REFERENCES

[1] Freake H. Curricular designs for general education at the UGC-supported universities in Hong Kong. In: Xing J, Ng PS, Cheng C,eds. General Education and the Development of Global Citizenship in Hong Kong, Taiwan and Mainland China. New York: Routledge, 2013:105-250.

[2] McMahon WW. Higher learning, greater good: The private and social benefits of higher education. Baltimore, MD: Johns Hopkins University Press, 2009.

[3] Pascarella ET, Terenzini PT. How college affects students: A third decade of research (Vol. 2). San Francisco, CA: Jossey-Bass, 2009.

[4] Partnership for 21st century skills. 21st Century skills, education & competitiveness: A resource and policy guide. Tucson, AZ: Partnership for 21st Century Skills, 2008.
[5] University Grants Committee. Hong Kong higher education, to make a difference, to move with the times. Hong Kong: University Grants Committee, 2004. URL: http://www.ugc.edu.hk/eng/doc/ugc/publication/report/policy_document_e.pdf.
[6] Arum R, Roksa J. Academically adrift: Limited learning on college campuses. Chicago, IL: University of Chicago Press, 2011.
[7] Jackling B, De Lange P. Do accounting graduates' skills meet the expectations of employers? A matter of convergence or divergence. Account Educ 2009;18(4-5): 369-85.
[8] Barrie SC. A research-based approach to generic graduate attributes policy. High Educ Res Dev 2004;23(3):261-75.
[9] Bath D, Smith C, Stein S, and Swann R. Beyond mapping and embedding graduate attributes: Bringing together quality assurance and action learning to create a validated and living curriculum. High Educ Res Dev 2004;23(3):313-28.
[10] Laird TFN, Niskode-Dossett AS, Kuh GD. What general education courses contribute to essential learning outcomes. J Gen Educ 2009;58(2):65-84.
[11] Association of American Colleges and Universities. College learning for the new global century: A report from the national leadership council for liberal education and America's promise (Leap). Washington, DC: AACU, 2007.
[12] Hughes C, Barrie S. Influences on the assessment of graduate attributes in higher education. Assess Eval High Educ 2010;35(3):325-34.
[13] Kilgo CA, Sheets JKE, Pascarella ET. The link between high-impact practices and student learning: Some longitudinal evidence. High Educ 2015;69(4):509-25.
[14] Pascarella ET, Blaich C. Lessons from the Wabash national study of liberal arts education. Change: The Magazine of Higher Learning 2013;45(2):6-15.
[15] Kuh GD, Jankowski N, Ikenberry SO, Kinzie J. Knowing What students know and can do: The current state of student learning outcomes assessment at U.S. colleges and universities. Champaign, IL: National Institute for Learning Outcomes Assessment, 2014.
[16] Engberg ME, Fox K. Exploring the relationship between undergraduate service-learning experiences and global perspective-taking. J Stud Aff Res Pract 2011;48(1):83-103.
[17] Padgett RD, Keup JR, Pascarella ET. The impact of first-year seminars on college students' life-long learning orientations. J Stud Aff Res Pract 2013;50(2):133-151.
[18] Pike GR, Kuh GD, McCormick AC. An investigation of the contingent relationships between learning community participation and student engagement. Res High Educ 2011;52(3):300-22.
[19] Shek DTL, Chung PPY, Leung H. Manufacturing economy vs. service economy: Implications for service leadership. Int J Disabil Hum Dev 2015;14(3):205-15.
[20] Hong Kong Education Commission. Learning for life, learning through life: Report proposals for the education system in Hong Kong. Hong Kong: Hong Kong Education

Commission, 2000. URL: http://www.e-c.edu.hk/eng/reform/annex/Edu-reform-eng.pdf.

[21] Jaffee D. Building general education with Hong Kong characteristics. Int Educ 2013; 42(2):41-59.

[22] The South China Morning Post Group Limited. Reaching out: Annual report. South China Morning Post Group Limited, 2006. URL: http://globaldocuments.morningstar.com/documentlibrary/document/95a73fc4a50b1821.msdoc/original.

[23] University Grants Committee. Aspirations for the higher education system in Hong Kong: report of the University Grants Committee. Hong Kong: University Grants Committee, 2010. URL: http://www.ugc.hk/eng/doc/ugc/publication/report/her2010/her2010-rpt.pdf.

[24] Chickering AW, Gamson ZF. Seven principles for good practice in undergraduate education. AAHE Bulletin 1987;39(7):3-7.

[25] The Hong Kong Institue of Education. Evaluation of general education foundation course pilot in 2011-2012: Final report. Hong Kong: The Hong Kong Insitution of Education, 2012. URL: http://libir1.ied.edu.hk/pubdata/ir/link/pub/12695%20S.pdf.

[26] Baldwin Cheng Research Centre for General Education. Study of the assessment of the effectiveness of the GE Program (2011). Hong Kong: Baldwin Cheng Research Centre for General Education, 2011. URL: https://www5.cuhk.edu.hk/oge/index.php/en/research/research-geeffectiveness/assessment-of-the-effectiveness-of-gefp.

[27] Shek DTL, Yu L, Wu FKY, Ng CSM. General Education Program in a New 4-Year University Curriculum in Hong Kong: Findings Based on Multiple Evaluation Strategies. Int J Disabil Hum Dev 2015;14(4):377–84.

[28] The Hong Kong Polytechnic University. Learning outcomes for Polyu graduates at undergraduate level: Policy and guidelines. Hong Kong: The Hong Kong Polytechnic University, 2012. URL: http://www.polyu.edu.hk/obe/institutional_policies/Learning_Outcomes_for_PolyU_Graduates_at_Undergraduate_Degree_Level.pdf.

[29] Shek DTL, Yu L, Chi X. Focus group evaluation of teachers' views on a new general education program in Hong Kong. Int J Disabil Hum Dev 2017; 29(1):67-74.

[30] Shek DTL, Yu L, Ngai J. Evaluation of a general education program in Hong Kong: Secondary data analyses based on student feedback questionnaire. Int J Disabil Hum Dev 2015;14(4):401-06.

[31] Shek DTL, Yu L, Wu FKY, Chai WY. General university requirements at Hong Kong Polytechnic University: Evaluation findings based on student focus groups. Assess Eval High Educ 2014;40(8):1017-31.

[32] Shek DTL, Law MYM. Evaluation of a subject on leadership and intrapersonal development: Views of the students based on qualitative evaluation. Int J Disabil Hum Dev 2014;13(4):435-41.

[33] Shek DTL, Yu L, Zhu X. Evaluation of a leadership and intrapersonal development subject for university students in Hong Kong: Findings based on two years. Int J Disabil Hum Dev 2016;15(1):101-09.

[34] Shek DTL, Sun RCF. Promoting psychosocial competencies in university students: Evaluation based on a one-group pre-test/post-test design. Int J Disabil Hum Dev 2012;11(3):229–34.

[35] Zimmerman DW. The reliability of difference scores in populations and samples. J Educ Meas 2009;46(1):19-42.

[36] Shek DTL, Sun RCF, Liu TT. Evolution and realms of service leadership and leadership models. Int J Disabil Hum Dev 2015;14(3):243-54.

[37] Siu AMH, Shek DTL. Validation of the interpersonal reactivity index in a chinese context. Res Soc Work Pract 2005;15(2):118-26.

[38] Lai FHY, Siu AMH, Shek DTL. Individual and social predictors of prosocial behavior among chinese adolescents in Hong Kong. Front Peditr 2015;(3)39:1-8.

[39] Li X, Bian C, Chen Y, Huang J, Ma Y, Tang L, Yan Q, Ye X, Tang J, Yu Y. Indirect aggression and parental attachment in early adolescence: Examining the role of perspective taking and empathetic concern. Pers Individ Diff 2015;86:499-503.

[40] Shek DTL, Siu AMH, Lee TY. The Chinese positive youth development scale: A validation study. Res Soc Work Pract 2007;17(3):380-91.

[41] Shek DTL, Ma CMS. Dimensionality of the chinese positive youth development scale: Confirmatory factor analyses. Soc Indic Res 2010;98(1):41-59.

[42] Kuh GD. The national survey of student engagement: Conceptual framework and overview of psychometric properties. Bloomington, IN: Indiana University, 2004.

[43] Pascarella ET, Seifert TA, Blaich C. Validation of the NSSE benchmarks and deep approaches to learning against liberal arts outcomes. Proceeding of 33rd Annual Conference of the Association for the Study of Higher Education (ASHE); 2008 Nov 5-8; Jacksonville: Florida; 2008.

[44] Shi Jh, Wen W. Tsinghua university undergraduate education survey report, 2010. Tsinghua Journal of Education 2012;33(1):6-16.

[45] National Survey of Student Engagement. Engagement indicators & high-impact Practices. National Survey of Student Engagement, 2015. URL: http://nsse.indiana.edu/pdf/EIs_and_HIPs_2015.pdf.

[46] Jaffee D. The general education initiative in Hong Kong: Organized contradictions and Emerging Tensions. High Educ 2012;64(2):193-206.

[47] Wong T, Blankenship DJ, Wong M. Programmatic assessment of student learning outcomes in general education: Best practices, resources and example. Proceeding of General Education and University Curriculum Reform: An International Conference in Hong Kong; 2012 Jun 12-14; Hong Kong; 2012.

[48] Kennedy KJ. Conceptualising quality improvement in higher education: Policy, theory and practice for outcomes based learning in Hong Kong. J High Educ Pol Manage 2011;33(3):205-218.

[49] Shek DTL, Yu L, Ma CMS. The students were happy, but did they change positively? Int J Disabil Hum Dev 2014;13(4):505-511.

[50] Ikenberry SO, Kuh GD. From compliance to ownership: Why and how colleges and universities assess student learning. In: Kuh GD, Ikenberry SO, Jankowski NA, Cain TR, Hutchings P, Kinzie J, eds. Using evidence of student learning to improve higher education. San Francisco, CA: Jossey-Bass, 2014:1-23.

[51] Maunder RE, Cunliffe M, Galvin J, Mjali S, Rogers J. Listening to student voices: Student researchers exploring undergraduate experiences of university transition. High Educ 2013;66(2):139-152.

[52] Tobolowsky BF. Sophomores in transition: the forgotten year. New Direct Higher Educ 2008;144:59-67.

[53] Anderson MW, Teisl MF, Criner GK, Tisher S, Smith S, Hunter ML, Norton SA, Jellison J, Alyokhin A, Gallandt E. Attitude changes of undergraduate university students in general education courses. J Gen Educ 2007;56(2):149-168.

[54] Kuh GD, Laird TFN, Umbach PD. Aligning Faculty Activities & Student Behavior: Realizing the Promise of Greater Expectations. Liber Educ 2004;90(4):24-31.

[55] Bowman NA, Green B. Understanding and addressing the challenges of assessing college student growth in student affairs. Res Pract Assess 2013;8:5-14.

[56] Shek DT L. Evaluation of the project P.A.T.H.S. using multiple evaluation strategies. In :Shek DLT, Sun RCF, eds. Development and evaluation of positive adolescent training through holistic social programs (P.A.T.H.S.). Singapore: Springer, 2013:53-67.

[57] Nelson KJ, Duncan ME, Clarke JA. Student success: The identification and support of first year university students at risk of attrition. Studies in Learning, Evaluation, Innovation and Development 2009;6(1):1-15.

In: Advances in Chinese Children … ISBN: 978-1-53617-870-8
Editors: Ariel Tenenbaum et al.

Chapter 17

PROMOTION OF SERVICE LEADERSHIP QUALITIES IN CHINESE UNIVERSITY STUDENTS: OBJECTIVE OUTCOME EVALUATION BASED ON SIX WAVES OF DATA

Hildie Leung, PhD,
Daniel TL Shek*, PhD, FHKPS, BBS, SBS, JP
and Li Lin, PhD
Department of Applied Social Sciences, The Hong Kong Polytechnic University, Hong Kong, PR China

ABSTRACT

Economies worldwide are shifting from manufacturing to service economies, resulting in a demand for new leadership qualities. The Hong Kong Institute of Service Leadership & Management (HKI-SLAM) proposed the Service Leadership and Management Model which highlights the importance of leadership competencies, moral character, and caring

* Corresponding Author's E-mail: daniel.shek@polyu.edu.hk.

dispositions as crucial leadership attributes in service economies. The Global Youth Leadership Programme (GYLP) was developed for students from The Hong Kong Polytechnic University and the Peking University, aiming at nurturing students' service leadership qualities. The present paper reports findings based on objective outcome evaluation utilizing six waves of data. Results showed that students had significant improvement over time on different outcome measures, including positive youth development attributes, service leadership competencies, and life satisfaction. The study provides evidence for the effectiveness of service leadership education and GYLP. Implications for nurturing service leaders and promotion of holistic development of students through leadership programmes are discussed.

INTRODUCTION

One of the most challenging and imperative objectives of tertiary education is to help students develop integrity and strength of character which prepare them for leadership (1). As future professionals, students should acquire qualities such as, "increased sensitivity and action, responsibility… directness and honesty, and high demands on themselves and others" (2). Similarly, the Council for the Advancement of Standards in Higher Education asserted that "regardless of differences in academic discipline, organizational affiliation, cultural background, or geographical location, students must be better prepared to serve as citizen leaders in a global community" (3). Hence, one common expectation is to nurture university students to be leaders. In a recent review of leadership theories over the past two decades, Meuser and colleagues (4) identified 49 leadership approaches/theories. Some of the more popular theories/approaches included transformational leadership, charismatic leadership, participative/shared leadership, and the trait approach to leadership.

Obviously, we have to ask whether existing leadership theories are deemed as effective and relevant in today's time and age. Satterwhite et al. (5) observed that our understanding of leadership has evolved in the past century as the challenges we face as a global community "have increased in complexity, size, scope, consequence. As a result of this contextual evolution, our definition of effective leadership is evolving as well" (5). This observation is concurred by Chung (6) in his latest article in the *South China Morning Post* where he spoke of the "economic complexity and challenges we face today". He argued that "the ones who will succeed in the next 30 years will be those who recognize that the economic growth of the past will not be replicated in the same way again" (para 13). This implies two things: 1) that global economies have changed over the years; and 2) that successful leaders are those who recognize these changes, and are equipped with the skillset that meets the needs of today's economy.

Indeed, economies worldwide are shifting from manufacturing to service economies. Service sectors are becoming increasingly contributive to nations' Gross Domestic Product (GDP). In 2014, the service constituted 79.7% in the US, 78.3% in the UK, 71.4% in Japan, 74.7% in Singapore, and 92.7% in Hong Kong (7). This economic shift poses new demands on the workforce, especially for that of desired leadership qualities. According to Shek and colleagues (8), while traditional manufacturing economies require leaders to be equipped with professional, hands-on knowledge, and skills, leaders are expected to be more "people-oriented" and demonstrate "soft skills" beyond hard skills in service economies. Individuals respect and prefer service leaders who are moral, caring, and willing to serve with empathy and integrity, rather than merely exerting power to exercise manipulation.

Against this background, The Hong Kong Institute of Service Leadership and Management (HKI-SLAM) under the leadership of Dr. Po Chung (co-founder of DHL International, Asia Pacific and Chairman Emeritus of DHL Express (Hong Kong) Ltd.) proposed the Service Leadership and Management Model which highlights the importance of leadership competencies, moral character, and caring dispositions as crucial leadership attributes in contemporary service driven society. According to the model, having leadership competence alone is not enough; moral character and caring dispositions are also vital to successful leadership. Chung (9) further proposed a holistic model which delineated 12 dimensions of an effective service leader. The dimensions are organized into four categories: *Doing* (e.g., possessing functional expertise, being physically healthy); *Thinking* (e.g., having emotional and cognitive competencies); *Growing* (i.e., being able to establish and maintain positive relationships with followers, and adopting the attitude of life-long learning); and *Being* (e.g., exercising compassion, morality, and spirituality).

In order to nurture students to become leaders, leadership programmes in tertiary education settings have proliferated since the eve of the 21st century. Binard and Brungardt (10) reported that there were over 600 campuses in the United States providing leadership training. In response to the longstanding question of whether leadership can be "taught", the authors investigated the impact of leadership programmes on various student outcomes. Findings revealed that students who participated in leadership programmes had improved in leadership behaviours (e.g., inspiring a shared vision, enabling others to act, modelling, encouraging others, and challenging the process), as compared with their counterparts who had never attended such collegiate leadership training.

Although collegiate leadership training has existed for a while, formal leadership programmes are still relatively new. It may be due to two main reasons. First, there is yet to be a consensus on a particular theory or approach about *how* to develop leaders (11). Second, the differentiation between "leader development" vs. "leadership development" remains clouded. Leader development activities target specifically on nurturing skills and traits of individuals "designated" as a leader or an emerging leader. This notion is somewhat in line with the elitist approach of leadership. In contrast, leadership development refers to nurturing intrapersonal, as well as leader traits and skills that would enable effective interpersonal interactions and facilitate leader-follower exchange (12).

Day et al. (13) pointed out that "leaders do not 'develop' in workshops or seminars but rather 'in the so-called white space between such leader development events' (p. 80). This "white space" may be certain trigger events that enable individuals to experience and construct a personally meaningful narrative about their own leadership (14). In line with the above perspectives, the Global Youth Leadership Programme (GYLP) was developed for students from The Hong Kong Polytechnic University and the Peking University, aiming at nurturing students' service leadership qualities, including leadership competencies, moral competencies, and caring disposition. The GYLP was designed such that students first attended a series of lectures where the concept of service leadership and psychological theoretical underpinnings were introduced. Existing leadership theories were also presented and students were guided to evaluate and compare and contrast different leadership theories while reflecting on the importance and relevance of the service leadership model in the present service economy. During the lectures, students were also given the opportunity to engage in personal reflection on their service leadership competencies (i.e., moral character, leadership competencies, and caring dispositions) and how they can apply these competencies in serving others.

Upon completion of the service leadership lectures, students were given the chance to gain hands-on experience and apply service leadership concepts, and reflect on their competencies through a wide-range of talks, presentations, experiential activities, and service in mainland China, Hong Kong, and Cambodia. For instance, during their initial trip to Beijing and Xi'an, students attended different talks regarding contemporary issues in China such as Chinese Foreign Policy, China's Five-Year Plan, and Minority Tribes in Western China. Students also engaged in dialogues with renowned community leaders and executives of large corporations.

Students took the self-initiative to conduct research in preparation of presentations during the "Youth Forum on Poverty in Hong Kong and Chinese Mainland" in Hong Kong. Students prepared presentations on the causes and government policies regarding poverty, and looked into what the young generation can do to alleviate poverty. They also engaged in an experiential activity of role-playing as a homeless, sleeping in the streets, and scavenging cardboard boxes to make money to buy food. Students generally reflected that they had positive experience about the programme, such as

> "Observing something bad happening around us urges me to think more about how to change the situation. And I felt a greater eagerness to take some actions" and "Leadership should be at the base of the spirit of service, so that one can become a valuable and admirable leader. Though I

am still a university student, I will try my best to prepare for the future in my position and serve the society".

Table 1. Detailed GYLP activities

Beijing and Xi'an Trip
• Opening ceremony
• Welcome lunch
• Service leadership lecture
• Talk: Foreign Policy of China
• Visit: Migrant worker community service center
• Visit: Organic farm
• Visit: African culture project
• Visit: Tencent office
• Leaders Dialogue Forum
• Visit: United Nation Development Programme
• Visit: Hong Kong Special Administrative Region Beijing Office
• Talk: 125 National Planning
• Visit: Museum of Qin Terracotta Warriors and Horses
• Talk: Development policy of Western China
• Talk: Chinese culture and society
• Visit: Deprived village of Shanxi
• Talk: Minority tribes in Western China
• Visit: Community walk in Muslim district
• Group presentation
• Visit: Great Wall of China
Hong Kong Trip
• Talk: Social welfare system in Hong Kong
• Visit: New Life Psychiatric Organization
• Visit: Hong Kong Christian Service Ethnic Minority Services
• Practical Dreamers seminar
• Talk: Environmental challenges of Hong Kong and Mainland in Global context
• Visit: Legislative council
• Experiential activity: Role-playing as homeless
• Youth Forum on Poverty in Mainland China and Hong Kong
• Youth Forum dinner
Cambodia Trip
• Preparation and conducting rural asset survey
• Visit: Slum area
• Cultural programme at learning village
• Talk: Social issues in Cambodia
• Orientation with local volunteers
• Service at local primary school and orphanage
• Visit: Village area
• Visit: Killing Fields Museum of Cambodia

Finally, during the Cambodia trip, students provided service to the needy. For instance, some students visited a village where farmers experienced the problem of drought and devised creative ways of irrigation to alleviate the problem. Another group of students visited a primary school where they organized vision screening projects and helped raise awareness of ocular health among the underprivileged in the area. A third group of students served in an orphanage housing children diagnosed with AIDS. The GYLP service leaders developed creative activities such as photography to allow the students to capture and express things in life that they felt grateful towards. Through different services, students demonstrated their service leadership competencies to understand the needs of different parties and applied leadership competencies, care, and moral character, alongside their discipline knowledge to propose solutions to the problems faced by the underprivileged. The detailed programme can be seen in Table 1.

In order to gain a better understanding of the effectiveness of the programme, objective evaluation outcome evaluation data were collected from students at six waves of data during different stages of the Programme. The present paper reports the findings arising from the evaluation study.

OUR STUDY

A total of forty-eight university students (37 females; Mage = 19.65 years, SD = 0.76) participated in the GYLP, in which 24 students were from The Hong Kong Polytechnic University and the other 24 students were from Peking University. The students were enrolled into the programme via application and interview. Besides students from Hong Kong and mainland China (n = 42, 87.5%), there were three Koreans (6.25%), one Taiwanese (2.08%), one Thai (2.08%), and one American (2.08%) joining the programme. The numbers of students participated in different trips varied because some students skipped one or two trips and some quitted the programme halfway due to other commitment (see Table 2). Finally, a total of 39 students completed all the assessments.

Table 2. Description of trips of GYLP

Trip	Time	Assessment time	No. of students
Mainland China trip	July 7-27, 2013	Pretest: July 8, 2013	47
		2nd test: July 12, 2013	48
		3rd test: July 25, 2013	47
Hong Kong trip	January 13-19, 2014	4th test: January 19, 2014	44
Cambodia trip	July 27 - August 6, 2014	5th test: July 24, 2014	41
		6th test: August 5, 2014	40

Table 3. Descriptive information of the variables of study

	Trip to Mainland China						Trip to Hong Kong		Trip to Cambodia			
	Baseline		2nd		3rd		4th		5th		6th	
	Mean (SD)	α	Mean (SD)	α	Mean (SD)	α	Mean (SD)	α	Mean (SD)	α	Mean (SD)	α
Positive youth development total score	$4.73(0.45)_a$	.90	$5.04(0.43)_b$	.90	$5.09(0.42)_{bc}$	.91	$5.02(0.45)_b$	.92	$4.95(0.54)_b$	.95	$5.15(0.40)_c$	.95
Cognitive-behavioral competence	$4.71(0.55)_a$	.82	$5.04(0.47)_b$	.81	$5.11(0.49)_{bc}$	.83	$5.01(0.60)_{bc}$	.88	$4.97(0.63)_b$	.93	$5.18(0.48)_c$	.93
Positive identity	$4.78(0.64)_a$	.78	$5.07(0.68)_b$	.83	$5.07(0.64)_b$	.78	$5.16(0.58)_{bc}$	.86	$5.23(0.55)_b$	.86	$5.23(0.55)_c$	.86
General positive youth development attributes	$4.72(0.45)_a$	.80	$5.03(0.42)_{bd}$	.80	$5.09(0.40)_c$	.81	$4.97(0.44)_d$	.85	$5.09(0.43)_{bd}$	.77	$5.09(0.43)_c$	.87
Life satisfaction	$4.17(0.82)_a$	.86	$4.78(0.82)_b$	.86	$4.78(0.62)_b$	.86	$4.76(0.80)_b$	.88	$4.91(0.66)_b$	.83	$5.15(0.61)_c$	.89
Self-leadership	$4.72(0.48)_a$	.61	$5.03(0.62)_b$	.84	$5.12(0.44)_{bc}$	.73	$5.05(0.57)_b$	.80	$5.01(0.64)_b$	.88	$5.26(0.49)_c$	.88
Caring disposition	$4.98(0.58)_a$	.86	$5.26(0.52)_{bc}$	.85	$5.20(0.51)_{bc}$	.87	$5.20(0.55)_{bc}$	.88	$5.16(0.60)_b$	.94	$5.30(0.47)_c$	.94
Moral Character	$4.66(0.49)_a$	.82	$4.94(0.42)_b$	.79	$5.08(0.43)_{bc}$	.87	$4.97(0.44)_b$	.81	$4.97(0.50)_b$	.89	$5.13(0.46)_c$	.90
Service leadership beliefs	$5.14(0.65)_a$	.91	$5.56(0.51)_b$	.89	$5.49(0.55)_b$	.94	$5.42(0.60)_b$	.94	$5.35(0.63)_b$	.96	$5.43(0.56)_b$	.96

Note: same subscript letter indicates no significant difference in mean level.

Instrument

The students were invited to respond to an identical objective outcome evaluation form at six time points, including baseline test before the service leadership class, posttest of service leadership class (i.e., 2nd test), posttest of mainland China trip (i.e., 3rd test), posttest of Hong Kong trip (i.e., 4th), pretest of Cambodian trip (i.e., 5th test), and posttest of Cambodian trip (i.e., 6th test). Due to the short duration, there was no pretest for the Hong Kong trip. This evaluation form includes ten positive youth development attributes, life satisfaction and service leadership qualities and beliefs. It has been repeatedly used in the evaluation of the subject "Service Leadership" with good psychometric properties (15, 16). Students completed the form in a self-administration manner. The internal consistencies of the scales used in this study were generally good (see Table 3).

Positive youth development

The items of positive youth development were selected from the Chinese Positive Youth Development Scale (CPYDS; 17) with modification to fit the context of the programme (31 items). These items assess social competence, cognitive competence, emotional competence, moral competence, behavioral competence, clear and positive identity, belief in the future, self-determination, spirituality, and resilience. According to Shek and Ma (18)'s factor analysis, there are four higher-order factors, including cognitive-behavioral competencies, positive identity, prosocial attributes, general positive youth development qualities. In this study, we tested students' changes of positive youth development on three higher order factors (i.e., cognitive-behavioral competencies, positive identity, and general positive youth development qualities) and positive youth development total score. Cognitive-behavioral competencies score includes the subscales of cognitive competence, behavioral competence and self-determination; positive identity score includes subscales of clear and positive identity as well as belief in future; general positive youth development qualities score includes the subscales of emotional competence, social competence, moral competence, resilience, and spirituality; positive youth development total score includes all of the subscales of positive youth development attributes. With negative items reverse coded, a higher score denotes a higher level of positive youth development.

Life satisfaction

Students reported their overall satisfaction with life via the five-item Satisfaction with Life Scale (SWLS) developed by Diener and associates (19). This scale has been repeatedly used in Chinese population (20). Mean scores were taken with higher scores indicating higher levels of life satisfaction.

Service leadership qualities and beliefs

Students reported their service leadership qualities and beliefs via a scale developed based on the service leadership model (16, 21). The scale assesses critical components of service leadership, including self-leadership, caring disposition and character strengths as well as service leadership beliefs. Mean scores were taken with higher scores indicating higher levels of service leadership qualities and stronger endorsement of service leadership beliefs.

Findings

Series of ANOVA analyses with time as repeated measure were conducted on the outcome variables. Time effect was significant on all outcome measures, which indicated that positive youth development, life satisfaction and service leadership qualities and beliefs changed positively during the programme participation. LSD post-hoc analyses were then used to understand the variation across different time points. We focused on the comparison between the baseline test and the subsequent tests, and that between the pretest and the posttest of one trip. The results were presented in table 3.

First, three components of positive youth development all changed positively over time (cognitive-behavioral competence: $F(5,31) = 5.57$, $p < .001$, $\eta^2_p = .47$; positive identity: $F(5,31) = 7.12$, $p < .001$, $\eta^2_p = .51$; general positive youth development qualities: $F(5,34) = 10.82$, $p < .001$; $\eta^2_p = .61$). For cognitive-behavioral competence, compared with the baseline test, the scores of all subsequent tests were higher (1st vs. 2nd: $p < .01$; 1st vs. 3rd: $p < .001$; 1st vs. 4th: $p < .001$; 1st vs. 5th: $p < .01$; 1st vs. 6th: $p < .001$). The score increased from the baseline test to the second test, maintained stable between the second test and the fifth test, and finally increased again from fifth test to the sixth test ($p < .05$). Similar pattern was observed in positive identity. Compared with the baseline test, the scores of all subsequent tests were higher (1st vs. 2nd: $p < .01$; 1st vs. 3rd: $p < .01$; 1st vs. 4th: $p < .001$; 1st vs. 5th: $p < .01$; 1st vs. 6th: $p < .001$). The score increased from the baseline test to the second test, maintained stable between the second test and the fifth test, and finally increased again from fifth test to the sixth test ($p < .01$). For general positive youth development qualities, compared with the baseline test, the scores of all subsequent tests were higher (1st vs. 2nd: $p < .001$; 1st vs. 3rd: $p < .001$; 1st vs. 4th: $p < .001$; 1st vs. 5th: $p < .01$; 1st vs. 6th: $p < .001$). The score kept increasing from the baseline test to the third test (2nd vs. 3rd: $p < .05$), but declined from the third test to the fourth test ($p < .05$). With no difference between the fourth test and the fifth test, the score increased from the fifth test to the sixth test ($p < .001$). Taking all positive youth development attributes as a whole, we found the time change as well ($F(5,34) = 10.72$, $p < .001$, $\eta^2_p = .61$). Compared with the baseline test, the scores of all the subsequent tests were higher (1st vs. 2nd: $p < .001$; 1st vs. 3rd: $p < .001$; 1st vs. 4th: $p < .001$; 1st vs. 5th: $p < .01$; 1st vs. 6th: $p < .001$). The total score increased from the baseline test to the second test, maintained stable from the second test to the fifth test, and finally increased again from the fifth test to the sixth test ($p < .01$). All these findings suggested that the programme was effective to promote positive youth development of students. As we found a decline in general positive youth development qualities from the third test to the fourth test, more effort is needed to maintain the programme benefits.

Second, time change occurred in life satisfaction ($F(5,34) = 11.60$, $p < .001$, $\eta^2_p = .63$). LSD post hoc analysis revealed that the score of baseline test was lower than all of the subsequent tests ($ps < .001$). In addition, there was no change from the second test to the fifth test, but with an increase from the fifth test to the sixth test ($p < .01$). Students' life satisfaction reached the highest point at the sixth test (6th vs. 4th: $p < .001$; 6th vs. 3rd: $p < .01$; 6th vs. 2nd: $p < .01$). These results suggested the programme was effective to boost students' life satisfaction.

Third, time changes occurred in service leadership qualities (self-leadership: $F(5,34) = 12.84$, $p < .001$, $\eta^2_p = .65$; caring disposition: $F(5,34) = 4.55$, $p < .01$, $\eta^2_p = .40$; moral character: $F(5,34) = 14.44$, $p < .001$, $\eta^2_p = .68$) and service leadership beliefs ($F(5,34) = 3.29$, $p < .05$, $\eta^2_p = .33$). For self-leadership, compared with the baseline test, the scores of all subsequent tests were higher (1st vs. 2nd: $p < .01$; 1st vs. 3rd: $p < .01$; 1st vs. 4th: $p < .01$; 1st vs. 5th: $p < .05$; 1st vs. 6th: $p < .001$). Specifically, the score increased from the baseline test to the second test ($p < .001$), maintained stable between the second test and the fifth test, and finally increased again from the fifth test to the sixth test ($p < .05$). Similar pattern was found in caring disposition, in which the score of baseline test was lower than the subsequent tests (1st vs. 2nd: $p < .01$; 1st vs. 3rd: $p < .01$; 1st vs. 4th: $p < .01$; 1st vs. 5th: $p < .05$; 1st vs. 6th: $p < .001$). Specifically, the score increased from the baseline test to the second test ($p < .01$), maintained stable between the second test and the fifth test, and finally increased again from fifth test to the sixth test ($p < .05$). Similarly, for moral character, the score of baseline test was lower than the subsequent tests (1st vs. 2nd: $p < .01$; 1st vs. 3rd: $p < .001$; 1st vs. 4th: $p < .001$; 1st vs. 5th: $p < .001$; 1st vs. 6th: $p < .001$). Specifically, the score increased from the baseline test to the second test, maintained stable between the second test and the fifth test, and finally increased again from fifth test to the sixth test ($p < .01$). Different pattern was observed in service leadership beliefs. Compared with the baseline, only the scores of second, third and sixth tests were higher (1st vs. 2nd: $p < .01$; 1st vs. 3rd: $p < .01$; 1st vs. 6th: $p < .05$). Specifically, the score increased from the baseline test to the second test, but then maintained stable from the second test to the final test. These findings suggested that the programme was effective to enhance service leadership qualities and maintain them at a relatively high level. However, it seems more difficult to boost the level of service leadership beliefs, probably because the baseline was quite high.

DISCUSSION

Student development in tertiary education refers to "the application of human development concepts in postsecondary settings so that everyone involved can master increasingly complex developmental tasks, achieve self-direction, and become interdependent" (22, p. 3). It is concerned with the development of the whole person and stimulation of positive growth in students (23). The GYLP is not merely a leadership development programme – it is a programme that targets holistic development among students. As evidenced by the 12 dimensions of an effective service leader, the Service Leadership and Management Model aims to nurture a holistic set of competencies, which would allow students to provide high-quality service in this interdependent world. The service leadership model coincides with existing wellness models targeting to enhance individuals' wellbeing. For instance, the empirically-based Model of Wellness (24) postulated that individuals' total wellness comprises of healthy development in five self domains, namely the Creative Self (e.g., being mentally active, emotional awareness and expressivity, control); Coping Self (e.g., stress management, a sense of self-worth, realistic beliefs); Social Self (e.g., connecting with others, having empathy, ability to trust and love); Essential Self (e.g., spirituality, self-care, gender and cultural identity); and Physical Self (e.g., exercising, eating healthily). Taken as a whole, our findings showed that the GYLP influenced the participants positively in many of the aforementioned dimensions and beyond. Students' positive youth development competencies including cognitive behavioral competencies, positive identity, and general positive youth development qualities significantly increased when comparing the 1st and 6th wave. Similarly, service leadership competencies, and life satisfaction also improved.

The present findings suggest that more programmes similar to GYLP should be developed which would benefit students in different ways. First, regarding employability and leadership challenges, Clarke (25) reported on the present "soft skills crisis", referring to the phenomenon where employers believed that young people are ill-prepared for the world of work, and lack soft skills such as communication, resilience, and the ability to work in teams. "Survey after survey is employers saying qualifications are important, but that just as important to us are so-called soft skills, character skills, the ability to get on with different people, to articulate yourself clearly, confidence, grit, self-control. They are saying we are not seeing enough of this in kids coming out of school" (26, para. 6). Therefore, contemporary leadership theories and development programmes should include components to equip graduates with the very much needed soft skills.

Second, compared with the general population, university students reported higher levels of psychological issues (27). In the US, suicide is the second lead cause to death of college students (28), and 14.9% of students reported having been diagnosed with a depressive disorder during their college studies (29). In Hong Kong, worrying trends in suicide have been observed. Since the start of 2015-2016 academic year, an alarming number of 22 young people have taken their lives. Experts have attributed the phenomenon to the high-pressure education system and low levels of resilience against problems and stress (30). Furthermore, the annual World Happiness report revealed that Hong Kong's ranking in the United Nations' global ranking of happiness dropped to its lowest ranking 75th among 156 countries and territories examined. "Hong Kong is losing a lot of competitiveness in terms of social conditions. We are trying our best to develop our economy at the expense of social life" (31). This further reiterates the dire need and essence of holistic student development. Educators should strive to develop programmes that aim to prepare students to become service leaders in this competitive arena; but not in the expense of the development of intrapersonal and interpersonal competencies, as well as general life satisfaction. The present findings are also consistent with the previous with evidence that Service Leadership education can help students develop effective service leadership qualities based on objective outcome, subjective outcome, and qualitative evaluation (e.g., 8, 32, 33) studies.

While the findings from the objective outcome evaluation of the GYLP provide evidence to support the effectiveness of the programme in nurturing students' service leadership, positive youth development competencies, and enhancing their life satisfaction, there are some limitations to the study. First, the evaluation was conducted using self-report assessment, which some scholars claimed may be subject to social desirability bias. However, according to Paulhus and Vazire (34), this is seldom a problem in research if well-established instruments are administered as in the case of our present study. The instruments we administered have been validated and widely used among tertiary students with high psychometric credibility. Second, respondents included only the participant themselves, thus providing us with a single source of evidence. Adopting a multi-informant approach to solicit data from participants' peers or family would provide additional support to corroborate with our findings.

Although there is no consensus within the literature on a particular method that is most effective in leadership development among tertiary students, findings from the objective outcome evaluation in the present study provide evidence to support the effectiveness of the GYLP, targeted to enhance tertiary students' service leadership, positive youth development competencies, and life satisfaction. Tertiary institutions globally may model after the GYLP in developing leadership programmes to prepare students to meet the challenges and needs in contemporary service economies. Highly autocratic, directive, and transactional leadership styles are dated (35). Service leaders should be equipped with leadership competencies, caring dispositions, and moral competence. As quoted by Simon Sinek (36), renowned expert in leadership and management:

> "The best leaders are those that understand the meaning of service, those who are willing to sacrifice for their own people."

ACKNOWLEDGMENTS

This paper and the GYLP are financially supported by the Victor and William Fung Foundation. This chapter is a revised and adapted version of an earlier published paper in the International Journal of Child and Adolescent Health 2018;11(1) issue with permission.

REFERENCES

[1] King PM. Character and civic education: what does it take? Educ Rec 1997;78(3):87-90.

[2] Valeeva RA, Koroleva NE, Sakhapova FK. Civic education of the technical university students in foreign language classes. Rev Eur Stud 2015;7(1):176-81.

[3] Council for the Advancement of Standards in Higher Education. CAS self-assessment guide for student leadership programs. Washington, DC: CASHE, 2012.

[4] Meuser JD, Gardner WL, Dinh JE, Hu J, Liden RC, Lord RG. A network analysis of leadership theory: the infancy of integration. J Manage 2016;42(5):1374-403.

[5] Satterwhite R, Miller WM, Sheridan K. Leadership for sustainability and peace: responding to the wicked challenges of the future. In: Sowcik M, Andernoro AC, McNutt M, Murphy SE. eds. Leadership 2050: critical challenges, key contexts and emerging trends. United Kingdom: Emerald Group, 2015:59-74.

[6] Chung P. Why China's economic boom will never be repeated. The South China Morning Post. URL: http://www.scmp.com/comment/insight-opinion/article/2025636/why-chinas-economic-boom-will-never-be-repeated.

[7] The World Bank. Gross domestic product ranking, 2015. URL: http://data.worldbank.org/data-catalog/GDP-ranking-table.

[8] Shek DTL, Sun RCF, Yu L, Ma CMS, Siu AMH, Leung H, Law MYM. Service leadership education and research at The Hong Kong Polytechnic University of Hong Kong: an overview. In: Promoting service leadership qualities in university students. Singapore: Springer, 2015:117-33.

[9] Chung P. Your second skin. Managing the 12 dimensions of your personal brand for the service age. Unpublished manuscript, 2015.

[10] Binard K, Brungardt C. Learning leadership: assessing students at the community college of Denver. J Leadersh Organ Stud 1997;4(4):128-40.

[11] Lunsford LG, Brown BA. Preparing leaders while neglecting leadership: an analysis of US collegiate leadership centers. J Leadersh Organ Stud 2016. doi:10.1177/1548051816662613.

[12] Day DV. Leadership development: a review in context. Leadersh Q 2001;11(4):581-613.
[13] Day DV, Fleenor JW, Atwater LE, Sturm RE, McKee RA. Advances in leader and leadership development: a review of 25years of research and theory. Leadersh Q 2014;25(1):63-82.
[14] Avolio BJ, Hannah ST. Developmental readiness: accelerating leader development. Consult Psychol J 2008;60(4):331-47.
[15] Shek DTL, Lin L, Leung H. Objective Outcome Evaluation of Service Leadership Education at The Hong Kong Polytechnic University. Paper presented at the International Conference on Service Leadership Education in Service Economies, Hong Kong, 2016 January 6-7.
[16] Shek DTL, Yu L, Ma CMS. The students were happy, but did they change positively?. Int J Disabil Hum Dev 2014;13(4):505-11.
[17] Shek DTL, Siu AMH, Lee TY. The Chinese positive youth development scale: a validation study. Res Soc Work Pract 2007;17(3):380-91.
[18] Shek DTL, Ma CMS. Dimensionality of the Chinese positive youth development scale: confirmatory factor analyses. Soc Indic Res 2010;98(1):41-59.
[19] Diener ED, Emmons RA, Larsen RJ, Griffin S. The satisfaction with life scale. J Pers Assess 1985;49(1):71-5.
[20] Sun RCF, Shek DTL. Life satisfaction, positive youth development, and problem behaviour among Chinese adolescents in Hong Kong. Soc Indic Res 2010;95(3):455-74.
[21] Chung P, Bell AH. The 25 principles of service leadership. Hong Kong: Lexingford Publishing, 2015.
[22] Miller TK, Prince JS. The future of student affairs. San Francisco, CA: Jossey-Bass, 1976.
[23] Patton LD, Renn KA, Guido FM, Quaye SJ, Evans NJ, Forney DS. Student development in college: Theory, research, and practice. San Francisco, CA: John Wiley, 2016.
[24] Myers JE, Sweeney TJ. eds. *Wellness in counseling: theory, research, and practice.* Alexandria, VA: American Counseling Association, 2005.
[25] Clarke M. Addressing the soft skills crisis. Strategic HR Rev 2016;15(3):137-9.
[26] Smith JL. Why soft skills are more important than a great CV. The Telegraph. Accessed 2015 Jan 6. URL: http://www.telegraph.co.uk/women/womens-business/11326058/Forget-the-CV-Why-soft-skills-are-more-important.html.
[27] Berger H, Franke GH, Hofmann FH, Sperth M, Holm-Hadulla RM. Mental health of students and its development between 1994 and 2012. Ment Health Prevent 2015;3(1):48-56.
[28] Wilcox HC, Arria AM, Caldeira KM, Vincent KB, Pinchevsky GM, O'Grady KE. Prevalence and predictors of persistent suicide ideation, plans, and attempts during college. J Affect Disorders 2010;27(1-3):287-94.

[29] American College Health Association. American college health association-national college health assessment spring 2008 reference group data report. J Am Coll Health 2009;57(5):477-88.

[30] Cheung E, Chiu P. Students at breaking point: Hong Kong announces emergency measures after 22 suicides since the start of academic year. The South China Morning Post 2016 Mar 12. URL: http://www.scmp.com/news/hong-kong/health-environment/article/1923465/students-breaking-point-hong-kong-announces.

[31] Lee D. Deep blue: Hong Kong tumbles to 75th in world happiness rankings, lowest since UN report debuted. The South China Morning Post 2016 Mar 17. URL: http://www.scmp.com/news/hong-kong/education-community/article/1926391/deep-blue-hong-kong-tumbles-75th-world-happiness.

[32] Shek DTL, Lin L. Evaluating service leadership programs with multiple strategies. In: promoting service leadership qualities in university students. Singapore: Springer, 2015:197-211.

[33] Shek DTL, Law MYM, Liu TT. Focus group evaluation of a service leadership subject in Hong Kong. Int J Disabil Hum Dev 2015;14(4):371-6.

[34] Paulhus DL, Vazire S. The self-report method. In: Robins RW, Fraley RC, Krueger RF. eds. Handbook of research methods in personality psychology. New York: Guilford, 2007:224-39.

[35] Shek DTL, Chung PPY, Leung H. Manufacturing economy vs. service economy: implications for service leadership. Int J Disabil Hum Dev 2015;14(3):205-15.

[36] Sinek S. Leaders eat last: why some teams pull together and others don't. London: Penguin, 2014.

SECTION TWO: ACKNOWLEDGMENTS

In: Advances in Chinese Children … ISBN: 978-1-53617-870-8
Editors: Ariel Tenenbaum et al.

Chapter 18

ABOUT THE EDITORS

Ariel Tenenbaum, MD is the director of the Center for Children with Chronic Diseases at the Hadassah-Hebrew University Medical Center at the Mount Scopus Campus, Jerusalem, Israel. He graduated the Hadassah-Hebrew University Medical School and after pediatric residency at the Department of Pediatrics at Mount Scopus Campus, he continued his work at the hospital as a senior pediatric consultant and teacher of medical students. In 2004 he was appointed the head of the new Israeli Down syndrome program in the hospital. In 2005 he started the pre-adoption clinic together with Professor Isaiah D. Wexler. In 2012 he opened the Hadassah Intellectual and Developmental Disability Multidisciplinary Evaluation Center in collaboration with the Ministry of Social Affairs. He co-founded the Disability Studies Center at the Hebrew University, where he teaches students from humanities and social studies. He was recently appointed as a child development consultant. In 2019 he was elected to the Israeli Pediatric Association Committee and serves as its scientific secretary. His main research topics are disabilities, adoption, chronic diseases and general pediatrics. He has published numerous book chapters, edited several books, and published dozens of scientific articles in international journals. E-mail: tene@hadassah.org.il

Daniel TL Shek, PhD, FHKPS, BBS, SBS, JP, is Associate Vice President (Undergraduate Programme), Chair Professor of Applied Social Sciences, and Li and Fung Professor in Service Leadership Education, The Hong Kong Polytechnic University, Hung Hom, Hong Kong, PRC, Changjiang Scholar (Changjiang Chair Professor), Advisory Professor of East China Normal University, and Honorary Professor of Kiang Wu Nursing College of Macau. He is Chief Editor of *Applied Research in Quality of Life*, past Consulting Editor of *Journal of Clinical Psychology* and *Journal of Youth Studies*, and editorial board member of *Social Indicators Research, International Journal of Adolescent Medicine and Health, International Journal of Disability and Human Development, Journal of Adolescent Health, Journal of Child and Family Studies* and *Children and Youth Services Review.* He has served in many government advisory bodies, including the Action Committee against Narcotics, Commission on Youth, Fight Crime Committee and Family Council. He has published numerous books, book chapters and more than 500 scientific articles in international refereed journals. E-mail: daniel.shek@polyu.edu.hk

Moon YM Law, BSW, MSW, DSW, RSW, is Assistant Professor of School of Social Sciences, Caritas Institue of Higher Education, Hong Kong, PRC. Before that, she worked as the Teaching Fellow of the Department of Applied Social Sciences at The Hong Kong Polytechnic University for ten years. She also worked as a frontline social worker in youth services to mentor young people and families for positive changes in their development. Furthermore, apart from providing training for teachers and social workers in Hong Kong and mainland China, she has taught different courses for university students, includes leadership, service learning, and counseling,. Her research interests include positive youth development, parenting, leadership, and Internet addiction. Her current research projects focus on positive youth development programs. Her work appears in *Journal of Pediatric and Adolescent Gynecology, International Journal of Adolescent Medicine and Health, International Journal of Disability and Human Development*, and books related to family, positive youth development, and leadership. E-mail: mlaw@cihe.edu.hk

Joav Merrick, MD, MMedSci, DMSc, born and educated in Denmark, is professor of pediatrics, Division of Pediatrics, Hadassah Hebrew University Medical Center, Mt Scopus Campus, Jerusalem, Israel and Kentucky Children's Hospital, University of Kentucky, Lexington, Kentucky United States and professor of public health at the Center for Healthy Development, School of Public Health, Georgia State University, Atlanta, United States, the former medical director of the Health Services, Division for Intellectual and Developmental Disabilities, Ministry of Social Affairs and Social Services, Jerusalem, the founder and director of the National Institute of Child Health and Human Development in Israel. Numerous publications in the field of pediatrics, child health and human development, rehabilitation, intellectual disability, disability, health, welfare, abuse, advocacy, quality of life and prevention. Received the Peter Sabroe Child Award for outstanding work on behalf of Danish Children in 1985 and the International LEGO-Prize ("The Children's Nobel Prize") for an extraordinary contribution towards improvement in child welfare and well-being in 1987. In 2017 appointed a Kentucky Colonel by the Commonwealth of Kentucky, the highest honor the governor can bestow to a person. E-mail: jmerrick@zahav.net.il

In: Advances in Chinese Children … ISBN: 978-1-53617-870-8
Editors: Ariel Tenenbaum et al.

Chapter 19

About the Center for Children with Chronic Diseases and Down Syndrome Center Jerusalem, Israel, Department of Pediatrics, Mt Scopus Campus, Hadassah Hebrew University Medical Center, Jerusalem, Israel

Chronic illnesses are common among children. These conditions last longer than a year and require continuous medical care and special needs. It is estimated that 10-20% of children in developed countries have one or more chronic condition. Advances in medicine and technology lead to an increase in the survival rate and longevity of children with chronic diseases and special needs. The severity of different chronic illnesses is variable, but there are many similarities. The child with a chronic illness faces physical, social, and emotional challenges. Therefore, medical care is not sufficient without rehabilitative service and emotional care for the child and his family.

Chronic illnesses are time and energy consuming. These children go through treatments, procedures and many healthcare visits. At home they often continue treatments as well, e.g., physiotherapy, breathing support machines and medications. This lifestyle may have detrimental effect on the child's social and emotional well-being, and similarly affect his parents and siblings.

CENTER FOR CHILDREN WITH CHRONIC DISEASES

The aim of the Center for Children with Chronic Diseases at the Hadassah-Hebrew University Medical Center at the Mount Scopus Campus, Jerusalem, is to enhance medical care, comfort and well-being of patients and their families in the hospital and beyond. The center provides integrated and comprehensive care for these patients. This includes extensive support services and helping their families cope with the burden of care.

Numerous pediatric specialty programs and medical divisions have been established in the center to care for specific chronic conditions; among them are cystic fibrosis, Down syndrome, diabetes mellitus, familial dysautonomia, neuromuscular diseases, rheumatic diseases, feeding disorders and metabolic diseases. All these programs include evaluation and support from common services in the center: Nursing, nutrition, psycho-social care, speech therapy, physiotherapy and more.

The center works as a "one stop shop" for these children; As many services as possible, under one roof, on the same visit. Centralizing the care enables parents to come to one location to receive care. The physicians and nurses coordinate the care of the children thereby alleviating some of the burden of care off the families.

Children who are included in the programs of the center usually need returning visits to various medical specialists, consultations by multidisciplinary health professionals and performing diagnostic tests e.g., blood work, x-rays and respiratory functions. Some children may need hospitalization or palliative care. The center can concentrate all diagnostic and follow-up testing, medical surveillance and treatment in the hands of an experienced staff who knows the child and his unique situation.

The center is situated close to the entrance of the hospital and the families can access it without going through the main hospital building. In the center there are ten rooms for consultations. In addition, there are dedicated rooms for tests, e.g., respiratory functions, blood tests, sweat test and more. There is a large space with eight beds for continuous treatments, for example intravenous immunoglobulins and biological medications. In this space several unique tests are performed as well, for example growth hormone test and allergy challenge tests. There is also a special room for procedures, in which children can go through painful treatments with appropriate anesthetics and surveillance.

A special classroom in the center is operated by the ministry of education. In the classroom, children can continue their studies or play and interact with other children, in arts and crafts and many other programs.

The center is surrounded by a large healing garden that is partially maintained by the children themselves.

Conclusion

In conclusion, we believe that the "all inclusive" model of a center for children with chronic conditions is beneficial for the children and their families in terms of health and quality of life, and that this model is currently the best service for them.

Contact

Ariel Tenenbaum, MD, Isaiah D Wexler, MD, PhD
Center for Children with Chronic Diseases, Department of Pediatrics,
Mt Scopus Campus, Hadassah Hebrew University Medical Center,
Jerusalem, Israel
E-mail: TENE@hadassah.org.il

In: Advances in Chinese Children … ISBN: 978-1-53617-870-8
Editors: Ariel Tenenbaum et al.

Chapter 20

About the Department of Applied Social Sciences, The Hong Kong Polytechnic University, Hung Hom, Hong Kong

The Department of Applied Social Sciences (APSS) of the Hong Kong Polytechnic University began as the Institute of Social Work Training in 1973 before it became the School of Social Work in the Hong Kong Polytechnic in 1977. In 2000, the department was renamed as the Department of Applied Social Sciences. It is now one of the largest social science departments in the Asia-Pacific region with a strong tradition of researching on and working with socially vulnerable groups through education, research and service in diverse areas incorporating social work, social policy and administration, psychology, sociology and philosophy.

Education

In education, we strive to nurture human service professionals who are knowledgeable, resourceful, caring, worldly but reflexive, and possess a strong commitment to social justice and responsibility. We also see them as practitioners and researchers who are able to integrate theory and practice, and develop appropriate indigenous knowledge that can meet the challenges of rapid social change in Chinese societies.

Research

In research, to respond to the constantly changing global socio-economic order and address the subsequently emerged local problems, the strategic foci of our research and social investigation have also been expanded to include migration and mobilities, family and life-span development, social economy, online communities/social media, disaster and risks reduction, applied philosophy and social work practices.

Community Service

In community service, we continue to collaborate with community partners to allow our students to understand better the different lifeworlds of our society, and design programmes and supportive services that are innovative, relevant and socially responsible.

Students

As to students in our department, we see it necessary for them to develop a global outlook while firmly grounded in Hong Kong. To this end, in recent years more than 200 full-time and part-time students as well as alumni have participated in the various study tours and exchange programmes we held in the Chinese Mainland and overseas, including the University of Nottingham, United Kingdom; University of Queensland, Australia; University of California at Berkeley, United States; Washington University at St. Louis,

United States; York University, Canada; Peking University and Yunnan University in China.

FACULTY AND TEACHING

In the 2019/20 academic year, the Department has around 200 members, including academic staff, part-time fieldwork instructors, research and project staff and administrative and supporting technical staff. The APSS offers many undergraduate and coursework and research postgraduate programmes.

In: Advances in Chinese Children … ISBN: 978-1-53617-870-8
Editors: Ariel Tenenbaum et al.

Chapter 21

ABOUT THE NATIONAL INSTITUTE OF CHILD HEALTH AND HUMAN DEVELOPMENT IN ISRAEL

The National Institute of Child Health and Human Development (NICHD) in Israel was established in 1998 as a virtual institute under the auspicies of the Medical Director, Ministry of Social Affairs and Social Services in order to function as the research arm for the Office of the Medical Director. In 1998 the National Council for Child Health and Pediatrics, Ministry of Health and in 1999 the Director General and Deputy Director General of the Ministry of Health endorsed the establishment of the NICHD.

MISSION

The mission of a National Institute for Child Health and Human Development in Israel is to provide an academic focal point for the scholarly interdisciplinary study of child life, health, public health, welfare, disability, rehabilitation, intellectual disability and related aspects of human development. This mission includes research, teaching, clinical work, information and public service activities in the field of child health and human development.

SERVICE AND ACADEMIC ACTIVITIES

Over the years many activities became focused in the south of Israel due to collaboration with various professionals at the Faculty of Health Sciences (FOHS) at the Ben Gurion University of the Negev (BGU). Since 2000 an affiliation with the Zusman Child Development Center at the Pediatric Division of Soroka University Medical Center has resulted in collaboration around the establishment of the Down Syndrome Clinic at that center. In 2002 a full course on "Disability" was established at the Recanati School for Allied Professions in the Community, FOHS, BGU and in 2005 collaboration was started with the Primary Care Unit of the faculty and disability became part of the master of public health course on "Children and society". In the academic year 2005-2006 a one semester course on "Aging with disability" was started as part of the master of science program in gerontology in our collaboration with the Center for Multidisciplinary Research in Aging. In 2010 collaborations with the Division of Pediatrics, Hadassah Hebrew University Medical Center, Jerusalem, Israel around the National Down Syndrome Center and teaching students and residents about intellectual and developmental disabilities as part of their training at this campus.

RESEARCH ACTIVITIES

The affiliated staff have over the years published work from projects and research activities in this national and international collaboration. In the year 2000 the International Journal of Adolescent Medicine and Health and in 2005 the International Journal on Disability and Human Development of De Gruyter Publishing House (Berlin and New York) were affiliated with the

National Institute of Child Health and Human Development. From 2008 also the International Journal of Child Health and Human Development (Nova Science, New York), the International Journal of Child and Adolescent Health (Nova Science) and the Journal of Pain Management (Nova Science) affiliated and from 2009 the International Public Health Journal (Nova Science) and Journal of Alternative Medicine Research (Nova Science). All peer-reviewed international journals.

National Collaborations

Nationally the NICHD works in collaboration with the Faculty of Health Sciences, Ben Gurion University of the Negev; Department of Physical Therapy, Sackler School of Medicine, Tel Aviv University; Autism Center, Assaf HaRofeh Medical Center; National Rett and PKU Centers at Chaim Sheba Medical Center, Tel HaShomer; Department of Physiotherapy, Haifa University; Department of Education, Bar Ilan University, Ramat Gan, Faculty of Social Sciences and Health Sciences; College of Judea and Samaria in Ariel and in 2011 affiliation with Center for Pediatric Chronic Diseases and National Center for Down Syndrome, Department of Pediatrics, Hadassah Hebrew University Medical Center, Mount Scopus Campus, Jerusalem.

International Collaborations

Internationally with the Department of Disability and Human Development, College of Applied Health Sciences, University of Illinois at Chicago; Strong Center for Developmental Disabilities, Golisano Children's Hospital at Strong, University of Rochester School of Medicine and Dentistry, New York; Centre on Intellectual Disabilities, University of Albany, New York; Centre for Chronic Disease Prevention and Control, Health Canada, Ottawa; Chandler Medical Center and Children's Hospital, Kentucky Children's

Hospital, Section of Adolescent Medicine, University of Kentucky, Lexington; Chronic Disease Prevention and Control Research Center, Baylor College of Medicine, Houston, Texas; Division of Neuroscience, Department of Psychiatry, Columbia University, New York; Institute for the Study of Disadvantage and Disability, Atlanta; Center for Autism and Related Disorders, Department Psychiatry, Children's Hospital Boston, Boston; Department of Pediatric and Adolescent Medicine, Western Michigan University Homer Stryker MD School of Medicine, Kalamazoo, Michigan, United States; Department of Paediatrics, Child Health and Adolescent Medicine, Children's Hospital at Westmead, Westmead, Australia; International Centre for the Study of Occupational and Mental Health, Düsseldorf, Germany; Centre for Advanced Studies in Nursing, Department of General Practice and Primary Care, University of Aberdeen, Aberdeen, United Kingdom; Quality of Life Research Center, Copenhagen, Denmark; Nordic School of Public Health, Gottenburg, Sweden, Scandinavian Institute of Quality of Working Life, Oslo, Norway; The Department of Applied Social Sciences (APSS) of The Hong Kong Polytechnic University Hong Kong.

Targets

Our focus is on research, international collaborations, clinical work, teaching and policy in health, disability and human development and to establish the NICHD as a permanent institute in Israel in order to conduct model research and policy.

Contact

Professor Joav Merrick, MD, MMedSci, DMSc
Director, National Institute of Child Health and Human Development,
Jerusalem, Israel.
E-mail: jmerrick@zahav.net.il

Chapter 22

About the Book Series "Public Health: Practices, Methods and Policies"

Public health is a book series with publications from a multidisciplinary group of researchers, practitioners and clinicians for an international professional forum interested in the broad spectrum of public health issues.

Books already published:

- Rubin IL, Merrick J, eds. *Environment and public health: Environmental health, law and international perspectives*. New York: Nova Science, 2014.
- Shek DTL, Siu AMH, Merrick J, eds. *Tomorrow's leaders: Service leadership and holistic development in Chinese university students.* New York: Nova Science, 2015.
- Siziya S, Mazaba ML, Merrick J, eds. *Arbovirus: Public health experience from Zambia.* New York: Nova Science, 2015.
- Obeng C, Obeng SG, Merrick J, eds. *Health issues in diverse cultures.* New York: Nova Science, 2015.
- Friedman BD, Merrick J, eds. *Public health, social work and health inequalities.* New York: Nova Science, 2015.

- Rubin IL, Merrick J, eds. *Environmental health disparities: Costs and benefits of breaking the cycle.* New York: Nova Science, 2016.
- Mazaba ML, Siziya S, Merrick J, eds. *Smoking and adolescence: International public health experiences*. New York: Nova Science, 2016.
- Merrick J, ed. Public health: *Some international perspectives*. New York: Nova Science, 2016.
- Greydanus DE, Merrick J. *Medical history: Some perspectives.* New York: Nova Science, 2016.
- Rubin IL, Merrick J, eds. *Public health: International aspects on environment and health.* New York: Nova Science, 2016.
- Shek DTL, Ma C, Lin L, Merrick J, eds. *Education in Hong Kong: Service leadership for university students.* New York: Nova Science, 2016.
- Shek DTL, Siu AMH, Leung H, Merrick J, eds. *Higher education in Hong Kong: Nurturing students to be caring service leaders.* New York: Nova Science, 2016.
- Marufu T, Siziya S, Mazaba ML, Merrick J, eds. *Measles: Epidemiology and control of measles in the Gweru urban district in Zimbabwe.* New York: Nova Science, 2016.
- Hegamin-Younger C, Merrick J, eds. *Caribbean adolescents: Misuse and abuse of alcohol.* New York: Nova Science, 2016.
- Greydanus DE, Merrick J. *Diabetes mellitus: A medical history journey.* New York: Nova Science, 2016.
- Rubin IL, Merrick J, eds. *Public health: An ecological framework for child environmental health interventions.* New York: Nova Science, 2017.
- Shek DTL, Chung P, Lin L, Merrick J, eds. *Service leadership education for university students.* New York: Nova Science, 2017.
- Shek DTL, Ma C, Merrick J, eds. *Leadership: Promoting leadership and intrapersonal development in university students.* New York: Nova Science, 2017.

- Shek DTL, Yu L, Merrick J, eds. *University students: Promoting of holistic development in Hong Kong*. New York: Nova Science, 2017.
- Chow R, Hollenberg D, Borean M, Merrick J, eds. *Alzheimer's disease: Awareness among young adults*. New York: Nova Science, 2017.
- Rubin IL, Merrick J, eds. *Resilience and health: A potent dynamic*. New York: Nova Science, 2018.
- Greydanus DE, Merrick J. *Medical history: Some new perspectives, Second edition*. New York: Nova Science, 2018.

CONTACT

Professor Joav Merrick, MD, MMedSci, DMSc
Director, National Institute of Child Health and Human Development, Jerusalem, Israel
E-mail: jmerrick@zahav.net.il

Section three: Index

INDEX

A

academic motivation, 232
academic performance, 59, 233, 251
administrative arrangement, 176, 180, 181, 182, 186, 187, 188, 189, 190
adolescent, vii, viii, ix, 3, 4, 6, 7, 8, 9, 35, 55, 56, 58, 59, 60, 70, 71, 72, 73, 74, 78, 79, 80, 81, 82, 83, 84, 91, 93, 94, 95, 100, 112, 115, 134, 143, 155, 159, 160, 168, 170, 171, 176, 177, 178, 183, 186, 194, 195, 198, 209, 210, 214, 215, 216, 227, 228, 229, 230, 232, 233, 234, 235, 245, 246, 247, 251, 263, 264, 311, 328, 334, 346, 348
adolescent behavior, 159, 232, 251
adolescent development, ix, 6, 9, 55, 56, 58, 70, 74, 78, 79, 91, 95, 134, 155, 160, 168, 170, 176, 177, 178, 183, 186, 194, 198, 215, 232, 233
adolescent problem behavior, 100, 112, 214, 233
adolescents, iv, viii, ix, x, 4, 6, 7, 8, 35, 55, 56, 57, 58, 60, 61, 65, 66, 67, 68, 70, 71, 72, 73, 74, 77, 78, 79, 80, 81, 82, 83, 85, 86, 87, 88, 89, 90, 91, 92, 93, 94, 100, 104, 112, 115, 126, 137, 142, 143, 144, 155, 158, 159, 171, 172, 176, 177, 178, 189, 194, 198, 210, 214, 215, 216, 225, 226, 228, 229, 232, 233, 234, 235, 242, 243, 245, 246, 247, 250, 252, 257, 260, 262, 263, 264, 298, 310, 329, 350
adolescents in Hong Kong, 56, 60, 61, 71, 74, 78, 81, 91, 92, 210, 310
adulthood, 6, 124, 128, 232, 269
adults, 35, 124, 126, 130, 132, 133, 156, 171, 225
advancement, 120, 124, 128, 243
adverse conditions, 150, 165, 205, 222, 241, 258, 279
advocacy, 335
age, 12, 13, 17, 18, 22, 23, 25, 26, 32, 33, 39, 40, 44, 56, 58, 59, 70, 78, 82, 87, 90, 92, 100, 105, 111, 117, 119, 124, 128, 131, 132, 133, 139, 233, 296, 314, 328

alcohol use, 171, 214, 250
anxiety, 125, 128, 142, 155, 232, 262
Asia, 8, 128, 138, 155, 228, 291, 315, 341
assessment, xi, 12, 13, 15, 22, 31, 32, 33, 35, 36, 139, 156, 234, 236, 289, 290, 291, 293, 294, 303, 305, 306, 308, 309, 310, 327, 330
assets, 78, 80, 215, 225, 234, 246, 270
atmosphere, 4, 7, 111, 148, 164, 203, 215, 218, 220, 226, 240, 256, 274, 277, 285
attitudes, 58, 60, 71, 149, 156, 165, 204, 225, 228, 233, 237, 240, 256, 257, 273, 275, 278, 284, 293
autism, 11, 12, 13, 14, 17, 18, 19, 20, 22, 24, 32, 33, 34, 35, 36
autism spectrum disorder (ASD), 12, 13, 14, 15, 16, 18, 31, 33, 34, 35, 36, 103
awareness, 150, 222, 241, 258, 268, 319, 325

B

behavior of children, 14
behavioral disorders, 246
behavioral problems, 250
behaviors, 11, 12, 13, 19, 20, 21, 23, 25, 26, 28, 29, 30, 33, 85, 87, 88, 158, 159, 171, 210, 215, 232, 233, 245, 246, 251, 284
beneficial effect, 307
benefits, 74, 85, 87, 88, 92, 95, 126, 158, 166, 167, 169, 179, 180, 181, 182, 183, 186, 187, 188, 189, 190, 198, 201, 209, 214, 216, 225, 226, 232, 235, 237, 238, 239, 241, 243, 244, 253, 254, 255, 257, 258, 259, 260, 262, 268, 271, 272, 273, 274, 275, 279, 280, 282, 283, 284, 285, 323, 350
birth control, 116, 119, 120, 125, 129, 131, 134
birth rate, 116, 129, 130, 131, 133
bonding, 150, 165, 166, 177, 201, 205, 221, 222, 225, 241, 250, 258

C

career development, 290
career prospects, 122
Caregiver Report, 13, 14, 16, 19, 33, 36
causal relationship, 101, 102, 110
challenges, 6, 53, 130, 138, 158, 216, 244, 251, 269, 285, 294, 295, 304, 311, 314, 318, 326, 327, 328, 337, 342
changing environment, 233
character traits, 59
child behavior, x, 99, 100, 101, 102, 103, 105, 109, 110, 111
child development, 110, 111, 133, 333
child rearing, 116, 131
childcare, 126, 129, 132, 135
childhood, 44, 79, 113
Childhood Autism Rating Scale (CARS), 14, 19, 20, 22, 26, 27, 29, 30, 32, 35
children, vii, viii, ix, x, xii, 3, 4, 7, 11, 12, 13, 14, 15, 16, 17, 18, 19, 20, 21, 22, 23, 24, 25, 26, 31, 32, 33, 34, 35, 36, 39, 40, 42, 43, 51, 52, 53, 72, 74, 79, 94, 99, 100, 101, 102, 103, 104, 105, 106, 110, 111, 112, 113, 115, 116, 120, 121, 122,124, 125, 126, 128, 129, 130, 131, 132, 133, 134, 135, 137, 159, 171, 172, 229, 245, 246, 247, 251, 319, 333, 334, 335, 337, 338, 339, 346, 347
China, viii, ix, x, 3, 5, 11, 34, 37, 38, 39, 40, 50, 52, 53, 54, 55, 77, 99, 115, 119, 122, 128, 129, 133, 137, 138, 139, 141, 142, 143, 144, 145, 152, 153, 155, 157, 158, 159, 160, 161, 162, 168, 169, 170, 171, 172, 175, 176, 177, 178, 179, 180, 189, 190, 191, 194, 195, 196, 197, 198, 199, 209, 210, 211, 213, 215, 216, 224, 225, 226, 229, 230, 231, 232, 233, 234, 235,

243, 244, 246, 247, 249, 251, 260, 263, 264, 267, 289, 292, 296, 299, 306, 307, 309, 313, 315, 317, 318, 319, 320, 321, 328, 330, 334, 343
Chinese adolescents, ix, x, 8, 55, 71, 77, 81, 82, 83, 92, 94, 142, 155, 158, 159, 171, 176, 189, 194, 210, 215, 227, 229, 233, 234, 235, 242, 245, 246, 247, 250, 263, 264, 298, 329
Chinese communities, 135, 143, 168, 177, 179, 214, 234
Chinese medicine, 38
chronic diseases, 333, 337
chronic illness, 337
cities, xi, 5, 38, 176, 189, 199, 213, 249, 251, 252, 260, 262
classes, 59, 272, 274, 275, 328
classroom, 148, 164, 203, 216, 218, 220, 240, 253, 256, 274, 277, 292, 339
classroom settings, 253
client satisfaction approach, 141, 144, 153, 156, 211, 248
cognition, 270
cognitive ability, 113
cognitive function, 20, 166
collaboration, 179, 333, 346, 347
college campuses, 308
college students, 286, 308, 326
colleges, 44, 308, 311
communication, 13, 19, 101, 106, 261, 292, 295, 299, 302
communication skills, 292
communities, 94, 130, 135, 142, 143, 168, 177, 179, 214, 234, 292, 342
community, 73, 94, 142, 150, 156, 166, 169, 173, 205, 222, 229, 242, 247, 258, 308, 314, 317, 318, 328, 330, 342
community service, 318, 342
comparative analysis, 41, 48, 54
compassion, 57, 79, 80, 150, 166, 205, 221, 222, 241, 258, 273, 275, 279, 316
competence, 74, 75, 79, 80, 94, 95, 149, 150, 165, 166, 177, 189, 191, 192, 193, 201, 205, 214, 218, 222, 225, 234, 241, 243, 250, 258, 268, 269, 270, 273, 279, 285, 292, 297, 298, 299, 300, 301, 302, 315, 320, 321, 323, 327
competitiveness, 271, 291, 308, 326
compulsory education, 121, 134
conception, 116, 120, 129, 131
confidentiality, 145, 236, 253
conflict, 102, 104, 106, 107, 108, 110, 270, 307
conflict of interest, 307
conflict resolution, 270
consensus, 235, 316, 327
consent, 59, 103, 108, 146
construct validity, 15, 34
consumption, 56, 57, 79
contraceptives, 120, 233
control group, 33, 306
correlation, 14, 16, 21, 22, 23, 24, 25, 26, 32, 56, 60, 70, 86, 87, 145, 147, 151, 163, 167, 182, 188, 200, 202, 208, 209, 223, 237, 238, 239, 243, 260, 276, 282, 297
correlation analysis, 61, 86, 163, 237
correlation coefficient, 14, 21, 22, 23, 24, 25, 26, 32, 202
correlations, 19, 32, 70, 106, 147, 153, 163, 182, 188, 206, 218, 219, 235, 238, 254, 276
cost, 144, 190, 229, 305
counseling, 134, 142, 329, 334
course content, 225, 268, 271, 272, 283, 284, 285
critical thinking, 226, 279, 289, 292, 293, 295, 301, 304, 305, 306
cultural beliefs, 125
cultural differences, 4, 5, 7, 215
cultural tradition, 305
cultural transformation, 116

cultural values, 129
culture, 36, 38, 56, 102, 117, 120, 121, 126, 127, 128, 131, 133, 134, 135, 229, 294, 305, 318
curricula, 144, 145, 159, 234, 291, 292, 293, 294, 303, 305, 306
curriculum, 142, 143, 148, 149, 160, 161, 162, 164, 165, 168, 177, 185, 186, 201, 203, 204, 209, 214, 220, 221, 224, 225, 226, 234, 238, 240, 245, 250, 252, 255, 256, 257, 261, 274, 277, 284, 285, 289, 291, 294, 295, 303, 304, 305, 308
cystic fibrosis, 338

D

data collection, 40, 59, 82, 103, 145, 200, 236, 296
data set, 105, 108
database, 40
delinquency, 78, 215, 232, 250
delinquent behavior, 245
demographic characteristics, 106
demographic factors, 78, 89, 90
dependent variable, 255, 259, 299
depressive symptoms, 142, 232, 247, 251, 264
depth, 92, 178, 190, 306
depth perception, 306
descriptive statistical analyses, 60, 61, 146, 237, 238
developmental assets, 78, 80, 215, 234, 246, 270
developmental disorder, 12, 17, 31, 35
developmental process, 233
dignity, 58, 62, 63, 64, 65, 66, 67, 68, 88, 91
disability, 335, 345, 346, 348
discrimination, 16, 22, 25, 32, 36
disorder, 12, 18, 34, 245, 326
disposition, 269, 270, 279, 317, 320, 322, 324
drug abuse, 53, 158, 171, 215
drugs, 39, 46

E

eating disorders, 232
economic boom, 328
economic change, 252
economic development, 269, 292
economic disadvantage, 59, 70, 72, 135
economic growth, 142, 215, 315
economic policy, 122, 128, 129
economic problem, 72
economic reforms, 38
education, ii, iv, 15, 17, 35, 44, 56, 70, 72, 75, 95, 103, 105, 106, 121, 124, 128, 129, 130, 133, 134, 137, 155, 169, 195, 198, 268, 269, 270, 284, 285, 286, 287, 288, 289, 290, 291, 292, 293, 294, 303, 305, 306, 308, 314, 326, 328, 330, 339, 341, 350
education reform, 293
educational attainment, 121, 124
educational opportunities, 116, 126, 131
educational practices, 293
educational programs, 291
educational psychologists, 18, 19
educators, 15, 17, 176
egocentrism, x, 6, 58, 77, 78, 79, 80, 81, 83, 84, 85, 86, 87, 88, 89, 90, 91, 92, 93, 94
emotional problems, 159
emotional well-being, 338
empathy, 78, 79, 270, 298, 302, 304, 315, 325
employers, 291, 293, 308, 326
employment, 105, 123, 124, 128, 129
employment opportunities, 124, 128
environment, x, 13, 32, 97, 99, 100, 101, 102, 103, 105, 108, 110, 111, 177, 268, 269, 306, 330, 350
environmental health disparities, ii, iv

environments, 33
evidence, 12, 15, 22, 24, 27, 31, 33, 34, 102, 110, 111, 153, 171, 179, 190, 215, 216, 228, 232, 233, 244, 247, 250, 257, 261, 263, 265, 275, 294, 295, 301, 304, 305, 308, 311, 314, 326, 327
experiential learning, 216, 225, 229, 261, 284, 287
externalizing behavior, 100, 232, 233, 246

F

familial dysautonomia, 338
families, 4, 15, 42, 70, 72, 102, 108, 110, 111, 112, 113, 116, 117, 119, 120, 123, 124, 125, 126, 127, 128, 130, 131, 132, 133, 134, 136, 137, 138, 165, 166, 221, 222, 334, 338, 339
family conflict, 133
family development, 116, 117, 118, 119, 123, 124, 134, 135, 246
family factors, 7, 245
family functioning, 72, 100, 101, 102, 103, 104, 105, 110, 113, 171, 247
family income, 42, 105, 110
family life, 59, 118, 125, 126, 131, 132, 133, 134
family meals, 101, 112
family mealtime environment, x, 99, 100, 101, 102, 103, 105, 110, 111
family members, 101, 102, 104, 117, 126, 132, 133
family planning, 120
family research, 1, ii, vii, viii, ix, x, 3, 4, 7, 115, 116, 131, 133, 139
feelings, 80, 85, 86, 87, 88, 92, 101, 154, 198, 201
fertility, 120, 121, 128, 138
fertility rate, 120, 121
financial, 57, 128, 177, 214, 215, 251, 269, 306, 307
financial support, 177, 214, 215, 251

G

general education, xi, 289, 290, 291, 292, 293, 294, 303, 305, 307, 308, 309, 310, 311
Global Youth Leadership Programme, 314, 316
grades, 67, 78, 92, 145, 147, 170, 239, 244, 253, 255, 259, 262
growth, 39, 51, 53, 207, 228, 264, 294, 295, 301, 304, 305, 306, 311, 325, 339

H

happiness, 57, 72, 74, 93, 252, 262, 326, 330
health, ii, iii, iv, v, vi, ix, xii, 37, 38, 40, 41, 42, 43, 44, 45, 46, 47, 50, 51, 52, 53, 54, 111, 142, 158, 159, 171, 172, 210, 215, 228, 233, 245, 246, 247, 251, 265, 268, 319, 329, 330, 335, 338, 339, 345, 348, 349, 350, 351
health care, ix, 37, 38, 39, 40, 41, 45, 47, 50, 51, 52
health care system, 52
health disparities, ii, iv
health education, 46, 51, 111, 142
health problems, 251
health promotion, ix, 37, 50, 54
health services, 53
health-promoting behaviors, 159
high school, x, 55, 58, 59, 61, 64, 70, 71, 72, 73, 80, 81, 91, 93, 156, 157, 158, 160, 161, 168, 170, 189, 246, 251, 253, 262, 264
high school students, 55, 58, 59, 61, 63, 64, 66, 70, 71, 72, 73, 80, 81, 91, 93, 156, 170, 251, 264

higher education, 72, 121, 122, 288, 290, 291, 292, 293, 303, 307, 308, 309, 310, 311
higher-order thinking, 290, 292
Hong Kong Education Commission, 293, 308
household income, 42, 105, 107
human agency, 118, 119, 136
human capital, 124
human capital theory, 124
human development, 4, 7, 56, 57, 118, 131, 136, 325, 335, 345, 348
human resources, 306
hypothesis, 58, 207, 208

I

identity, 56, 82, 112, 132, 133, 234, 250, 304, 320, 321, 323, 325
imitation, 21, 23, 25, 26, 28, 29, 30
immigrants, 119
immigration, 123, 126, 129
in transition, x, 115, 119, 136, 311
income, 43, 72, 105, 108, 116, 127
information technology, 122
informed consent, 16, 200, 272, 296
institutions, 291, 292, 306, 327
instructor quality, 176, 187, 188, 190, 209, 235, 238, 239, 243, 268
integration, 172, 196, 328
integrity, 139, 270, 314, 315
internal consistency, 12, 14, 15, 16, 22, 31, 147, 162, 163, 181, 202, 219, 237, 238, 254
internalizing, 112, 232, 233, 243, 245, 246
interpersonal interactions, 316
interpersonal relations, 72, 79, 92
interpersonal relationships, 72, 79
interpersonal skills, 293
intervention, 5, 6, 13, 14, 33, 143, 144, 155, 228, 245, 251, 265
intervention research, 5, 6
intrapersonal development, iv, 144, 156, 295, 309, 310, 350
issues, 50, 80, 91, 134, 156, 158, 159, 179, 198, 216, 232, 233, 234, 245, 246, 251, 287, 317, 318, 326, 349

J

job performance, 173
job satisfaction, 173
job training, 124
junior high school, 59, 61, 63, 66, 71
junior secondary schools, xi, 145, 160, 168, 198, 213
juvenile delinquency, 214

L

labor force, 116, 121, 124, 126, 127, 129, 131, 132, 133
labor force participation, 122, 124
leadership, iv, vi, xi, 51, 144, 156, 211, 265, 267, 268, 269, 270, 271, 273, 275, 279, 282, 283, 284, 285, 286, 287, 288, 290, 292, 293, 295, 297, 298, 300, 302, 304, 307, 308, 309, 310, 313, 314, 315, 316, 317, 318, 319, 320, 321, 322, 324, 325, 326, 327,328, 329, 330, 334, 349, 350
leadership development, 285, 288, 316, 325, 327, 329
leadership style, 284, 327
learning, 5, 15, 113, 148, 169, 177, 179, 189, 201, 203, 215, 216, 225, 226, 229, 235, 240, 256, 261, 269, 277, 284, 285, 287, 288, 290, 291, 292, 293, 294, 295, 299, 301, 302, 303, 304, 305, 306, 307, 308, 310, 311, 316, 318, 334
learning behavior, 169
learning environment, 226, 229

learning outcomes, 235, 290, 291, 293, 294, 295, 303, 304, 305, 306, 308, 310
learning styles, 216, 294
liberal education, 291, 292, 308
life course, 116, 117, 118, 119, 124, 125, 127, 129, 130, 131, 132, 133, 134, 136, 138
life cycle, 118, 131, 132, 136
life satisfaction, 74, 210, 215, 252, 262, 314, 320, 321, 322, 324, 325, 326, 327, 329
lifelong learning, 290, 293, 295, 299, 301
Likert scale, 60, 82, 83, 104, 146, 148, 149, 150, 151, 162, 164, 165, 166, 167, 181, 203, 204, 205, 206, 207, 218, 219, 220, 221, 222, 223, 237, 240, 241, 242, 254, 256, 257, 258, 273, 274, 298, 299
longitudinal evaluation, 234, 295, 307
longitudinal study, 8, 100, 195, 228, 233, 245, 295

M

majority, 152, 161, 164, 166, 168, 182, 189, 198, 203, 217, 243, 249, 255, 261, 268, 275
management, 41, 45, 46, 50, 52, 102, 110, 135, 154, 156, 234, 253, 271, 287, 327
manufacturing, 122, 292, 313, 315
marriage, 68, 69, 70, 116, 124, 125, 128, 129, 130, 131, 132, 135, 136, 137, 138, 296
married couples, 128
materialism, ix, x, 6, 55, 56, 57, 58, 59, 60, 61, 67, 68, 69, 70, 71, 73, 74, 77, 78, 80, 81, 82, 84, 86, 87, 89, 90, 91, 92, 93, 94, 143, 177, 215, 228, 229, 269, 287
materialistic beliefs, 55, 58, 59, 60, 61, 62, 63, 64, 65, 66, 70, 71, 72, 73, 78, 82, 84, 85, 86, 88, 91
materials, 5, 24, 142, 160, 169, 191, 192, 199
matter, viii, 85, 87, 88, 113, 172, 272, 308
measurement, 36, 50, 73, 94, 113, 156, 224
measurements, 4, 38
median, 24, 25, 26, 32, 41, 43, 105, 124, 125
medical, 38, 41, 45, 46, 50, 51, 333, 335, 337, 338, 350
mental health, 110, 142, 155, 158, 159, 171, 176, 215, 246, 251, 252, 264
Merrill–Palmer Revised Scales of Development (MPR), 19, 20, 22, 26, 27, 28, 32
meta-analysis, 155, 171, 229
mineral resources, 252
models, 55, 57, 78, 80, 101, 136, 153, 233, 270, 284, 310, 325
money and success education (MS), iv
moral development, 58, 73, 93
moral reasoning, 292
motor behavior, 21, 23, 25, 26, 28, 29, 30
multiple regression, 61, 70, 147, 152, 153, 163, 167, 188, 202, 219, 223, 238, 255, 260, 274
multiple regression analyses, 56, 61, 147, 152, 153, 168, 188, 202, 208, 238, 244, 255, 274, 282, 283
multiple regression analysis, 70, 163, 167, 219, 223, 260
multivariate analysis, 147
multivariate analysis of variance (MANOVA), 86, 147, 151, 187, 237, 239, 244, 255, 259
mutuality, 104, 106, 107

N

neuromuscular diseases, 338
nutrition, 39, 53, 246, 338

O

objective outcome evaluation, xi, 143, 155, 160, 172, 177, 189, 190, 194, 195, 196, 199, 228, 229, 244, 247, 264, 286, 288, 295, 304, 313, 314, 321, 327, 329
opportunities, 111, 119, 124, 126, 134, 178, 191, 193, 214, 269
overall satisfaction, 142, 146, 148, 176, 180, 181, 182, 184, 187, 188, 189, 201, 203, 237, 253, 254, 257, 259, 322

P

P.A.T.H.S., x, xi, 5, 8, 141, 143, 144, 145, 152, 153, 154, 155, 156, 157, 158, 159, 160, 161, 168, 170, 172, 175, 176, 177, 180, 183, 189, 190, 191, 192, 193, 194, 195, 196, 197, 198, 199, 200, 201, 209, 210, 211, 213, 214, 215, 216, 224, 225, 227, 228, 229, 230, 231, 232, 234, 235, 236, 242, 243, 245, 247, 248, 250, 251, 261, 263, 264, 265, 311
parental care, 100
parental control, 104, 107
parent-child relationship, 127
parenthood, 116, 124, 129, 130, 131, 132, 135
parenting, ii, 72, 100, 101, 102, 103, 104, 105, 107, 108, 109, 110, 111, 112, 113, 126, 127, 128, 130, 132, 133, 134, 135, 138, 334
parenting styles, 104, 110, 111, 126, 133
parents, 7, 13, 43, 59, 72, 74, 75, 81, 95, 100, 102, 103, 104, 105, 106, 108, 111, 113, 116, 121, 125, 126, 130, 131, 133, 135, 137, 156, 216, 229, 251, 253, 262, 338
participants, 5, 6, 15, 17, 18, 19, 22, 25, 26, 32, 33, 59, 60, 71, 100, 103, 106, 108, 111, 141, 144, 146, 148, 149, 150, 151, 152, 153, 154, 160, 169, 170, 172, 176, 177, 178, 179, 180, 181, 182, 183, 184, 185, 186, 187, 188, 189, 190, 191, 192, 193, 195, 196, 198, 199, 200, 201, 203, 204, 205, 206, 207, 209, 211, 214, 215, 221, 225, 232, 233, 234, 235, 236, 237, 238, 239, 240, 241, 242, 243, 244, 249, 253, 254, 255, 256, 257, 258, 259, 260, 261, 262, 271, 272, 273, 274, 275, 277, 278, 279, 281, 282, 283, 284, 285, 296, 300, 301, 325, 327
pedagogy, 216, 225, 226, 261, 284, 293
peer influence, 72, 78, 264
perceived self-performance, 163, 164, 176, 187
performance test, 12, 13, 15, 16, 18, 19, 22, 24, 26, 31, 32, 33
permission, viii, 34, 52, 73, 93, 112, 135, 142, 154, 171, 191, 210, 227, 245, 263, 286, 307, 328
personal choice, 128
personal computers, 56
personal development, 209, 250, 290, 295, 305
personal qualities, 234
personal views, 226
personality, 112, 156, 271, 330
personhood, 229
pervasive developmental disorders (PPDs), 12, 17, 35
policy, 117, 121, 122, 123, 137, 139, 142, 144, 153, 170, 173, 176, 179, 195, 225, 229, 308, 318, 348
population, 4, 12, 14, 31, 34, 43, 61, 81, 84, 103, 111, 113, 119, 136, 137, 138, 143, 159, 160, 251, 252, 322, 326
positive attitudes, 178, 232, 238, 244
positive correlation, 14, 20, 189
positive development, 57, 161, 189, 214, 233, 252, 260, 270, 301

positive feedback, 5, 169, 189
positive influences, 168
positive relationship, 92, 169, 217, 316
positive youth development (PYD), ii, x, 5, 8, 57, 73, 74, 78, 80, 94, 95, 141, 142, 143, 153, 155, 156, 159, 168, 169, 170, 171, 172, 173, 175, 176, 177, 178, 183, 186, 189, 194, 195, 198, 201, 209, 210, 211, 214, 215, 216, 225, 226, 227, 228, 229, 230, 232, 233, 234, 235, 242, 243, 245, 246, 247, 249, 250, 261, 263, 264, 265, 269, 297, 298, 310, 314, 320, 321, 322, 323, 325, 327, 329, 334
positive youth development (PYD) approach, 176, 250, 263
positive youth development program, x, 5, 8, 74, 95, 141, 155, 156, 170, 172, 173, 175, 194, 195, 198, 210, 211, 228, 229, 230, 245, 247, 249, 250, 251, 261, 263, 264, 334
preparation, viii, 146, 148, 154, 170, 191, 201, 209, 216, 226, 227, 244, 253, 261, 263, 275, 284, 286, 317
preschool, x, 18, 35, 99, 100, 101, 102, 103, 104, 105, 110
preschool children, x, 35, 99, 102, 104, 110
prevention, 5, 51, 74, 94, 142, 155, 159, 172, 177, 178, 214, 228, 230, 233, 245, 247, 251, 335
primary caregivers, 16
primary function, 120
primary school, 45, 100, 318, 319
principles, 60, 62, 63, 64, 65, 66, 67, 68, 82, 83, 84, 85, 88, 145, 177, 288, 309, 329
problem behavior, 105, 110, 177, 210
problem solving, 289, 295, 300, 304
professional development, 219, 225
professional growth, 163, 167, 222, 223, 224
professional teacher, 80
professionalism, 146, 148
professionals, 12, 13, 14, 17, 18, 111, 122, 138, 160, 314, 338, 341, 346
program benefits, 182, 189, 190, 201, 214, 232, 235, 237, 238, 239, 241, 244, 254, 255, 258, 259, 260, 262, 273, 275, 276, 279, 280, 282, 283
program content, 142, 144, 145, 146, 147, 148, 151, 152, 153, 154, 158, 160, 161, 162, 163, 164, 167, 168, 169, 176, 182, 187, 189, 198, 199, 200, 201, 202, 203, 206, 207, 208, 209, 214, 217, 218, 220, 223, 224, 225, 226, 235, 237, 238, 239, 240, 243, 244, 250, 253, 254,255, 256, 259, 260, 261, 273, 274, 276, 277, 282, 283, 284, 285
program effectiveness, 5, 142, 144, 145, 146, 147, 149, 150, 151, 152, 153, 158, 161, 162, 163, 165, 167, 168, 169, 170, 198, 199, 200, 201, 202, 205, 206, 207, 208, 209, 216, 217, 218, 219, 221, 222, 223, 224, 225, 226, 227, 235, 236, 238, 239, 243, 285
program instructors, 182, 186, 198, 199, 200, 201, 202, 203, 204, 206, 207, 208, 209, 237, 238, 240, 244, 254, 257, 278, 285
program quality, 176, 181, 182, 183, 186, 187, 188, 189, 219, 223, 232, 236, 243, 253, 285
project, ix, x, 37, 38, 39, 40, 41, 50, 51, 52, 54, 112, 143, 144, 153, 159, 160, 161, 162, 166, 168, 169, 170, 175, 177, 178, 179, 186, 189, 190, 192, 193, 196, 197, 198, 199, 209, 210, 213, 214, 216, 225, 228, 230, 234, 249, 250, 251, 252, 253, 254, 255, 257, 260, 261, 262, 263, 264, 265, 292, 293, 295, 311, 318, 343
Project P.A.T.H.S., x, 5, 8, 143, 145, 155, 156, 157, 158, 159, 160, 161, 170, 172, 177, 180, 183, 189, 190, 194, 195, 196, 210, 211, 213, 214, 215, 216, 228, 229,

234, 236, 243, 245, 247, 248, 250, 251, 264, 265
psychiatric disorder, 159, 171
psychological development, 142
psychological stress, 264
psychological well-being, 8, 72, 228, 251
psychology, 112, 136, 330, 341
psychometric properties, 12, 14, 15, 16, 21, 31, 33, 35, 36, 74, 94, 199, 201, 202, 243, 310, 321
psychosocial development, 81
public health, 53, 335, 345, 346, 349, 350
public service, 346

Q

quality control, 40
quality improvement, 310
quality of life, 74, 95, 172, 233, 247, 248, 265, 335, 339
quantitative research, 306
questionnaire, 18, 25, 59, 104, 141, 180, 181, 200, 306, 309

R

reasoning, 94, 290, 293, 298, 304
reciprocity, 21, 23, 25, 26, 28, 29, 30
recognition, 101, 116, 130, 131, 186, 250
recommendations, viii, 201
reform, 53, 290, 292, 293, 309
regression, 56, 61, 69, 70, 86, 152, 168, 188, 208, 224, 239, 244, 282, 283
reliability, ix, 11, 12, 14, 15, 16, 17, 18, 22, 23, 30, 31, 32, 33, 35, 36, 59, 106, 146, 147, 163, 181, 202, 218, 219, 227, 236, 237, 238, 254, 297, 298, 310
researchers, 4, 5, 6, 13, 14, 18, 19, 40, 58, 131, 144, 153, 170, 214, 232, 261, 262, 291, 292, 306, 311, 342, 349
resilience, 134, 150, 165, 166, 205, 218, 222, 225, 241, 258, 264, 268, 279, 321, 326
resources, 127, 133, 134, 142, 179, 191, 192, 233, 252, 310
response, 27, 29, 60, 83, 84, 118, 132, 156, 162, 187, 218, 234, 237, 243, 259, 291, 296, 316
risk, 8, 17, 51, 57, 125, 128, 133, 143, 158, 159, 172, 177, 198, 228, 233, 247, 251, 264, 311

S

school, 6, 20, 36, 44, 45, 58, 59, 61, 71, 78, 81, 82, 100, 108, 124, 143, 145, 154, 155, 158, 159, 160, 161, 162, 169, 170, 171, 172, 177, 178, 179, 180, 187, 189, 191, 192, 193, 199, 200, 202, 203, 204, 205, 206, 207, 209, 215, 216, 217, 224, 228, 229, 230, 232, 234, 235, 236, 247, 250, 251, 252, 253, 261, 262, 264, 296, 326
school climate, 235, 251, 264
school culture, 251
school performance, 215, 216
schooling, 216
science, 136, 195, 228, 245, 246, 341, 346
secondary school students, xi, 71, 158, 177, 231, 232, 249, 251, 252, 261
secondary schools, xi, 59, 81, 142, 143, 145, 158, 160, 162, 168, 169, 177, 178, 180, 189, 198, 213, 216, 232, 234, 250, 251, 252, 253, 263
secondary students, 5, 143, 215, 232, 234, 236, 243, 244
self-awareness, 149, 166, 205, 207, 225, 239
self-confidence, 149, 150, 166, 205, 215, 222, 241, 258, 268, 279
self-control, 326

self-efficacy, 225, 234, 250, 270
self-esteem, 215
self-improvement, 270
self-reflection, 169, 183, 186, 190, 192, 193, 226
self-regulation, 110, 113, 270
self-report data, 80
self-reports, 77, 80
self-worth, 325
service leadership, iv, vi, xi, 55, 115, 211, 267, 268, 269, 270, 271, 272, 275, 282, 283, 284, 285, 286, 287, 288, 308, 310, 313, 315, 316, 317, 318, 319, 320, 321, 322, 324, 325, 326, 327, 328, 329, 330, 334, 349, 350
service leadership competencies, 314, 317, 319, 325
services, viii, 120, 134, 135, 144, 154, 156, 268, 319, 334, 338, 342
social behavior, 59, 112
social benefits, 307
social care, 338
social change, 117, 119, 136, 342
social circle, 78
social class, 137
social competence, 80, 149, 150, 165, 177, 205, 215, 218, 222, 234, 241, 250, 258, 279, 321
social construct, 118
social context, 118, 131, 132, 159, 172
social desirability, 71, 80, 227, 327
social development, 112, 118, 251
social environment, 119, 304
social programs, 8, 194, 311
social psychology, 58, 71, 81
social relations, 119, 270
social relationships, 119
social responsibility, 169, 269, 291, 292
social roles, 119, 125
social services, 195
social skills, 159, 166, 201
social structure, 117
social support, 159, 171
social units, 117
social welfare, 105, 134
social workers, 160, 201, 203, 209, 252, 334
socialization, 93, 116
socializing agent, 101
society, 6, 116, 120, 121, 133, 150, 166, 205, 216, 222, 242, 243, 258, 275, 280, 291, 293, 315, 318, 342, 346
socio-demographic, ix, 55, 56, 60, 71, 73, 86, 91, 92, 93, 94
soft skills, 291, 315, 326, 329
standard deviation, 22, 106, 147, 163, 182, 202, 206, 218, 255, 276, 301
structure, 73, 94, 105, 117, 119, 122, 132, 235, 285, 293, 294
student achievement, 230, 292, 294, 306
student development, 284, 298, 299, 305, 306, 326
student enrollment, 292
student-centered pedagogy, 216, 293
style, 5, 79, 100, 101, 102, 103, 104, 105, 107, 108, 110, 111, 112, 113, 126, 226, 293, 305
subjective outcome evaluation, x, xi, 141, 143, 144, 145, 152, 153, 154, 155, 158, 160, 161, 162, 167, 168, 169, 172, 176, 179, 181, 182, 187, 189, 190, 194, 195, 196, 198, 199, 206, 209, 211, 213, 217, 224, 227, 229, 230, 231, 232, 234, 235, 236, 237, 238, 243, 244, 247, 253, 254, 255, 260, 264, 267, 271, 272, 273, 282, 286, 287, 288, 304
subjective outcome evaluation instrument, 153, 243
substance abuse, 100, 143, 172, 177, 214, 232
suicide, 176, 177, 194, 210, 251, 326, 329
suicide attempts, 176, 194, 210
symptoms, 12, 13, 16, 176, 232, 233, 246

T

teacher perception, 84, 85, 86, 87
teacher support, 230
teacher training, 179, 195, 199, 210
teachers, x, 5, 18, 24, 74, 75, 77, 80, 81, 82, 83, 84, 86, 87, 88, 90, 91, 92, 93, 95, 142, 150, 160, 161, 162, 165, 166, 169, 170, 180, 186, 187, 189, 190, 191, 192, 193, 199, 201, 203, 205, 209, 216, 217, 221, 222, 224, 226, 241, 252, 256, 258, 261, 309, 334
teaching experience, 82, 164, 180, 183, 191, 220, 226
teaching quality, 235
teaching strategies, 273
techniques, 40, 113, 191, 306
technological advances, 56
technology, 196, 269, 337
television viewing, 101, 102, 104, 105, 107, 108
tertiary education, 314, 316, 325
testing, 18, 22, 32, 36, 105, 339
test-retest reliability, 12, 15, 16, 17, 18, 22, 32
The Psycho-Educational Profile-3rd edition (PEP-3), 11, 13, 14, 15, 16, 19, 22, 23, 24, 27, 30, 31
Tin Ka Ping Foundation, 143, 154, 160, 170, 177, 191, 209, 215, 227, 234, 245, 263
Tin Ka Ping P.A.T.H.S. Project, x, xi, 5, 141, 143, 144, 145, 152, 153, 154, 160, 161, 170, 172, 176, 177, 180, 191, 192, 193, 195, 196, 209, 210, 211, 213, 224, 227, 230, 231, 232, 234, 235, 236, 242, 243, 245, 263
Tin Ka Ping Positive Adolescent Training through Holistic Social Program, 143
training, x, 8, 15, 17, 18, 44, 45, 80, 133, 134, 145, 160, 162, 169, 172, 175, 176, 177, 178, 179, 180, 181, 182, 183, 184, 185, 186, 187, 189, 190, 191, 192, 194, 195, 196, 199, 210, 211, 218, 226, 229, 230, 251, 261, 264, 294, 311, 316, 334, 346
training program, x, 160, 169, 172, 175, 176, 178, 179, 180, 181, 182, 183, 184, 185, 187, 189, 190, 191, 192, 194, 195, 196, 199, 210, 211, 226, 229, 230, 264
training programs, 160, 169, 178, 179, 181, 189, 190, 194, 195, 199, 226
treatment, 12, 14, 35, 41, 44, 45, 46, 50, 51, 155, 233, 339

U

undergraduate education, 288, 289, 290, 292, 293, 294, 309, 310
unique features, 31, 78, 128, 226
United States, 4, 14, 24, 27, 33, 34, 37, 74, 95, 115, 142, 172, 194, 210, 215, 229, 263, 291, 294, 316, 335, 342, 348
universities, 159, 270, 290, 293, 294, 299, 303, 305, 306, 307, 308, 311
university education, 269, 285, 291
urban, 38, 39, 137, 176, 350

V

validation, 15, 18, 27, 34, 35, 94, 113, 155, 310, 329
validity, ix, 11, 12, 13, 14, 15, 16, 17, 18, 19, 20, 21, 22, 24, 25, 26, 31, 32, 33, 35, 36, 60, 236, 247
variables, 41, 68, 69, 70, 89, 101, 102, 105, 107, 108, 110, 111, 188, 202, 218, 255, 282, 320, 322
violent behavior, 158

W

welfare, 59, 135, 318, 335, 345
well-being, 6, 8, 72, 74, 95, 96, 112, 135, 171, 198, 215, 228, 247, 251, 287, 288, 335, 338
workers, 15, 123, 172, 201, 203, 209, 230, 253
workforce, 292, 315
working hours, 124

Y

young adults, 171, 198, 351
young people, 56, 57, 61, 78, 80, 92, 142, 198, 246, 251, 261, 263, 269, 285, 326, 334